Creative Arts-Based
with Ado~~.~~

Creative Arts-Based Group Therapy with Adolescents provides principles for effective use of different arts-based approaches in adolescent group therapy, grounding these principles in neuroscience and group process practice-based evidence. It includes chapters covering each of the main creative arts therapy modalities—art therapy, bibliotherapy, dance/movement therapy, drama therapy, music therapy, and poetry/expressive writing therapy—written by respected contributors who are experts in the application of these modalities in the context of groups. These methods are uniquely effective for engaging adolescents and addressing many of the developmental, familial, and societal problems that they face. The text offers theory and guiding principles, while also providing a comprehensive resource for group therapists of diverse disciplines who wish to incorporate creative arts-based methods into their practice with teens.

Craig Haen, Ph.D., RDT, CGP, LCAT, FAGPA treats children, adolescents, and adults in private practice. He is Faculty at New York University and Lesley University, and Co-Founder of the Kint Institute. His books include *Handbook of Child and Adolescent Group Therapy* and *Engaging Boys in Treatment: Creative Approaches to the Therapy Process.*

Nancy Boyd Webb, DSW, LICSW, RPT-S is a leading authority on play therapy with children and adolescents who have experienced loss and traumatic bereavement. Dr. Webb is a clinical social worker and Distinguished University Professor Emerita at Fordham University Graduate School of Social Service, where she held an Endowed Chair in Child Welfare Studies and founded, directed, and taught in the Post-Master's Certificate Program in Child and Adolescent Therapy for 22 years. Dr. Webb has published 15 previous books.

Creative Arts-Based Group Therapy with Adolescents

Theory and Practice

Edited by Craig Haen and
Nancy Boyd Webb

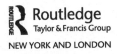
Routledge
Taylor & Francis Group

NEW YORK AND LONDON

First published 2019
by Routledge
52 Vanderbilt Avenue, New York, NY 10017

and by Routledge
2 Park Square, Milton Park, Abingdon, Oxon, OX14 4RN

Routledge is an imprint of the Taylor & Francis Group, an informa business

© 2019 Taylor & Francis

Library of Congress Cataloging-in-Publication Data
Names: Haen, Craig, editor. | Webb, Nancy Boyd, 1932– editor.
Title: Creative arts-based group therapy with adolescents : theory and
     practice / edited by Craig Haen and Nancy Boyd Webb.
Description: New York, NY : Routledge, 2019. | Includes bibliographical
     references and index.
Identifiers: LCCN 2018040184 | ISBN 9781138572515 (hbk) |
     ISBN 9781138572546 (pbk) | ISBN 9780203702000 (ebk)
Subjects: | MESH: Art Therapy | Adolescent | Psychotherapy, Group |
     Creativity
Classification: LCC RJ505.A7 | NLM WM 450.5.A8 | DDC
     616.89/165600835—dc23
LC record available at https://lccn.loc.gov/2018040184

ISBN: 978-1-138-57251-5 (hbk)
ISBN: 978-1-138-57254-6 (pbk)
ISBN: 978-0-203-70200-0 (ebk)

Typeset in Minion
by Apex CoVantage, LLC

At the time of writing this book, some 2,000 children have been separated from their parents by the federal government and are being held in camps at the borders of the United States.

This book is dedicated to those young people, and to adolescents and their parents everywhere. May there one day be a time when the forces that work to tear families apart no longer are supported by powerful systems.

Contents

Editors

Craig Haen, Ph.D., RDT, CGP, LCAT, FAGPA is Editor of the book *Engaging Boys in Treatment: Creative Approaches to the Therapy Process* (2011), and Co-Editor of the *Handbook of Child and Adolescent Group Therapy* (2017) and *Clinical Applications of Drama Therapy in Child and Adolescent Treatment* (2005). He has a private psychotherapy practice where he works with children, adolescents, adults, and families in White Plains, NY. He serves as Adjunct Faculty in the Department of Applied Psychology and the graduate drama therapy program at New York University, and in the expressive therapies doctoral program at Lesley University, teaching courses in both clinical practice and research. He is also Co-Founder and Training Director of the Kint Institute, which offers a Post-Master's Certificate Program in the arts and trauma treatment in New York City.

Dr. Haen has extensive experience providing group work to children and adolescents in shelters, community centers, hospitals, residential facilities, schools, and on Native American reservations. He has presented trainings and published clinical papers internationally. In addition, he is a Fellow of the American Group Psychotherapy Association, where he co-chairs the Community Outreach Task Force, a group that responds to trauma events and training needs in the U.S. and abroad.

Nancy Boyd Webb, DSW, LICSW, RPT-S is a leading authority on play therapy with children who have experienced loss and traumatic bereavement. Dr. Webb is a clinical social worker and Distinguished University Professor Emerita at Fordham University Graduate School of Social Service, where she held an Endowed Chair in Child Welfare Studies and founded, directed, and taught in the Post-Master's Certificate Program in Child and Adolescent Therapy for 22 years until her retirement in 2008. She taught clinical practice at Fordham for 30 years.

Dr. Webb is a prolific author and scholar in the areas of child therapy, trauma, and bereavement, and has published 14 books on these topics since 1991, including third editions of *Helping Bereaved Children* and *Social Work Practice With Children*, and a fourth edition of *Play Therapy With Children and Adolescents in Crisis*. Dr. Webb presents frequently as a keynote speaker and workshop leader at professional conferences, and she also conducts staff training and consultation and offers individual and group supervision. She has received numerous honors, including Smith College's Day-Garrett Award, the Clinical Practice Award of the Association for Death Education and Counseling, and the designation of Distinguished Scholar by the National Academies of Practice in Social Work.

Contributors

Wendy Allen
Naropa University
Boulder, CO

Mark Beauregard
New York Creative Arts Therapists, PLLC
Brooklyn, NY

Robyn Flaum Cruz
Lesley University
Cambridge, MA

Angel Duncan
Neuropsychiatric Research Center of Southwest Florida
Evolution Research Group
Fort Myers, FL

Paula Kingwill
Freelance Dramatherapist
Eastern Cape, South Africa

Heidi Landis
Claremont International High School
New York, NY

Reina Lombardi
Florida Art Therapy Services, LLC
Fort Myers, FL

Kristin Long
Institute for Expressive Analysis
New York, NY

Terry Marks-Tarlow
Insight Center
Los Angeles, CA

Katrina Skewes McFerran
The University of Melbourne
Melbourne, Australia

Dawn Morningstar
Drexel University
Philadelphia, PA

Lesley Palmer
Freelance Dramatherapist
Cape Town, South Africa

Sian Palmer
Freelance Dramatherapist
Johannesburg, South Africa

Laura Santner
South Beach Psychiatric Center
Brooklyn, NY

Nancy S. Scherlong
Wellness Metaphors
Norwalk, CT

Elly Scrine
National Music Therapy Research Unit
University of Melbourne,
Melbourne, Australia

Zipora Shechtman
Professor (Emerita), Haifa University
Haifa, Israel

Camilla Stanger
Goldsmiths University
London, United Kingdom

T. Thomas
Lesley University
Cambridge, MA

Britton Williams
New York–Presbyterian Hospital
New York, NY

Denise Wolf
Drexel University
Philadelphia, PA

Foreword

Social work has long been considered both an art and a science, applied theory and creative innovation. Nevertheless, my profession is far from the only field in which those characteristics come into play. Although I've worked with adolescents in one manner or another for more than 44 years, my wife Dale, an art teacher, beats me when it comes to actual time spent with teens. She has worked with countless teenage groups, teaching them to create art for nearly 40 years in one high school classroom.

Despite our professional credentials, in four decades of marriage our conversations are rarely academic. Without any intention to minimize formal studies or scholarship, we've never had a discussion about research findings or evidence-based practice protocols. Our conversations veer more toward what it's like to be in close quarters with groups of teenagers. I tell her stories and share my writings about my work with teen groups, and she tells me about her classes and shows me photos of her students' artwork—drawings, paintings, ceramics, murals, parade banners, and play scenery. We exchange war stories and laugh and shake our heads about the myriad challenges, surprising moments, and unforeseen outcomes in working with this unpredictable population of young people.

This book reinforces what it takes to be successful in both my and Dale's work with adolescents: trusting relationships, competence, and a passion for the job. In addition, most of the authors in this collection embrace the triadic relationship between group worker, group members, and the artistic process, and they have an inclination toward creative experimentation and natural play, as opposed to unyielding conformity to prescribed evidence-based protocols.

Group Work Is Messy

When my wife and I talk about our passion for the work, we also share stories about colleagues who respect and appreciate what we do and those who are judgmental, often wishing that our kids would quiet down and be more orderly. Too often, group workers are faced not only with getting a creative arts group started but also getting buy-in from those in formal positions of authority. For example, in one group a social work intern struggled mightily to develop a knitting group for homeless teen mothers in a residential setting (Rebmann, 2006). After many long weeks of surreptitious knitting circles, which at best were met with ambivalence by her supervisor, her perseverance started to pay off:

> At this time, my supervisor poked her head into the living room looking for me. She saw the mass of yarn on the floor and the girls all around me practicing. This was it. This was the moment of truth. Would I be called out and punished for going behind her back? Would I fall back into my own pattern of acting from a place of disempowerment? "Wow!" she exclaimed excitedly as I approached her, "are they really into it?" I asked if we could move into her office, as I was afraid of being reprimanded for my disobedience in

front of my clients. To my great surprise she was very enthusiastic about the whole intervention. I took a risk and explained to her what had been going on and how eager the girls had been to learn. My supervisor responded by sanctioning the [knitting] lessons and offering for the program to pay for supplies.

(p. 19)

Although, as cited repeatedly in this collection, research has demonstrated that group therapy is at least as successful as individual therapy, group therapists who utilize the creative arts often must apply extra effort to getting their work sanctioned, particularly when there is a lack of institutional support. Consequently, in addition to developing direct practice skill, we need to embrace the roles of *advocate* and *itinerant educator*. This requires teaching-on-the-go. But what does this have to do with creative arts-based group work with adolescents?

I believe strongly that group work with adolescents requires consistent and persistent advocacy for the method. A proactive stance mitigates defensiveness when unschooled critics question the approach and discount the value of a method that vibrates, makes noise, and rarely sits still. This is unnerving for many. Therefore, an essential part of a group worker's role is to be a knowledgeable and proud group educator to parents, school personnel, agency administrators, and others.

Being an itinerant educator or roaming teacher requires the ability and will to demystify group work—to help those within earshot of a kids' group to better understand "what is going on in there" amid the noise, movement, and seeming chaos. Incorporating the role of itinerant educator into your professional identity makes you, by definition, a missionary for this work (Malekoff, 2009). We must all contribute to building institutional support for our groups—for ourselves and for one another.

Context Counts

Co-editors Craig Haen and Nancy Boyd Webb open this collection with a tribute to the over 2,000 Latinx children that were forcibly separated from their parents on a hot Texas plain as they attempted to cross over the border from Mexico to the United States to escape the violence and poverty of their homelands in places such as El Salvador, Guatemala, and Honduras. These migrant children, some infants and toddlers, were placed in settings such as abandoned Walmart department stores and tent cities. Once inside these strange places, they were contained in smaller areas subdivided by chain-link fences that appeared as makeshift cages. Some were transported by federal government officials to facilities thousands of miles away with no clear sense of what was happening to them and whether or when they would be reunited with their parents.

Despite our having made it to the twenty-first century, it often feels as if we are suspended in a medieval zeitgeist when the concept of childhood did not even exist. It is times like these that the term *humane treatment of children* is an oxymoron. Those of us who work with children, adolescents, and their parents must never lose sight of the fact that *context counts* or fail to factor in the *situational surround* in our work—and not only when front page news stories enter our consciousness, but also when much quieter events closer to home impact our group members' day-to-day lives.

The arts-based group work practices presented herein contain tools to help teenagers heal emotional hurts, cope with psychosocial challenges, and overcome the impact of traumatic handling. Although not a direct focus of this book, the tools can also be used to advance effective citizenship and social justice. Unquestionably, part of our job as group workers is to promote our young group members' capacity to become socially conscious, active participants in community affairs so that they might one day change the world in ways that we have failed to.

On March 24, 2018, I was proud to stand with the youth leaders from Parkland, Florida, and other youth activists across the United States in their *March for Unity*, following the mass shooting at Marjory Stoneman Douglas High School that took the lives of 17 students and teachers. As one of the student activists said on a news broadcast, "Every voice matters." They demonstrated that fact by extending their reach to youth survivors beyond Parkland and broadening the frame to include gun violence in all domains.

Think for just a moment about the authenticity of these social-justice youth warriors compared to the failure of government to take appropriate action about guns. Group workers can help to cultivate the capacity in young people to make a difference. And then we can follow or get out of their way. As Haen and Boyd Webb state early on in this text, "Group work, at its best, has the potential to shape a generation."

Nondeliberative Practice

In addition to the discussion of specific creative arts presented in this book, there are the artful activities that grow spontaneously out of the living together that a group does. These are the creative applications, the group member- and worker-initiated innovations that can be cultivated and brought to life in the group, contributing to a growing sense of groupness and rich history of experience together. The expressive activities illustrated herein, although well grounded in theory, also have a spontaneous and unpredictable quality, mirroring adolescent group members themselves. "Like the sorcerer's apprentice, they can get out of hand and do their own thing," as opposed to interventions that are more calculated and predictable (Middleman, 1981, p. 190).

Social group work scholar Norma Lang (2016) distinguished between *deliberative*, verbal, linear, rational, and planned practice that is cognitively directed and *nondeliberative*, nonverbal, circular, intuitive, visceral, organic, spontaneous, creative, inventive, actional, and holistic practice that is inspired by a more innovative spirit. Lang speaks of groups using activities and creative arts that *sidestep into a parallel reality*, where analogs serve as manageable equivalents of one's life situation. I include two illustrations of activities here to encourage readers to stretch the lessons of this book beyond the media presented.

In a program for LGBTQ youth known as ArtThrust, a twenty-first-century feminist-based social practice art form (Northington, 2018),

> *students were divided into pairs and took turns making plastic armatures of their bodies with cling wrap and clear packaging tape. It took multiple layers to create*

a body cast. At that point, the cast was cut off the student with scissors then reassembled and painted.

One student, Alley, processed internally while she worked quietly on her piece. Her sculpture was a beautiful dancing figure. Part of the body was translucent from the clear plastic that showed through part of the body. Alley used red, blue, and yellow paint on the limbs, and glass stones on the arms. No one knew the depth of the content behind the work until she shared her artist statement.

She wrote, in part, "The positioning of the limbs in a sort of Fighting Dance was meant to show the way that I greet life. Sometimes with a fight, other times more smoothly but no less challenging. The glass stone represents my shell, tough, but not unmovable."

(pp. 145–146)

When a challenging life event is replayed in another medium, it can create an analogic form that allows group members the occasion to discover their own solutions (Abbas & Sulman, 2016), as the following example further illustrates.

Dario was a small fourteen-year-old boy in an indoor rock climbing group in New York City for adolescents who had lost a parent to AIDS. He never spoke about his mother, who had died several months before. But he climbed like a pro. At the top of the climbing wall was a bell. Each group session he was first on the wall, scaled it in seconds, rang the bell, then stayed at the top until the bell was silent again. Then he rappelled down and did it again and again. One afternoon, after his tenth time up, he stayed at the top of the wall with his hand in the bell. After much pleading from the other members, he finally lowered himself down, with tears in his eyes. Worker: "You really like to ring the bell." Dario: "It makes me feel my Mom. Like every time I ring it she is touching me. She was magic when she would hug me. She's up there somewhere and this bell is how I reach her."

(Wright, 2016, p. 180)

Although the rock climbing illustration does not reflect the use of creative arts media per se, it speaks directly to some of the same benefits presented in this collection that are derived from painting, drawing, dance, drama, poetry, music, and more. To me it reflects the notion of *life as art*. I include this illustration to encourage readers to absorb all that is provided herein and then to stretch a bit to apply the lessons learned to other activities that may spark creativity and action in another realm, whether up the side of a mountain, in a knitting circle, in the kitchen, or on a ball field.

Conclusion

In her chapter on "Music Therapy in Adolescent Groups," Katrina Skewes McFerran writes: "In our best moments, we transcend any particular theoretical orientation and integrate everything that [we know], both consciously and unconsciously, into the encounter." This collection is a welcome antidote to manuals that advocate strict adherence to practices that leave little room for mutual aid and spontaneity. This text does not discount the value of research evidence and the practice protocols that they generate, nor does it worship them. It advocates for incorporating the best evidence and timeworn practice guidelines in order to inform one's own clinical judgment and leave room for innovation and invention using the creative arts.

—Andrew Malekoff
Executive Director and CEO, North Shore
Child and Family Guidance Center
Editor-in-Chief, *Social Work With Groups,*
A Journal of Community and Clinical Practice

References

Abbas, S., & Sulman, J. (2016). Nondeliberative crisis intervention in disaster zones: Social group-work using guided artwork with child survivors. *Social Work with Groups, 39*(2/3), 118–128.

Lang, N. (2016). Nondeliberative forms of practice in social work: Artful, actional, analogic. *Social Work with Groups, 39*(2/3), 97–117.

Malekoff, A. (2009). Gatekeepers, gatecrashers and gateways in group work with kids: A mystery story. *Social Work with Groups, 32*(3), 193–208.

Middleman, R. (1981). The use of program: Review and update. In S. L. Abels & P. Abels (Eds.), *Social work with groups proceedings, 1979* (pp. 187–205). Louisville, KY: Committee for the Advancement of Social Work with Groups.

Northington, T. (2018). ArtThrust teen empowerment program: Teaching youth to fly against resistance. *Social Work with Groups, 41*(1/2), 139–150.

Rebmann, H. (2006). There's a lot of yelling in knitting: The impact of parallel process on empowerment in a group setting, *Social Work with Groups. 29*(4), 5–24.

Wright, W. (2016). A punch, a stitch, a bell: The power of nondeliberative practice in social group work. *Social Work with Groups, 39*(2/3), 170–182.

Preface

The Stresses and Challenges Facing Adolescents in the Second Decade of the Twenty-First Century

This book demonstrates the positive role of creative arts therapy groups in helping adolescents deal with the many stresses that impinge on their daily lives. Before presenting these therapeutic approaches, however, the editors believe that we must first review some of the numerous and serious challenges facing adolescents in the second decade of the twenty-first century. While everyone realizes that the period of adolescence is typically stormy and chaotic, the developmental struggle of today's teenagers is further complicated by the barrage of *external stressors* that interact with their internal developmental changes and serve to complicate their passage from childhood to adulthood.

Epidemiological data show that mental health problems have always been an endemic part of adolescence (Hagell & Maughan, 2017), with the proportion of teenagers with a psychiatric diagnosis at any given time estimated to be about one in five (Costello, Copeland, & Angold, 2011). Comorbidity, or the presence of more than one disorder, is extremely common (Kessler et al., 2012). Fewer than half of American adolescents with mental health issues will receive treatment of any kind during their teen years (Costello, He, Sampson, Kessler, & Merikangas, 2014). Buntin (2017) captured the emotions common to this stage of life when she wrote:

> Great loneliness, profound isolation, a cataclysmic, overpowering sense of being misunderstood. When does that kind of deep feeling just stop? Where does it go? At fifteen, the world ended over and over and over again. To be so young is a kind of self-violence. No foresight, an inflated sense of wisdom, and yet you're still responsible for your mistakes. It's a little frightening to remember just how much, and how precisely, I felt.
>
> (Buntin, 2017, p. 105)

This chapter discusses some of the major stressors that are prevalent in the everyday lives of teenagers in the second decade of the twenty-first century and that may interfere with typical adolescent development between the ages of 13 and 20 years. This is not a comprehensive list, but one that highlights some of the challenges confronting teens in their struggle to assume a new identity within a changing world that contains many dangers and difficulties. It is important for therapists to be aware of these struggles to better facilitate and support teens as they attempt to deal with them.

Stressful Challenges for Adolescent Development

1. **Violence** in Schools and Communities as Evidenced in Shootings, Gang Warfare, and Domestic Violence.

2. The Compelling Influence of **Technological Media** That Dominates the Lives of Young People and Competes With Social Interactions.
3. **Substance Abuse.** The Presence of Drugs, Alcohol, and Vaping as Methods for Dealing With Stress, Avoiding Feelings, and Attempting to Feel Good.
4. The **Pressures to Succeed** in Multiple Realms, Such as Academics, Sports, Music, and Performance.
5. The Experiencing of **Anxiety and Major Depression,** Which Can Contribute to Suicidal Thoughts and Behavior.

Some or all these factors can weigh heavily on a teenager and have a negative influence on his or her development. We present them not as evidence that the cards are stacked against adolescents, but as the reality of daily life with which youth today must cope. Many young people are resilient and manage to get through their teen years relatively unscathed, while others struggle to find their way and require therapeutic interventions to assist them.

The Presence of Guns and Violence in Everyday Life

The social environment in 2018 and 2019 includes the harmful prevalence of violence, with possible traumatic effects on the victims and observers, and a resulting absence of a sense of safety among all. This violence may occur at home, in the community, and/or in schools. In the month of January 2018, there were at least 11 episodes of gun violence on school property in the United States (Blinder & Victor, 2018). This was followed by the school shooting in Parkland, Florida, in February 2018, which resulted in 17 deaths. Because of the activism of the teen survivors in arguing for gun control following the Florida shooting, the issue is one about which all American citizens are aware, and there are varied opinions about steps necessary to prevent similar tragedies. Adolescents have led marches, spoken forcefully on television, and been determined to change current gun legislation that allows the purchase of firearms by 18-year-olds without any background checks.

Since the earlier killings of 26 children and staff members at Sandy Hook Elementary School in Newtown, Connecticut, in 2012, about two-thirds of American schools now conduct active shooter drills (Blinder & Williams, 2018), in which students practice hiding from imaginary mass murderers, but the passage of gun legislation on a national level has not occurred. Currently, some American legislators are recommending that teachers should be armed, but there is understandable disagreement about this. This possibility can increase anxiety and lead to psychological problems for some young people who no longer consider school a safe place. For teens who live in homes where family tensions and violence are common, and for those in communities where gangs and shootings are an ever-present reality, violence in their schools means that no place is safe. It is understandable that some youth will themselves decide to join gangs as a source of belonging and a perceived means of self-protection.

The Influence of Technology on the Lives of Adolescents

Teens spend a fair amount of their time involved with social media and playing video games, with 90% reportedly using the internet daily and 22% being online nearly constantly (Belfort & Miller, 2018). Facebook is the most popular social media site among American teens ages 13–17 years (Calancie, Ewing, Narducci, Horgan, & Khalid-Khan, 2017), with Instagram and Snapchat also used by many (though as with any trends, adolescent rates of participation in these platforms could well change by the time this book is published). Teenage girls use social media sites—particularly visually oriented ones—for sharing more frequently than their male counterparts do (Krämer et al., 2017). Boys are more likely than girls to own gaming consoles and play video games (Belfort & Miller, 2018). For example, one popular game, *Fortnite Battle Royale*, is a third-person shooter game in which the players air-drop out of a flying battle bus, then fight to survive as the play space slowly shrinks to force people into combat. This involves playing alone or teaming up with peers, building massive forts, collecting weapons, battling against other players, and trying to be the last person alive in the game. Anecdotally, many parents are reporting that this game has consumed much of their adolescent's free time, particularly as the ability to play on squads with peers capitalizes on the power of social influence.

A recent review of existing research conducted by the APA Task Force on Violent Media concluded that "there is an effect of violent video game use on aggression," which causes a "decrease in positive outcomes such as pro-social behavior, empathy, and sensitivity to aggression" (Calvert et al., 2017, p. 141). These findings were evident in numerous studies and especially applicable to older children, adolescents, and young adults. Although the task force did not find sufficient evidence to evaluate whether there is a direct link between violent video games and criminal aggression, they did conclude that playing violent games is a risk factor for subsequent aggression. It remains to be seen whether and to what extent these findings will affect future use of this popular recreational outlet. In July 2018, the World Health Organization announced that it was adding Gaming Disorder to its disease classification manual.

On the one hand, technology and social media can provide forms of connection for adolescents marginalized because of race, sexual orientation, or other differences (Belfort & Miller, 2018). They have generally opened teens to a wider sense of cultural integration, reflected in the now-normative blending of formerly distinct musical genres into a mainstream style that combines elements of hip hop, dance music, rock, and pop. Contemporary teens are generally more socially conscious and engaged in activism, more embracing of difference, and less likely to conform to traditional gender norms. At the same time, they appear more risk-averse, at times less autonomous, and subject to the paradox of feeling always connected through social media, yet more emotionally alone. This sense of isolation is reflected by both data showing that today's adolescents have fewer conversation partners than previous generations and in teens' artwork, which depicts greater solitude and distance from peers (Gardner & Davis, 2013). However, the ubiquity of technology in the lives of contemporary teenagers has significant ramifications for development.

One way in which the proliferation of technology has instituted a cultural transformation is in teens rarely having to sit with themselves or tolerate moments of downtime that are a typical part of life (e.g., waiting in line, making conversation in a car ride), instead remaining connected to their devices. The frequency of sharing photos on Instagram, keeping up streaks on Snapchat, and posting events in real time has led to a notable shift from *being* to *doing*, one that often precludes self-reflection and digesting of events before communicating about them (Gardner & Davis, 2013). It also reflects a move from sustained focus on one task to multi-tasking as normative behavior. In this condition, minimal attention is given to the task at hand, while the brain prioritizes incoming stimuli with a level of hyper-alertness that parallels the processing of trauma (Music, 2017).

Some adolescents find the lure of social media difficult to resist, and the time they spend on it can interfere with homework, sleep, and physical activity. Social media is Elkind's (1967) theory of the *imaginary audience* (teens' notion that they are constantly being observed and judged by others) writ large—reinforcing self-evaluation through comparing oneself to the highly composed presentation of others' lives and achieving approval through comments and likes (Underwood & Ehrenreich, 2017). In addition, these platforms can change the frequency, imme-diacy, and intensity of peer interactions while providing mechanisms for cyber-bullying and sexting, among other dangers (Nesi, Choukas-Bradley, & Prinstein, 2018). For the majority of young people who engage in average use of video games and social media, there has been little quantifiable negative impact, but factors such as family support, poverty, and other stressors can heighten the effect. In general, youth who are more at-risk offline tend to also be at greater risk online (Martínez-Ferrer, Ruiz, & Ochoa, in press; Music, 2017).

Exposure to pornography also occurs online. Teens may turn to various forms of media for guidance and relief from stress and, in the process, may come across an array of pornographic displays that often portray males dominating and abus-ing females during sexual interactions that are centered on physical discharge of impulses, rather than on emotional connection. According to Jones (2018), boys typ-ically first view pornography when they are about 13 years old, and girls when they are 14. Often this occurs through seeing a porn clip on a friend's phone, or by find-ing the website Pornhub, which contains millions of free short videos that serve as 'how-to guides' about sex for many adolescents. This content is more readily available than ever (with an estimated 40% of children ages 10–17 years having been exposed), providing what Lemma (2017) termed *immediacy without mediation*, or immediate gratification without having to wait. Ongoing exposure to internet pornography is thought to contribute to belief in rape myths and to reinforce the idea that the goal of heterosexual engagement is to please the male partner (Orenstein, 2016).

Interviews with teenagers refer to their wishes for sex education classes that give details about anatomy, intimacy, and healthy relationships, but relatively few schools deal with these matters effectively, in a way that balances teaching about both pleasure and risk. According to Jones (2018), the World Health Organization recommends that educators should openly discuss the influence of pornography on sexuality beginning in late elementary school and through high school. In the absence of information about healthy sex, adolescents continue to be influenced by narrow and negative portrayals on pornographic websites.

Substance Abuse: The Use of Drugs, Alcohol, and Vaping

Teens in the second decade of the twenty-first century are surrounded by an array of alcohol and other substances and, if their parents were addicted, they may not have received effective responsiveness in their growing years to normal needs for love and attention. Under these circumstances, many youths develop a tendency to mistrust adults and to believe that they must take care of themselves. They also may develop dependency on drugs and alcohol, following their parents' example (Straussner & Donath, 2015; Straussner, & Fewell, 2015). Adolescents who have had mental health disorders demonstrate higher rates of both alcohol (10%) and drug (15%) abuse, with the most robust correlations being for teens who have been diagnosed with anxiety and behavior disorders (Conway, Swendsen, Husky, He, & Merikangas, 2016).

Those adolescents who grow up in families that have healthier relationships with drugs and alcohol may experiment with substances to conform to peer pressure or simply to try something for relaxation. Daily use of marijuana is reported to be close to 6% among 12th graders, and research shows that 25–50% of these daily users will become addicted (Pathway to Prevention, 2015). Many teens did not like the taste of traditional cigarettes and instead opted for e-cigarettes. However, in 2017 e-cigarettes were eclipsed by a vape product known as 'Juul' (Barshad, 2018). This is a tobacco device that mimics the nicotine effects of a cigarette and is available in different flavors. It is small, looks like a USB drive, and is rechargeable. Originally developed to wean adult addicts off cigarettes, it has become popular among teens, who carry their Juuls with them in school, where group use is common. There actually has been a decline in the use of alcohol and tobacco among contemporary teens (Malekoff, 2014; Pathway to Prevention, 2015), but the increase in vaping has created great concerns due to the unknown long-term effects of this form of nicotine intake on the lungs.

Multiple Pressures to Succeed

The lives of many adolescents are dominated by school activities that include academics plus extra-curricular sports and other obligations that are time-consuming and demanding. Teens may put pressure on themselves to succeed, and their parents also often contribute to this expectation for success. Many adolescents feel overscheduled and overwhelmed, with all their free time occupied and little room for rest or recreation. Likewise, the volume of homework given in most American schools exceeds the amount that studies have shown produces academic benefit, and is connected to greater stress, physical illness, and a lack of life balance (Fernández-Alonso, Álvarez-Díaz, Suárez-Álvarez, & Muñiz, 2017; Galloway, Conner, & Pope, 2013). In addition, homework can widen the gap between highly successful students who live in supportive home environments and those who lack these advantages (Fernández-Alonso et al., 2017). Robinson ("Q and A" with Sir Ken Robinson, 2018) presented the situation as follows:

> In the United States, more than eight out of ten teenagers experience extreme or moderate stress during the school year, including headaches, loss of sleep, anger and irritability. The main causes include anxieties about academic performance, the pressures of testing and parental pressures to excel at school and get into a good college.
>
> (p. F11)

The result, as Bruni (2015) noted, is that adolescents are often now oriented to a premature set of easily definable goals designed for gaining entry to the best college, already committed to what they will study when they get there. Such an approach, what Gardner and Davis (2013) called *the packaged self*, foreshortens the exploration of interests and identity that is a hallmark of this stage of development. It can result in teens being so focused on getting into college that they can end up feeling lost when they arrive there, having given little thought to what happens beyond admission (Bruni, 2015). The false belief that one can master life by cultivating an impressive resume does a disservice not only to teens who enact it, but also to those adolescents who have not locked on their passions and career goals and who come to believe that not knowing these things—which, a generation ago, was the norm—makes them deficient.

Likewise, not all individuals have the native ability to excel in academics, and those who do not may suffer from insecurities and feelings of inadequacy. A sense of disconnection and lack of school belonging have been found to negatively impact mental health in young people (Allen & Kern, 2017). The next section discusses unfortunate outcomes for adolescents who push themselves beyond their abilities or who become chronically frustrated or hopeless due to academic challenges.

Anxiety, Depression, and Suicidal Thoughts and Behavior

Anxiety and stress are inevitable in daily life, and some degree of anxiety can serve to motivate positive behavior. However, when anxiety becomes excessive it can seriously interfere with normal functioning and lead to problems such as substance abuse, social isolation, and depression. Most notably, anxiety is among the least addressed adolescent mental health problems, with only about 41% of teens with anxiety disorders receiving some form of treatment (Costello et al., 2014).

Adolescence is a developmental period characterized by marked increases in depression, with the prevalence of major depression in teens being between 5% and 10%. The rate among females is between two and three times the rate in males, and the rate among older adolescents is twice that of younger teens (Avenevoli, Swendsen, He, Burstein, & Merikangas, 2015; Straus, 2007). Comorbid anxiety and depression is also more common among older adolescents compared to younger ones (Harvey, 2014). Depression manifests in various symptoms such as irritability, a sense of hopelessness, somatic complaints, social isolation, and substance abuse. It often goes unrecognized in adolescents, as the outward signs may be regarded as 'just a phase.' Some parents and teachers regard depression as a sign of weakness that can be overcome with willpower. However, depression is a treatable illness that, when left unaddressed, can lead to suicidal behavior, the second leading cause of death of adolescents in the U.S. (Heron, 2017). Unfortunately, depressive episodes are highly recurrent, and 66% of depressed adolescents will have another episode before age 18 (Swartz, 2018).

Sleep

A final, often-overlooked problem area that has strong associations with the onset of depression, anxiety, and substance abuse is sleep deprivation (Harvey, 2014). Lack of sleep seems to be related to many of the aforementioned stressors, and most adolescents are not getting the nine hours of sleep their bodies need to be fully functioning. According to the UCLA Sleep Disorders Center (n.d.), puberty induces a shift in circadian rhythms that causes the body to start releasing the hormone melatonin, which induces sleepiness, about two hours later during adolescence. This shift, known as *sleep phase delay*, is one reason that the American Academy of Pediatrics (2014) urged later school start times for adolescents, a recommendation that most schools have not heeded. Delayed start times have been generally linked to increased sleep duration for teens, with the strength of this correlation most robust for boys (Paksarian, Rudolph, He, & Merikangas, 2015).

Stress levels and sleep seem to have a reciprocal relationship, so that that more stressed adolescents are, the less sleep they get, and vice versa (DeSilva Mousseau, Lund, Liang, Spencer, & Walsh, 2016). Sleep is also connected to academic performance, as the more tired teens are during the day, the less well they do in school (Hysing, Harvey, Linton, Askeland, & Sivertsen, 2016). Use of screens at nighttime, or just having an electronic device nearby (as many adolescents fall asleep with their phones) can impact sleep duration and quality (Music, 2017). Recent preliminary evidence suggests that the blue light emitted by electronic devices at night can further alter the body's circadian rhythms, contributing to more sustained sleep loss (Green, Cohen-Zion, Haim, & Dagan, 2017). Lack of sleep is problematic for all teens, but for some the consequences can indeed be dire, as sleep disturbances have been found to double one's risk of suicide (Ahmedani et al., 2017).

The Potential of the Arts

Adolescence has been noted to be one developmental period in the life cycle in which creativity peaks (Lilly, 2014). Increased interest in metaphor, symbolism, and multiple layers of meaning, as well as a capacity for abstraction and imagining possibilities for the self, are hallmarks of this stage. At the same time, there is evidence to suggest that today's teens have less facility of imagination than those of previous generations.

In a study focused on the impact of modern technology on children and adolescents, Gardner and Davis (2013) gathered data from semi-structured interviews with veteran teachers, focus groups with professionals working with teens, and individual interviews with 123 young people ages 10–20 years. These interviews with American participants were complemented by a mixed-method study in Bermuda. The researchers also conducted a systematic comparison of 354 creative products (pieces of visual art and fiction writing) produced by adolescents between 1990 and 2011.

Among their findings was that contemporary adolescents seemed to be exhibiting a reduction in creativity, specifically in their capacity for imagination (Gardner & Davis, 2013). While teens' artwork reflected a trend toward greater complexity and sophistication over time, their fiction showed decreased use of *genre play* (diverging from realist perspectives), more frequent reliance on mundane plots, fewer characters that differed substantially from the author, and fewer settings that reflected different time periods and cultures. In short, the stories had become more conventional, characterized by less creative elaboration, fewer novel approaches, and reduced perspective-taking; put simply, they showed a decline in imagination.

Whether this decline is reflective of external stressors or, as Gardner and Davis (2013) suggested, linked to increased reliance on technology, the data suggest that the arts are not only potentially curative, but also vital for today's teenagers. Recently, researchers Trevarthen and Panksepp (2017) argued that approaches that focus on play, the body, and the arts deserve more attention within psychotherapy for their potential to effect more rapid progress in young people than purely cognitively focused approaches. They advocated: "To restore resilience, one must restore *joie de vivre*. And as we will see, there is no better vehicle for that than natural play—the engagement that children themselves devise to pass the living moment" (p. 31).

Summary

Of course, not every adolescent experiences *all* the negative influences of these various challenges and stresses in everyday life. Different individuals respond differently to the same circumstances, with many factors determining the outcomes for teens who must confront these challenges. Biology impacts behavior, and an individual's genetics may shape certain responses such as the onset of depression, since children of a depressed parent are three times as likely to develop Major Depressive Disorder (Swartz, 2018). Support systems within the family or in the community, socioeconomic status, and one's membership in dominant or marginalized groups significantly affect the development of children into adulthood, thereby perpetuating or negating other influences on adolescents. A young person's social environment and peers play an important role in introducing and maintaining certain behaviors. For example, it appears that support from peers can help to provide a buffer for teens who perceive a lack of adult support in their lives, leading to better emotional, psychological, and social well-being (Ciarrochi, Morin, Sahdra, Litalien, & Parker, 2017).

This overview is intended to set the stage for understanding the complex lives of adolescents. The examples in the chapters to come demonstrate the great variety of positive and negative behaviors that adolescents present in public, with detailed illustrations of how some of the less adaptive responses can be modified through participation in creative arts therapy groups. As will be illustrated by numerous contributors, adolescents require specialized approaches that are developmentally responsive and capitalize on age-related drives toward peer connection. Likewise, as readers will come to know, the arts are well-suited to addressing the complex challenges facing contemporary teenagers.

The chapters in **Section I** will locate creative arts-based group approaches within the current psychotherapy and neuroscience research landscapes, and offer practice guidelines for implementation. **Section II** will cover each of the major creative arts therapy modalities, with a special focus on providing tools and practice considerations to adolescent group therapists. As many of the authors remind readers, each creative arts therapy approach has its own advanced training. While ethical guidelines reinforce not practicing beyond the scope of one's competency, treating teenagers often calls for a willingness to favor creative experimentation and integrative approaches over rigid methodology (Haen, 2017), and many adolescent therapists are already utilizing the arts within their groups. With the understanding that the arts are core elements of human culture that do not belong to one set of professionals, the contributors aim to enhance ethical practice by guiding readers with knowledge supported by research, theory, and real-world experience.

Section III will focus on a range of problem areas that are characteristic of adolescent experience and that transcend diagnoses and cultural differences. The contributors will illustrate how creative arts-based techniques and approaches can be used to address these challenges, which are part of the sometimes treacherous, sometimes thrilling terrain of adolescent group work. Ultimately, this book offers hope: that by drawing on the power of the arts, professionals can make a real difference in the lives of the teenagers with whom they come in contact. As Woolfolk (2015) so eloquently suggested, "Art can frighten us, ennoble us, and educe reverence, joy, sadness, or pity. But in its capacity to depict and elicit hope, it may be unsurpassed" (p. 189).

Nancy Boyd Webb and Craig Haen

References

Ahmedani, B. K., Peterson, E. L., Hu, Y., Rossom, R. C., Lynch, F., Lu, C. Y., . . . Simon, G. E. (2017). Major physical health conditions and risk of suicide. *American Journal of Preventive Medicine, 53*(3), 308–315.

Allen, K.-A., & Kern, M. L. (2017). *School belonging in adolescents: Theory, research and practice.* New York, NY: Springer.

American Academy of Pediatrics. (2014). Policy statement: School start times for adolescents. *Pediatrics, 134*(3), 643–649.

Avenevoli, S., Swendsen, J., He, J.-P., Burstein, M., & Merikangas, K. R. (2015). Major depression in the national comorbidity survey-adolescent supplement: Prevalence, correlates, and treatment. *Journal of the American Academy of Child & Adolescent Psychiatry, 54*(1), 37–44.

Barshad, A. (2018, April 8). The Juul is too cool. *The New York Times*, p. ST1.

Belfort, E. L., & Miller, L. (2018). Relationship between adolescent suicidality, self-injury, and media habits. *Child and Adolescent Psychiatric Clinics of North America, 27*, 159–169.

Blinder, A., & Victor, D. (2018, January 24). A school attack every other day. *The New York Times*, p. A-1.

Blinder, A., & Williams, T. (2018, January 25). Tears in a cockpit: When a school shooting hits close to home. *The New York Times*, p. A-12.

Bruni, F. (2015). *Where you go is not who you'll be: An antidote to the college admissions mania.* New York, NY: Grand Central Publishing.

Buntin, J. (2017). *Marlena: A novel.* New York, NY: Henry Holt.

Calancie, O., Ewing, L., Narducci, L. D., Horgan, S., & Khalid-Khan, S. (2017). Exploring how social networking sites impact youth with anxiety: A qualitative study of Facebook stressors among adolescents with an anxiety disorder diagnosis. *Cyberpsychology: Journal of Psychosocial Research on Cyberspace, 11*(4), article 2.

Calvert, S. L., Dodge, K. A., Nagayama Hall, G. C., Fasig-Caldwell, L. G., Galloway, D. P., Applebaum, M., . . . Hedges, L. V. (2017). The American Psychological Association Task Force assessment of violent video games: Science in the service of public interest. *American Psychologist, 72*(2), 126–143.

Ciarrochi, J., Morin, A. J. S., Sahdra, B. K., Litalien, D., & Parker, P. D. (2017). A longitudinal person-centered perspective on youth social support: Relations with psychological wellbeing. *Developmental Psychology, 53*(6), 1154–1169.

Conway, K. P., Swendsen, J., Husky, M. M., He, J.-P., & Merikangas, K. R. (2016). Association of lifetime mental disorders and subsequent alcohol and illicit drug use: Results from the National Comorbidity Survey-Adolescent Supplement. *Journal of the American Academy of Child & Adolescent Psychiatry, 55*(4), 280–288.

Costello, E. J., Copeland, W., & Angold, A. (2011). Trends in psychopathology across the adolescent years: What changes when children become adolescents, and when adolescents become adults? *The Journal of Child Psychology and Psychiatry, 52*(10), 1015–1025.

Costello, E. J., He, J.-P., Sampson, N. A., Kessler, R. C., & Merikangas, K. R. (2014). Services for adolescents with psychiatric disorders: 12-month data from the National Comorbidity Survey-Adolescent. *Psychiatric Services, 65*(3), 359–366.

DeSilva Mousseau, A. M., Lund, T. J., Liang, B., Spencer, R., & Walsh, J. (2016). Stressed and losing sleep: Sleep duration and perceived stress among affluent adolescent females. *Peabody Journal of Education, 91*(5), 628–644.

Elkind, D. (1967). Egocentrism in adolescence. *Child Development, 38*(4), 1025–1034.

Fernández-Alonso, R., Álvarez-Díaz, M., Suárez-Álvarez, J., & Muñiz, J. (2017). Students' achievement and homework assignment strategies. *Frontiers in Psychology, 8*(286). doi: 10.3389/fpsyg.2017.00286

Galloway, M., Conner, J., & Pope, D. (2013). Nonacademic effects of homework in privileged, high-performing high schools. *The Journal of Experimental Education, 81*(4), 490–510.

Gardner, H., & Davis, K. (2013). *The app generation: How today's youth navigate identity, intimacy, and imagination in a digital world*. New Haven, CT: Yale University Press.

Green, A., Cohen-Zion, M., Haim, A., & Dagan, Y. (2017). Evening light exposure to computer screens disrupts human sleep, biological rhythms, and attention abilities. *Chronobiology International, 34*(7), 855–865.

Haen, C. (2017). An integrative perspective on group therapy. In C. Haen & S. Aronson (Eds.), *Handbook of child and adolescent group therapy: A practitioner's reference* (pp. 193–202). New York, NY: Routledge.

Hagell, A., & Maughan, B. (2017). Epidemiology: Are mental health problems in children and young people really a big deal? In N. Midgley, J. Hayes & M. Cooper (Eds.), *Essential research findings in child and adolescent counselling and psychotherapy* (pp. 14–31). London: Sage.

Harvey, A. G. (2014). Transdiagnostic mechanisms and treatments for youth with psychiatric disorders: An opportunity to catapult progress? In J. Ehrenreich-May & B. C. Chu (Eds.), *Transdiagnostic treatments for children and adolescents: Principles and practice* (pp. 15–31). New York, NY: Guilford.

Heron, M. (2017, November 27). Deaths: Leading causes for 2015. *National Vital Statistics Reports, 66*(5). Hyattsville, MD: National Center for Health Statistics. Retrieved from www.cdc.gov/nchs/data/nvsr/nvsr66/nvsr66_05.pdf

Hysing, M., Harvey, A. G., Linton, S. J., Askeland, K. G., & Sivertsen, B. (2016). Sleep and academic performance in later adolescence: Results from a large population-based study. *Journal of Sleep Research, 25*(3), 318–324.

Jones, M. (2018, February 7). What teenagers are learning from online porn. *The New York Times Magazine*. Retrieved from www.nytimes.com/2018/02/07/magazine/teenagers-learning-online-porn-literacy-sex-education.html

Kessler, R. C., Avenevoli, S., McLaughlin, K. A., Green, J. G., Lakoma, M. D., Petukhova, M., . . . Merikangas, K. R. (2012). Lifetime co-morbidity of DSM-IV disorders in the US National Comorbidity Survey Replication Adolescent Supplement (NCS-A). *Psychological Medicine, 42*(9), 1997–2010.

Krämer, N. C., Feurstein, M., Kluck, J. P., Meier, Y., Rother, M., & Winter, S. (2017). Beware of selfies: The impact of photo type on impression formation based on social networking profiles. *Frontiers in Psychology, 8*(188). doi: 10.3389/fpsyg.2017.00188

Lemma, A. (2017). *The digital age on the couch: Psychoanalytic practice and new media*. New York, NY: Routledge.

Lilly, F. R. (2014). Creativity in adolescence. In T. P. Gullotta & M. Bloom (Eds.), *Encyclopedia of primary prevention and health promotion* (pp. 1057–1065). New York, NY: Springer.

Malekoff, A. (2014). *Group work with adolescents: Principles and practice* (3rd ed.). New York, NY: Guilford.

Martínez-Ferrer, B., Ruiz, D. M., & Ochoa, G. M. (in press). Are adolescents engaged in the problematic use of social networking sites more involved in peer aggression and victimization? *Frontiers in Psychology*. doi: 10.3389/fpsyg.2018.00801

Music, G. (2017). *Nurturing natures: Attachment and children's emotional, sociocultural and brain development* (2nd ed.). New York, NY: Psychology Press.

Nesi, J., Choukas-Bradley, S., & Prinstein, M. J. (2018). Transformation of adolescent peer relations in the social media context: Part 2—Application to peer group processes and future directions for research. *Clinical Child and Family Psychology Review*. Advance online publication. doi: 10.1007/s10567-018-0262-9

Orenstein, P. (2016). *Girls & sex: Navigating the complicated new landscape*. New York, NY: HarperCollins.

Paksarian, D., Rudolph, K. E., He, J.-P., & Merikangas, K. R. (2015). School start time and adolescent sleep patterns: Results from the US National Comorbidity Survey—Adolescent Supplement. *American Journal of Public Health, 105*(7), 1351–1357.

Pathway to Prevention. (2015). Teen drug and alcohol statistics 2014/2015. Retrieved from www. pathwaytoprevention.org/statistics/

Q. and A. with Sir Ken Robinson. (April 8, 2018). *The New York Times*, F11.

Straus, M. B. (2007). *Adolescent girls in crisis: Intervention and hope*. New York, NY: Norton.

Straussner, S. L. A., & Donath, R. (2015). Children and teens with substance-abusing parents. In N. B. Webb (Ed.), *Play therapy with children and adolescents in crisis* (4th ed., pp. 79–98). New York, NY: Guilford.

Straussner, S. L. A., & Fewell, C. H. (2015). Children of parents who abuse alcohol and other drugs. In A. Rupert, D. Mayberry, J. Nicholson, M. Göpfert & M. V. Seeman (Eds.), *Parental psychiatric disorder: Distressed parents and their families* (3rd ed., pp. 138–153). Cambridge: Cambridge University Press.

Swartz, K. (February 24, 2018). *Adolescent depression: Diagnosis, treatment, and community education*. Keynote presented at the 2018 Duvall Family Studies conference, Sarasota, FL.

Trevarthen, C., & Panksepp, J. (2017). In tune with feeling: Musical play with emotions of creativity, inspiring neuroaffective development and self-confidence for learning in company. In S. Hart (Ed.), *Inclusion, play and empathy: Neuroaffective development in children's groups* (pp. 29–54). London: Routledge.

UCLA Sleep Disorders Center (n.d.). Sleep and teens. Retrieved from www.uclahealth.org/sleep-center/body.cfm?id=63&iirf_redirect=1

Underwood, M. K., & Ehrenreich, S. E. (2017). The power and the pain of adolescents' digital communication: Cyber victimization and the perils of lurking. *American Psychologist, 72*(2), 144–158.

Woolfolk, R. L. (2015). *The value of psychotherapy: The talking cure in an age of clinical science*. New York, NY: Guilford.

Section 1
Overview

1
Engaging Adolescents in Group Work
Principles for Effective Practice

CRAIG HAEN AND NANCY BOYD WEBB

Many years ago, I (Haen, 2007) sat in the circle of an adolescent boys' group I was leading that took place in a boarding school. It was the start of a new cycle, and several members were entering the group for the first time. A new 16-year-old member walked into the room. He stopped, pointed at me, and yelled, "You're a child molester! You're a child molester!" The room froze in silence, all eyes on me: waiting to see how I might handle this moment.

Internally, in a few seconds that seemed to stretch for minutes, so many feelings and associations percolated—my own experiences of being called "gay" when I was younger, my desire to be liked by my peers as a teenager, my masculine adult need to overpower—and so many urges toward action rose up, chiefly to authoritatively set limits and make my shame go away. Fortunately, I was able to not act on any of those impulses. Instead, what emerged from my lips was a chuckle. I turned toward this new member and said, "Thank you, no one's ever greeted me quite that way before. Come, sit down and join us."

This boy's distinctive entry that first session evolved into a weekly ritual that was marked by his entering the group and loudly calling me whatever new and terrible thing he could think of. Eventually, his testing of our relationship and the boundaries of the group space gave way to him bravely disclosing his childhood molestation by his uncle. While he might have found his way to this disclosure eventually, our contention is that his trajectory was eased by that initial meeting and my thankfully being able to suppress my pull to act out of urgency, and instead welcoming his whole self into the space.

As in the previous clinical vignette, we have rarely received as sharp an education on being therapists as we have from our adolescent patients, and facilitating groups with them maximizes both the challenges and the potential. Despite the many fine writings that exist on clinical work with adolescents, few have the capacity to convey the visceral experience of being in a room full of teenagers. They can be angry, passive, confrontational, sarcastic, and unwilling to admit their need for any kind of help or therapy. They can also be charming and sweet, but often their positive characteristics are overshadowed by a 'chip-on-their-shoulders' stand-offish attitude that leads to conflict with parents, teachers, and other adults, and in turn causes the youth to feel misunderstood and isolated. This age group is perhaps most illustrative of Siegel's (2010) analogy depicting mental health as a river bordered by two banks: one marked by rigidity and the other by chaos. Within each adolescent group exist teens who tend to reside on one or the other end of that river, as well as members who flip between banks, sometimes multiple times in the course of a single session.

The group leader's education by adolescents often comes in the form of ongoing calls for authenticity (of expression, of presence, and of regard) on the part of the leader, as well as a wariness of the typical techniques that therapists employ (Edgette, 2006). Adolescent patients can present challenging requests and questions, primitive dynamics and behaviors, and mischievous attempts to derail the therapeutic process. As Phillips (2011) reminded, "Their development depends on their need to frustrate us [therapists]" (p. 189). It is therefore quite understandable that some practitioners avoid working with adolescents out of discomfort. A social work student once reflected her reluctance to work with teens by asking, "Why should I go overboard trying to help kids, when they only resent my efforts and don't see any need for help?"

Practitioners who successfully engage with adolescents have found ways to look beyond their surface presentations of bravado, because they realize that those outside personas are often armor intended to shield their more vulnerable interiors, and they may not know productive ways of interacting with others when they are upset. Teenagers also have the potential to take risks and to form meaningful connections that allow for a degree of change that is not always possible in individual treatment. It is true that I (CH) have at times felt a pull toward canceling my adolescent groups before sessions began, and have often left those same sessions feeling exhilarated by the process.

While there are existing guidelines for effective group practice with adults, many authors (Donald, Rickwood, & Carey, 2014; Lee et al., 2014; Shechtman, 2014) have contended that adolescent patients require different approaches and a distinct set of clinical skills, and that it is inappropriate to assume that findings from adult research and practice can simply be applied to therapy with young people. For this reason, theorists have outlined differential models of group development for adolescents, and researchers have started to identify differences in group process. For example, Dies (2000), highlighting the adolescent need for autonomy, proposed that groups of teens evolve in the following fashion: *initial relatedness; testing the limits; resolving authority issues; working on self; moving on.* Likewise, Shechtman and Leichtentritt (2010) established the importance of bonding between adolescent members and group leaders, which was found to be a significant predictor of outcomes for youth. While it is now well established that the quality of the therapeutic relationship is solidly connected to outcomes in group therapy, this correlation is even more robust with young people (Burlingame, Whitcomb, & Woodland, 2014).

Acknowledging that there may be considerable barriers to engaging teens in effective practice, we endeavor in this chapter to outline a set of principles for conducting creative arts-based group therapy with adolescents that is informed by the practice and supervision of such groups over many years. These principles are intended to be integrative and transdiagnostic, applicable to a wide range of adolescent groups regardless of therapist theoretical orientation or patient symptom categories. They are grounded in practice but supported by various streams of research. While they address the use of the arts as a core method of treatment, the principles outlined may be applied equally to a range of treatment approaches. Many of the chapters to follow illustrate wise and successful interventions, and this chapter serves as an introduction to highlight and frame these approaches.

Embracing Adolescent Development

Many authors (e.g., Malekoff, 2014; Steinberg, 2014) have outlined stages of adolescent development and have articulately captured this time period, which is marked by vast physiological and psychological change. We will not reiterate these stages here, except to highlight the significance of the fact that teenage selves are in forward motion (Karkou & Joseph, 2017), immersed in a process of evolving and becoming. As Kaduson (2016) noted, "What is unique about the stage of identity is that it is a synthesis of earlier stages and an anticipation of later ones" (p. 335).

Effective clinical work with adolescents involves accepting and supporting developmental processes, rather than viewing them as barriers to more mature modes of engagement (Haen & Weil, 2010). In doing so, the group leader expects certain limitations while capitalizing on the possibilities inherent to neuroplasticity, which makes teenagers particularly primed for learning and change (Jensen & Nutt, 2014). These principles are oriented to welcoming adolescent identity in its fullness, shaping and channeling resistant energy rather than attempting to confine or limit it. They offer ways of drawing on and fostering group dynamics to effect change. However, as a precursor, we begin with a discussion of effective leadership.

The Position of the Leader

Hurster (2017) noted that group leaders working with adolescents have to balance a number of roles in relationship to the members, including parent, teacher, therapist, and model. These roles call on the creativity and flexibility of therapists to a degree that working with adults often does not (Aronson, 2002), and group leadership skills are particularly critical to effective outcomes in adolescent groups (Shechtman, 2017). Hurster wrote:

> The group therapist with youth is compelled to be at once a model for identification, a limit-setter, an educator and resource for information, a container and creator of a safe environment, a facilitator of identity play, and always therapeutically engaged in encouraging clarity of emotional expression, thoughtful choices, and the exercise of free will.
>
> (p. 69)

It is not only normal, but frequently necessary, for adolescents to test the leader's trustworthiness through acting out and pushing boundaries. In doing so, they are often seeing how much of their whole selves they can bring to the group process. Will only their civil and compliant parts be welcome, or can the group leader see and embrace them in all their messiness (Haen, 2011)?

As Brady (2017) captured, subversion is a key feature of adolescence, ranging from mild forms of questioning the status quo to more dangerous attempts to overthrow the world of adults through destructive or violent behavior. Such subversion presages the development of an autonomous self that determines teens' personal ideologies and what is important to them (Kaduson, 2016). In groups, attacks on the leader are often initial test-runs at dealing with conflict with peers (Grover, 2017). The leader's receiving of these moments without defensiveness, and with an eye toward setting both firm and reasonable limits while also facilitating reflection about what's happening (either in the moment, or later when affect has become more manageable), can pave the way for teens being able to communicate with one another more effectively.

As such, it is part of healthy group development that adolescent members coalesce to claim more control over what happens in the group, allowing leaders to gradually step back. Manassis (2012) framed this as movement from dictatorship to democracy. The leader's abilities to balance seriousness with playfulness and humor (Malekoff, 2014) and to model responsible authority may be especially important when the leader is from a dominant cultural group and the members are primarily from nondominant groups (Haen, 2015b), or in settings such as hospitals and residential facilities where there is already a vast power differential between group members and staff (Creeden & Haen, 2017).

Adolescents often necessitate an openness from group leaders, as primary role models, that other populations do not. With teens, a more distanced therapeutic style is not conducive to effective practice, and so group leaders must be willing, from a stronger, self-aware place, to participate alongside the members without taking center stage. They also should be willing to try to answer members' genuine questions (those not intended solely to provoke) about them thoughtfully and with some transparency, giving consideration to the potential therapeutic purposes for doing so (Aronson, 2002). For example, teens struggling with sexual identity development often benefit from being able to ask an adult about sex, sexuality, and sexual orientation, and from having these questions responded to with sincerity (Rofofsky, Kalyanam, Berwald, & Krishnakumar, 2017).

Ultimately, the group leader's capacity to be present and to use their presence to engage teens can have a significant bearing on the success of groups (Himelstein, 2017). For example, implementation of creative arts-based approaches requires asking adolescent members to voyage into the unknown, which can at times be frightening for young people, especially if uncertainty became coupled with fear during past trauma. As such, it is important that leaders scaffold the experience for the group. Experiential techniques are likely to fail if the group leader does not present them with enthusiasm and an inviting approach (Gillam, 2018).

Wilson (2017) asserted the importance of therapists taking up the position of being a 'possibilist' in the face of the hopelessness that can pervade the lives of many adolescents. He wrote:

> To take a calculated risk in practice requires an attitude that welcomes uncertainty in the belief that such a step will bring with it a degree of hope and new possibility. This attitude of spirited practice is like the 'feel' a musician brings to his playing; it is something beyond technique, something that conveys an emotional engagement with the music, transcending mere repetition of the notes. It has soul.
>
> (p. 47)

Group Planning

The task of creating a group for adolescents involves planning and collaboration with practitioners in locales where referrals are generated. Often these come from the school setting, and many groups occur in schools. Others may be held in outpatient clinics, inpatient hospital units or residential programs, or various community settings. Teens who have been identified as having difficulty with peers or family members and/or in adapting to the school environment may be referred to a social worker, counselor, or creative arts therapist who conducts groups. It then becomes the challenge for that practitioner to determine the structure of the proposed group in terms of member selection, size, open format (in which new members can join frequently) or closed format (in which membership is fixed), duration and frequency of sessions, and the types of activities to include (Finneran, Nitza, & Patterson, 2017). Some groups are organized around shared experiences—such as parental divorce, substance abuse prevention, or traumatic exposure—or diagnoses. Others may consist of mixed group membership without a common theme, except for the fact that the teens are exhibiting problematic behaviors that have concerned an adult.

Prior to reaching out to the adolescent for an exploratory interview, the leader must decide certain factors about the proposed group. Among these are the group's gender composition (whether single or mixed gender), age range of participants, and whether the group will be open-ended or time-limited. These decisions will be guided by the leader's goals for the group, which may be modified once the sessions begin and the members express their wishes and concerns about the purpose of the group.

Burlingame et al. (2014) reported that, of the many elements involved in conducting a group, pre-group preparation has the strongest connection to treatment outcomes. Even in short-term settings in which a formal screening interview is not possible, taking a few minutes to prepare a teenager for entering a group can help to alleviate anticipatory anxiety. During a pre-group interview, the group worker assesses the teen's ability to participate in a group, orients them about what to expect, begins to foster a therapeutic alliance with them and their parents, and may establish goals for participation (Pojman, 2017). This process often includes some contracting about shared agreements for what it means to be a member of this particular group (Dumais, 2017). Rutan and Shay (2017) cautioned: "We believe the single biggest error group therapists can make in leading open-ended therapy groups is not having a clear set of group agreements that members accept before entering the group" (p. 227).

The following considerations can help guide a leader during the screening interview:

- Introduce the group as an option for the adolescent's participation.
- Emphasize that the group will consist of peers who have similar experiences and who can provide support and understanding to one another.
- Describe the group as an evolving process that will include both verbal and nonverbal activities (Malekoff, 2014); therefore, it is not primarily a talking group, but one in which experiential activities will be part of the process.

- Normalize and address fears about participating, including the common one that by focusing on and addressing problems things will get worse (Weitkamp, Klein, Hoffmann, Wiegand-Grefe, & Midgley, 2017).
- Share with them that when parents know their teenager is talking to an adult about their problems, they often back off a bit and give them a little more room to breathe.

Tri-partite Structure for Sessions

It is often helpful to organize sessions using a three-part structure consisting of Warm-Up, Action, and Closure (Haen, 2015b). This structure can guide interventions and serve as a map for leaders during a tumultuous group. The Warm-Up is intended to transition the members from the world outside of session to being part of a working group. As such, warm-ups should be based on an intuitive reading of what the members are bringing into the room psychologically and how that energy might be channeled (Emunah, 2005). Groups that are dysregulated benefit from warm-ups that help to structure and orient them; groups that are disengaged benefit from warm-ups that introduce playfulness and vitality in order to enliven them.

Action refers to the working phase, in which the main therapeutic work within the group is conducted. This work may evolve out of themes generated during the Warm-Up, be targeted to specific needs or therapeutic goals for the group or its members, or be guided by contributions from the teens (Dean & Landis, 2017). The Action stage is one of immersion in both group and creative processes (Moon, 1998).

Closure is intended to help the adolescents reflect on the work of the session, integrate the experience, and separate from one another. Dean and Landis (2017) divided Closure into both Transition, disengaging from the creative space (through de-roling, putting materials away, or shifting from moving around the room to sitting back in a circle), and Sharing, which involves verbally reflecting on the creative process that took place, also known as *post-enactment processing* (Wiener, 2017). They offered a helpful set of reflective questions that can be used for eliciting individual, interpersonal, and whole-group experiences. These include:

- What was it like to create this?
- What drew you to this color/picture/character?
- What have you learned about your partner?
- What stands out to you most about what you/we created today?

(Dean & Landis, 2017, p. 134)

Principles for Effective Practice

Based on the vagaries of adolescent development and on group dynamics, as previously discussed, we offer the following principles for leading creative arts-based groups with adolescents:

- Utilize brief exposure.
- Maximize the interpersonal rewards.

- Develop the group as a complex system.
- Play with paradox and perception.
- Work the edge.
- Facilitate movement between experience and reflection.
- Engage with the future as much, if not more, than the past.

The theory and aims of each principle will be discussed, and each will be accompanied by suggested techniques and/or clinical vignettes.

Principle 1: Utilize Brief Exposure

Group leaders should not fail to appreciate how anxiety-provoking entering a therapy group can be. The very qualities that make groups effective for teenagers also make them potentially triggering as they activate ambivalence around being seen and feeling exposed and vulnerable (Haen, 2015b). As Elkind (1967) first suggested, many adolescents already navigate the world with an *imaginary audience*, the sense that they are continually being watched by others, a notion that seems to have increased with the prominence of social media (Alter, 2017). Psychotherapy groups, especially in the beginning stages, can exacerbate feeling exposed, without the anonymity of the internet as a shield. Groups can also provoke fears in teenagers that by complying they will be sacrificing their autonomy and right to say "No."

The arts can help to mitigate the vulnerability of being in a group, allowing members to participate on their own terms and to disown the expression if necessary to save face. Nevertheless, most teenagers have had their participation in therapy chosen for them and may at first have difficulty viewing the group as anything other than a consequence, and the leader as a stand-in for the parent who decided they should attend (Berg, Landreth, & Fall, 2018). The adolescent rhythm of expression is often, therefore, one of brief exposure: expression followed by retreat (Haen & Weil, 2010; Kline, 2009). Leaders can capitalize on this rhythm by implementing an initial structure, whether through process or activity, that invites brief moments of sharing without requiring elaboration or going deeper. Once teenagers begin to sense that they will not be zoomed in on, nor prompted to "tell me more about that," they often acquire ownership over the process. This ownership fosters trust and eventually gives way to greater moments of sharing, engagement, emotional risk taking, and openness to different kinds of leader interventions.

Warm-ups that use brief exposure also differentiate the group process from that of traditional or stereotypic therapy approaches, which adolescents are often primed to reject. Rather than a rote check-in, for example, teens might be asked to give a "*thumbs up, middle, or down*" for how their day is going, or to scale their week between 1 and 10, with 1 being "*the worst week of my life*," 5 being "*a pretty normal, 'nothing-new' sort of week*," and 10 being "*best week ever*." They might be invited to sum up how they are feeling in a simple sound and movement. Or they might be asked to offer a color or a metaphor (e.g., a type of weather) to describe their present state.

Grover (2017) advocated for the use of symbolic communication, particularly with guarded and anxious adolescents. He suggested that the indirectness of such communication can serve to lower defensiveness, create interpersonal connections, and foster group identity. Likewise, Riley (2001) emphasized how artistic creations can offer safe forms of exposure:

> Creating an art statement is a projection of self, it is safe, it can be justified intellectually, it is not understood by an adult unless explained, and that explanation is controlled by the adolescent. Art expressions 'fit' the teen process.
>
> (p. 143)

In one technique that capitalizes on brief exposure, the leader places a chair in the center of the circle. The group members are given a series of sentences to complete. In order to answer, they are invited to come up and sit in the chair. After they complete the sentence, they return to their seat. Sentences are targeted toward the group members and their most pressing concerns. For example: "*The worst thing about school today was . . .*," "*Something people often misunderstand about me is . . .*," "*One decision I wish I could take back is . . .*" or "*Sometimes I wish that . . .*" For each, many possible answers are welcomed, but at no point does the leader ask the teens to elaborate. Within activities that use brief exposure, group members often end up revealing more about themselves than they would otherwise, as the structure allows them to feel in control of what they are choosing to share.

Principle 2: Maximize the Interpersonal Rewards

Recent research on the adolescent brain has established a basis for the risky decisions teenagers often make. Neuroscientists have attributed such behavior to the reward-seeking centers of the brain developing before those areas responsible for cognitive control, as well as the adolescent brain's sensitivity to increased levels of dopamine and oxytocin (see Marks-Tarlow & Haen, this volume; Steinberg, 2014). This combination of factors makes the act of thinking through decisions, as well as resisting attraction to easily attainable gratification through heightened sensation and peer approval, a more effortful process for teenagers. More often than not they act as "ingenious and committed pleasure seekers" (Phillips, 2011, p. 194).

For a generation of adolescents whose daily interactions are permeated by technology, sitting in a room and connecting interpersonally with others can seem blandly old-fashioned, requiring sustained engagement in a mode of being that is becoming increasingly unfamiliar (Twenge, 2017). Group leaders would therefore do well to capitalize on adolescent drives toward social reward and novelty by emphasizing the playful, humorous, and surprising aspects of group. The point is not about entertaining so much as it is about creating the conditions that allow for mutuality. As such, Malekoff (2017), asserted that "Activity is more than a 'tool,' more than programmed content, more than 'canned' exercises, and more than a mechanistic means to an end" (p. 259). Instead, he advocated that activities in the group, particularly those that grow spontaneously out of leader–member collaboration, can contribute to "a growing sense of groupness and rich history of experience together" (p. 260).

While predictability can create some degree of safety within groups, folding in elements of novelty and surprise will help to draw teens in. Techniques that surprise can shake up staid therapeutic routines and effect change by encouraging playful experimentation and interpersonal risk taking (Eberhart & Atkins, 2014). Based on extensive infant–caregiver observation, Stern (2010a, 2010b) identified *vitality affects* as nonverbal exchanges on a bodily level that reflect aliveness, connection, and a sense of moving somewhere. The arts can offer forms of vitality through which members feel an expansive sense of connectedness to others, to the universe, or to spirituality (Davies, 2015).

Improvisational activities lend themselves particularly well to surprise because of their inherent spontaneity and uncertainty. In one activity, three group members are selected to leave the room with one leader, while the rest of the group remains with a co-leader. While out of the room, the group of three is asked to select something about one of them that the group doesn't know. They then come back into the room and sit in three chairs facing the group and, in a variation of the TV game show *To Tell the Truth*, each introduces themselves and shares the identified 'secret' as if it were their own (e.g., Person A: *"My name is Stacy, and I am afraid of clowns."* Person B: *"My name is Mark, and I'm afraid of clowns"* . . .). Group members can then ask questions of the panel (e.g., *"Person C, how long have you had this fear?"* *"Person A, describe the scariest clown you've ever seen."*), who respond as though the topic is true for them. At the end, the group votes on which of the three people is telling the truth.

By engaging with youth culture and themes that naturally draw teens in, leaders can also maximize the interpersonal rewards. McFerran (2010) provided an example of listening to a song that group members identify with and then engaging them in lyric substitution. Similarly, using movie characters, memes, or other pop culture content that adolescents are interested in can allow for exchanges that are rewarding. The focus is not on the group leader appearing cool, as adolescents' developmental push is to separate from adults (Berg et al., 2018); instead, orienting to youth culture can create a hook that captures teens' attention.

In analyzing conversational turn-taking in an adolescent group, Arias-Pujol and Anguera (2017) found that an effective leader worked to stimulate conversation between members early in the group and intervened to draw out the more inhibited teens. Creating connections through the use of *bridging* (e.g., *"Tony, how do you relate to Leila's drawing?"*) or actively encouraging *subgrouping* (e.g., *"Asha, I have the feeling you're not the only one who this song speaks to. Who else in here knows something about feeling lonely?"*) can help to forge resonant interpersonal connections that work against isolation (Gantt & Agazarian, 2010; Ormont, 1990) and to prime the adolescent social engagement system (Gray & Porges, 2017). By underscoring connections within the group and the experience of feeling joined by others, leaders can maximize the interpersonal rewards.

For example, using brief exposure, a leader might ask all those who have had a similar experience to the one a member is describing to raise their hand. Then, that member can be encouraged to look around the room and see how many others relate. Validation can be similarly supported by snapping one's fingers (as in a poetry café) or gently tapping one's feet to underscore that someone is heard. Group members can be asked to "try on" the gesture or movement made by another member and describe what it feels like from the inside. Likewise, making the process visible to members by, for example, having conversations aloud with co-leaders regarding decision points in the session can help to demystify what's happening and reduce the power dynamic so that teens can gradually take ownership of the group.

Techniques that directly facilitate interpersonal connections can be especially effective. Riley (2001) suggested that members be invited to make a 'gift drawing' for a partner as an interpersonal exercise. Haen (2015b) described the use of a mock game show called "Guess Who Said It," in which one member leaves the room and then returns to guess which group members delivered three compliments about them while they were out. Creeden and Haen (2017) outlined a version of this game called Secret Affirmations in which members close their eyes and are touched on the shoulder in response to prompts such as: "*Tap three people in the group who you think are brave*" or "*Tap one person who you would go to if you needed advice about a difficult situation*."

Principle 3: Develop the Group as a Complex System

Building a group with teens hinges on promoting a sense of 'we' among its members so that they can begin to see the group as a balance of autonomous yet interconnected individuals. Using the language of 'we' is helpful for establishing a mode of operations for how to be a group member (e.g., "*When someone goes out on a limb in group, we join them by sharing some of our own feelings so we don't leave them hanging.*"). The backdrop to this sense of 'we' is the *group climate*, the general emotional atmosphere in the group that connotes a sense of acceptance, tolerance of differences, and freedom of being. Shechtman and Gluk (2005) found climate to be the most frequently valued therapeutic factor by children (except angry boys, who reportedly valued it least).

In a dance/movement therapy group, as an example, group development might be reflected in an initial move toward attuned synchronicity, with members moving in concert more often, followed by an eventual branching out into greater individuality—with group members responding to and supporting one another's movements and also elaborating upon them in their own individual forms of expression (Panagiotopoulou, 2018). This kind of group dynamic is similar to what Sawyer (2018) observed in his studies of jazz groups and improv theater companies, where he identified a dynamic interaction between individual contributions and group-level creativity. In these groups, individual members contribute to the emergent performance in ways that are unpredictable to them at the time. They make offerings and trust that these offerings will be enhanced or developed by the group. It is only later that they can look back and assign meaning to what they contributed. These observations make sense in the context of group psychotherapy in the way that one member's expressed affect or verbal content, when shared, opens the door to another member responding to or 'riffing' off of this sharing.

Because of the aforementioned observations, Sawyer (2007) likened the groups he studied to *complex systems*. Within chaos theory, complex systems are identified as developing in a nonlinear fashion, with small changes at the individual level reaping large changes at the macro (or group) level. Despite the seeming randomness of their component processes, there is a larger order that emerges in these systems due to a self-organizing tendency that emanates from the interaction of individual parts (or group members). As complex systems develop and strengthen, there is movement from simplicity to greater complexity, and toward balance between individuality and connectedness (Siegel, 2012; Stark, 2017).

While human beings can be understood as complex systems, so too can groups of people. While initial group development focuses on establishing a group identity (or a sense of 'we'), subsequent development might be noted in the group members' ability to feel both connected and differentiated (a balancing of 'we' and 'me'; Haen & Weil, 2010). This balance develops as members are able to increasingly think about the thoughts, feelings, and intentions of others, and not just react to them. This ability, known as *mentalization*, often goes hand in hand with a shift from an individual to a relational focus (Arias-Pujol & Anguera, 2017) and is sustained within a group atmosphere characterized by "curiosity, forgiveness, respectful disagreement, and reflection" (Malberg & Midgley, 2017, p. 155).

Group leaders can support the development of the group as a complex system by shifting from the initial use of interventions that support group cohesion to those that promote increased differentiation of members, welcome a range of opinions and expressions, and encourage mentalization. Group projects, such as a mural or patchwork quilt, in which individual components are combined to create a greater whole, reflect this dynamic, as do the performing of improvisational scenes, movement pieces, or songs that require collaboration between members.

There is some evidence to suggest that healthier groups are ones that resemble an *ensemble*, a working group like the ones Sawyer (2018) studied in which there is a sharing of roles among members. Within ensembles, different members take the focus at different points in time, and there is a spirit of collaboration that values individual contributions as they contribute to the greater group purpose (Chasen, 2011; Haen, 2014, 2015a). Group leaders can encourage ensemble-building by inviting members to take on new roles and explore behavior patterns that may not come naturally—so shy members are drawn out and more expressive members encouraged to observe at various points.

One adolescent outpatient group that had been meeting for several months was composed of a diverse set of members. The teens, while generally connected to one another, rarely mentioned or dealt with their differences. In one group session, they were invited to bring in a song that had meaning to them; predictably, their choices represented a range of genres, from rap and electronica, to pop and country. The group was encouraged to think of this as an exercise in being open to music that might not appeal to them and to look deeper, beyond their initial reactions. Each song was played in turn, and members were given notepads on which they were encouraged to write lyrics that stood out to them. They were also invited to speculate on what the artist was trying to convey. After each song was played, the member who brought it was encouraged to say a few words about what it meant to them personally. They then were asked to listen as group members called out lyrics they'd written down and shared thoughts about its message. A range of interpretations about what the songs meant was encouraged.

Principle 4: Play With Paradox and Perception

Paradox is one of the quintessential characteristics of adolescence. This stage of life is both the healthiest human developmental period, in which the immune system is quite effective, and also a time when mortality rates are at their height (Shatkin, 2017). Likewise, teens can be apathetic or exquisitely passionate depending on the subject (Malekoff, 2014), capable of deep connection and also jarring self-absorption. And, as humans in transition, adolescents are both mature and immature, seeming to vacillate between extremes intellectually, emotionally, and behaviorally.

Playing with paradox can help to engage adolescents who often think in extremes to be more specific about their emotions and reactions. Asking about the "best" and "worst" aspects of an experience, a setting, or the group itself and inviting group members to express those through drawing, sculpting clay, singing, role play, or movement can entice adolescents to offer content that invites deeper exploration, as well as engaging other group members, who see themselves reflected in their peers' creations (Riviere, 2005). I (CH) have also used self-created cards that offer either stark statements about basic core beliefs (e.g., "*I don't think my parents can ever understand me*" or "*It's not possible to find true love*") or dilemmas representing extreme choices (e.g., "*Would you rather be able to see the future but have no one believe you, or never be able to anticipate what's coming next?*" or "*Would you rather be the parent of a teenager who's having unprotected sex with multiple partners or the parent of a teenager who's drinking every day?*") to stimulate discussion or artistic responses.

Because teenagers are in the process of establishing identity, they are frequently hyper-focused on how they come across to others and who they are in relationship to peers. Increased knowledge of identity factors such as race, gender, and socioeconomic status have also led to being more conscious of how they get judged by others before they've had a chance to say a word. At the same time, they are often unaware of the various aspects of self that they unwittingly communicate. A prime value of groups is the opportunity to gain a better sense of these parts of self in action, as research suggests that group members tend to re-enact with others their relational patterns from life outside session (Goldberg & Hoyt, 2015). Understanding this natural curiosity about perceptions, leaders can focus the group both on how they see one another and also on how others are often not what they appear or are assumed to be. These represent important lessons for young people who are quick to judge others by initial impressions or who defensively reject possibilities for connection based on superficial characteristics.

The arts are an effective venue for fostering perspective-taking. Two-sided drawings, boxes that can be decorated on the outside and within, or two chairs placed one behind the other can be used to explore who one is perceived to be on the outside versus who they are on the inside. Riley (2001), for example, suggested teens be invited to create art pieces showing how old they think their parents see them being, versus how old they would like to be seen as. Cruz (2011) described an integrated arts activity with high-risk adolescents in which they posed for two photos of themselves: one wearing professional attire and the other in 'street' clothes. They then cut the photos down the center, mounting the two sides together. This integrated picture was used as a stimulus for writing about their two sides. Likewise, teens might explore through song, movement, or role play the feelings they tend to show versus those they tend to hide.

Groups are a natural venue for teens receiving input in real time through their interactions with others, as well as the chance to implement those new understandings in the moment (Rutan & Shay, 2017). Some group-based models with adolescents focus on peers giving constructive feedback to one another. While there is a certain value in that, often the feedback is of a behavioral nature and therefore offers the young person receiving it little they can integrate on an emotional level, beyond initial defensiveness. However, giving adolescents the opportunity to experientially explore how their peers see them can help cement new ideas about themselves. A well-curated collection of art postcards, for example, can provide opportunities for intra- and interpersonal exploration. Group members might be asked to choose an image that shows how they feel in their family, at school, or in the group and to share these with one another. However, as the group becomes more cohesive, they might also be invited to choose an image that represents something they see in the person sitting on their left. They can then be asked to show the image to that person and describe why they chose it.

In an adolescent crisis shelter, the most popular activity in group was a board game called Loaded Questions. *Within the game, members write responses to a question read aloud on sheets of paper. The leader collects the various answers and reads them to the group. One member, whose turn it is, guesses who wrote each response. Because of the game structure, members often wrote surprising things about themselves under the guise of fooling the person who was guessing. In one group a dominant male member who was often overtly concerned about appearing invulnerable used the game to reveal closely held secrets, such as the fact that he often cried in his bed at night and missed his grandmother. The game-like element provided the opening to share these things while passing them off as 'just part of the game.'*

Principle 5: Work the Edge

For adolescents, who are often subject to heightened affect, a prime goal of treatment is the regulation of emotion (see Lombardi & Duncan, this volume). The capacity for emotion regulation has been found to be closely connected to improvement in a range of disorders that are common during the teen years, including anxiety, depression, substance use and eating disorders, and borderline personality disorder (Sloan et al., 2017). However, as Weisz (2015) noted, there has been little effort to test whether evidence-based treatment approaches for young people are effective in promoting emotion regulation.

The amount of emotion one can handle while still remaining regulated is referred to as the *window of tolerance* (Weber & Haen, 2016). The width of the window of tolerance fluctuates for each individual throughout the day based on mood and circumstances, including who is present at the time, but some people are also naturally more open than others. Ogden (2017) wrote, "If our windows are wide enough, we can tolerate and be present with the uncertainty and novelty inherent in play and creative endeavors without arousal reaching extremes of hyper- or hypoarousal" (p. 93).

As such, group leaders can foster change by sustaining the right level of tension within the group, particularly in regard to emotion. Landy (2008) offered a distancing model that can be useful for arts-based group facilitators. He referred to *overdistance* as a lack of feeling, where the primary mode is cognitive, and *underdistance* as an excess of emotion. The balance between these two states, one of both feeling and reflection, he labeled *aesthetic distance*. Leaders can facilitate movement between the poles of affect and cognition in order to keep group members within their window of tolerance. Music and rhythm are particularly effective tools for providing external regulation, as they underlie the attuned caregiving provided in secure parent–child holding environment (McGrath, 2017).

Emunah (1994) discussed the importance of facilitating either emotional expression or containment in various moments. Expressive interventions have a spontaneous, somewhat unpredictable quality (for both leaders and members). They offer choice, invite individuality, widen the group's focus, draw attention to the here-and-now, and are meant to engage affect. By contrast, containing interventions tend to be planned, predictable, repetitive, and sometimes familiar to the group. They are aimed at narrowing the focus and drawing attention to the leader and rules. They might engage members in one action and are intended to promote cognition and reflection (Prendiville & Howard, 2017).

However, if groups only remain safely within their window of tolerance, the sessions may go "well," but it is unlikely that change will result. As Sawyer (2007) noted, progress in ensembles often happens "at the edge of chaos" (p. 15), in which there is a balancing of freedom and structure. Likewise, Stark (2017) advocated that complex systems evolve as a result of optimal stress—interventions that push at the edge of what the system can handle, thereby stimulating change. Learning to work the growth edge of groups with teens, with the ultimate goal of widening the window of tolerance, is an important facilitation skill.

Working the edge might include exposing them to new experiences while supporting them to hang in there through uncertainty. It might also mean encouraging the group to stay with difficult emotional material for a bit longer before shifting away from it. Group leaders, too, can often feel as though they are working at the edge of their own window of tolerance, just moments away from being rendered tongue-tied, overpowered, or subject to a coup occurring (Haen & Weil, 2010). By walking the edge and adhering to the age-old mantra to "trust the process," leaders may find themselves nurturing undeveloped parts of their teenage group members, parts that are newly emergent and full of potential (Fosha, 2017).

In a group for teens who were all coping with divorce, the leader passed out pencils and small pieces of paper. The members were challenged to write something on the paper that they'd have difficulty sharing out loud in the group. The leader collected the pieces in a bowl and mixed them up. He then asked them to move around the space; as they did so, he pulled out each paper and read it aloud. The members were asked to hear it and pause in a frozen sculpt showing how they would feel if the secret read aloud was their own. In this group, members wrote things like: "I don't even really miss my dad," "I actually kind of like having two bedrooms and getting two birthday parties," and "My dad doesn't know my mom cheated on him, but I do." They had the chance to hear it read aloud without anyone knowing whose it was, and to see all the group members embody the secret. Following that session, there was a noted increase in cohesion and self-disclosure in the group.

Principle 6: Facilitate Movement Between Experience and Reflection

One reason for using the arts within group treatment is their potent capacity to engage group members in the present moment (Stern, 2010b). Past events can be brought into a here-and-now process, making them a "live, present-tense phenomenon" (Moon, 1998, p. 176), and family dynamics and relational patterns can be accessed so that "processes may develop more quickly, and are made visible, more tangible and available for working on" (Waller, 2015, p. 44). Improvisational art forms, in particular, foster an atmosphere of "doing, then thinking" (MacLeod, 2016, p. 219), or experience followed by reflection. This approach, which stands in contrast to the traditional group therapy dictum of "talking, not action" may be just right for adolescents. The movement from experience into reflection is one that Yalom and Leszcz (2005) referred to as the *self-reflective loop*, which allows for making meaning of here-and-now experience from a cognitive place.

Reflective dialogue need not be saved for the Closure phase of session; instead, therapists might think about oscillating between experience and reflection as a natural rhythm within the group. Reflecting on what it feels like from moment to moment to be engaged experientially can help members track their internal process in a more observant way. Giving words to that experience can deepen it and encourage another level of here-and-now engagement (Fosha, 2017).

Currie (2011) described Mapping Anger, a technique in which angry adolescents are asked, after a moment in which they were triggered during the group, to draw a simple map showing the rise and fall of their anger. Using percussion instruments, often in collaboration with other group members, they are asked to play the map, putting physiological reactions into musical form. Currie noted how the experiential components of the exercise often result in group members showing greater curiosity and reflectiveness about their own anger.

Principle 7: Engage With the Future as Much, If Not More, Than the Past

Identity formation is a primary developmental task of the teen years, particularly during early and middle adolescence. Past linear models conceived of adolescence as a period of exploration in which teens consider who they are in relationship to their various cultural, ethnic, peer, and affinity groups, and then commit to a specific identity. However, more recent research suggests an ongoing dialectic between exploration and commitment (Verkuyten & Fleischmann, 2017). As such, identity formation might be best viewed as a continuing process of identity consolidation while examining that identity in light of new information and experiences. Friendships and romantic relationships with peers can help to reinforce sense of identity in both positive and negative ways (La Greca & Lai, 2014).

If adolescents can be supported in staying open to possibilities, groups can effectively foster identity by serving as interpersonal laboratories in which members can explore themselves as individuals while also having new relational experiences. It can be difficult, however, for teens to imagine that their present circumstances will not go on forever—that there will be a time when their life is not the way it currently feels. Rachman (1989) wrote about the tendency for adolescents to adopt a premature or fixed role identity to reduce anxiety resulting from role confusion. He advocated for the importance of groups being a place in which teens can engage in experimenting with various parts of self.

Techniques that encourage a sense of self-in-transition can help to reinforce for teens that they are evolving, rather than fixed, entities. Past, present, and future drawings, poems or songs, sentence-completion activities with prompts such as "*Yesterday, I . . . /Today, I . . . /Tomorrow I will . . .*" or "*I used to be . . . /But now . . .*" that lead to artistic responses, and exploration of identity through questions such as "*I am . . . /I am not . . . /I wish to be . . .*" can all foster this sense of movement (Long & McKechnie, 2008; Taylor & Abell, 2005). Likewise, arts-based approaches that help teens to conceptualize themselves as composed of many parts, and that invite underdeveloped parts of self to be expressed, allow for expansion of identity (Straus, 2017). Engaging with these parts through role play, storytelling, or letter writing can help teens to see greater possibilities, following the truism that humans have to first imagine something in order to become it.

The capacity to envision a future is theorized to correlate with increased self-control, as adolescents who have a sense of future are better able to delay gratification and plan for goal attainment (Brier, 2015). Doing so can also help to expand one's sense of time, while an exclusive focus on the past (e.g., "*what you did to get yourself into group*" or "*what you've learned from your mistakes*") can encourage rumination, which exacerbates internalizing conditions such as depression, anxiety, and trauma (La Greca & Lai, 2014). Ideally, the adolescent's vision of a future self gives way to his or her developing a sustained sense of agency to become what they have imagined (Bendicsen, 2013; Moon, 1998).

Blaustein and Habib (2017) used techniques of asking group members to write a future biography or to pair up with a partner to conduct a mock interview in which they discuss their life 30 years into the future (*What is their family like? Where do they work? What was their proudest accomplishment?*). Dean and Landis (2017) wrote about reunion scenes in which the group imagines being reunited several years into the future at an imagined location of their choosing. They enter the scene as their future selves, sharing how their lives are now, discussing memories of one another, and perhaps giving advice to the teenagers of the day. Being asked to write letters to their present self from their future self, to create an image of themselves in a future job, or to gaze into an imaginary crystal ball to share one thing they see for a fellow group member in the future can also be effective interventions.

Research shows that the identity formation process is nearly identical for most teens, regardless of gender or ethnicity; however, sociocultural factors, tied as they are to larger experiences of oppression and marginalization, influence the outcome (Hoff et al., 2017). Artistic expression can act as a form of resistance against oppression, channeling the adolescent desire for subversion into effective action (Scrine & McFerran, 2018) and helping group members to transcend current circumstances. In one meaningful project in an adolescent crisis shelter, group members wrote letters to an imagined future resident, offering advice on their stay there and providing a picture to serve as a calming image for that person when she or he is feeling hopeless. Other adolescents have created books about their own traumas to communicate to future group members what they've learned and to offer others a sense that they aren't alone.

In a group for immigrants, many of whom were refugees, the members began the session by using their bodies to create group sculptures representing 'home' and 'family.'

They then paired off and created short improv scenes or movement pieces in which they expressed their personal sense of feeling caught between two places and two cultures. After processing the experience of both creating and watching these emotional performances, the members talked about their desire to integrate what they loved about their countries of origin with what was positive about their new home. They were offered paper and invited to create personalized flags that contained cherished pieces of each cultural identity. These pieces, which the group members were quite proud of, were eventually used as part of an art exhibition in the lobby of a state office building. At the exhibition opening, one member of the group shared with a reporter how validated she felt to have her work displayed in a government building and seen by the many people who came there each day for important matters, and how relieving it was to know she didn't have to cut off part of who she was in order to acculturate—that there was room for all of her.

Conclusion

The principles in this chapter and the ideas presented are intended to be resources for group leaders who take on the formidable business of supporting teens on their path to adulthood. Taken together, they are intended as a guide rather than a recipe. Ultimately, each group process is unique—a co-creation of the teens and adults who enter the group room each session. As Nitsun (2014) reminded us, detectable shifts often result not from the complex and dramatic moments within groups, but from the seeds that get planted along the way.

> I have been struck that the most meaningful sessions are sometimes those in which something relatively simple happens. . . . My sense is that at these times the group functions as a refuge—a refuge from the madness of the outside world and a refuge from their inner distress and perplexity.
>
> (p. 132)

Providing refuge to adolescents is so vital in turbulent times and its positive influence can be far-reaching. Group work, at its best, has the potential to shape a generation.

References

Alter, A. (2017). *Irresistible: The rise of addictive technology and the business of keeping us hooked.* New York, NY: Penguin.

Arias-Pujol, E., & Anguera, M. T. (2017). Observation of interactions in adolescent group therapy: A mixed methods study. *Frontiers in Psychology, 8*(1188). doi: 10.3389/psyg.2017.01188

Aronson, S. (2002). The group treatment process. In S. Aronson & S. Scheidlinger (Eds.), *Group treatment of adolescents in context: Outpatient, inpatient, and school* (pp. 37–54). Madison, CT: International Universities Press.

Bendicsen, H. K. (2013). *The transformational self: Attachment and the end of the adolescent phase.* London: Karnac.

Berg, R. C., Landreth, G. L., & Fall, K. A. (2018). Group counseling with adolescents. In *Group counseling: Concepts and procedures* (2nd ed., pp. 181–190). New York, NY: Routledge.

Blaustein, M., & Habib, M. (2017). Trauma-impacted children and adolescents. In C. Haen & S. Aronson (Eds.), *Handbook of child and adolescent group therapy: A practitioner's reference* (pp. 389–403). New York, NY: Routledge.

Brady, M. T. (2017). Subversiveness in adolescence. *Contemporary Psychoanalysis, 53*(3), 346–361.

Brier, N. (2015). *Enhancing self-control in adolescents: Treatment strategies derived from psychological science.* New York, NY: Routledge.

Burlingame, G. M., Whitcomb, K., & Woodland, S. (2014). Process and outcome in group counseling and psychotherapy: A perspective. In J. DeLucia-Waack, C. R. Kalodner & M. T. Riva (Eds.), *Handbook of group counseling and psychotherapy* (2nd ed., pp. 55–67). Thousand Oaks, CA: Sage.

Chasen, L. R. (2011). *Social skills, emotional growth and drama therapy: Inspiring connection on the autism spectrum.* London: Jessica Kingsley.

Creeden, K., & Haen, C. (2017). Groups in residential settings. In C. Haen & S. Aronson (Eds.), *Handbook of child and adolescent group therapy: A practitioner's reference* (pp. 229–239). New York, NY: Routledge.

Cruz, J. (2011). Breaking through with art: Art therapy approaches for working with at-risk boys. In C. Haen (Ed.), *Engaging boys in treatment: Creative approaches to the therapy process* (pp. 177–194). New York, NY: Routledge.

Currie, M. (2011). Doing anger differently: Working creatively with angry and aggressive boys. In C. Haen (Ed.), *Engaging boys in treatment: Creative approaches to the therapy process* (pp. 197–217). New York, NY: Routledge.

Davies, A. (2015). Early years: Experiences with others. In A. Davies, E. Richards & N. Barwick (Eds.), *Group music therapy: A group analytic approach* (pp. 91–99). New York, NY: Routledge.

Dean, M. E., & Landis, H. (2017). Creative arts-based approaches with adolescent groups. In C. Haen & S. Aronson (Eds.), *Handbook of child and adolescent group therapy: A practitioner's reference* (pp. 124–136). New York, NY: Routledge.

Dies, K. G. (2000). Adolescent development and a model of group psychotherapy: Effective leadership in the new millennium. *Journal of Child and Adolescent Group Psychotherapy, 10*(2), 97–111.

Donald, I. N., Rickwood, D. J., & Carey, T. A. (2014). Understanding therapeutic change in young people—A pressing research agenda. *Journal of Psychotherapy Integration, 24*(4), 313–322.

Dumais, D. (2017). Operating instructions: The group contract. In C. Haen & S. Aronson (Eds.), *Handbook of child and adolescent group therapy: A practitioner's reference* (pp. 30–39). New York, NY: Routledge.

Eberhart, H., & Atkins, S. (2014). *Presence and process in expressive arts work: At the edge of wonder.* London: Jessica Kingsley.

Edgette, J. S. (2006). *Adolescent therapy that really works: Helping kids who never asked for help in the first place.* New York, NY: Norton.

Elkind, D. (1967). Egocentrism in adolescence. *Child Development, 38,* 1025–1034.

Emunah, R. (1994). *Acting for real: Drama therapy process, technique, and performance.* New York, NY: Routledge.

Emunah, R. (2005). Drama therapy and adolescent resistance. In A. M. Weber & C. Haen (Eds.), *Clinical applications of drama therapy in child and adolescent treatment* (pp. 107–120). New York, NY: Brunner-Routledge.

Finneran, K. R., Nitza, A., & Patterson, K. W. (2017). Planning for groups. In C. Haen & S. Aronson (Eds.), *Handbook of child and adolescent group therapy: A practitioner's reference* (pp. 9–19). New York, NY: Routledge.

Fosha, D. (2017). Something more than "'something more' than interpretation": Accelerated Experiential Dynamic Psychotherapy (AEDP) works the experiential edge of transformational experience to transform the internal working model. In S. Lord (Ed.), *Moments of meeting in psychoanalysis: Interaction and change in the therapeutic encounter* (pp. 267–292). New York, NY: Routledge.

Gantt, S. P., & Agazarian, Y. M. (2010). Developing the group mind through functional subgrouping: Linking systems-centered training (SCT) and interpersonal neurobiology. *International Journal of Group Psychotherapy, 60*(4), 514–545.

Gillam, T. (2018). *Creativity, wellbeing and mental health practice.* Cham, Switzerland: Palgrave Pivot.

Goldberg, S. B., & Hoyt, W. T. (2015). Group as social microcosm: Within-group interpersonal style is congruent with outside group relational tendencies. *Psychotherapy, 52*(2), 195–204.

Gray, A. E. L., & Porges, S. W. (2017). Polyvagal-informed dance/movement therapy with children who shut down: Restoring core rhythmicity. In C. A. Malchiodi & D. A. Crenshaw (Eds.), *What to do when children clam up in psychotherapy: Interventions to facilitate communication* (pp. 102–136). New York, NY: Guilford.

Grover, S. (2017). Depressed adolescents. In C. Haen & S. Aronson (Eds.), *Handbook of child and adolescent group therapy: A practitioner's reference* (pp. 311–321). New York, NY: Routledge.

Haen, C. (2007). "Make me wanna holler": Dramatic encounters with boys from the inner-city. In V. A. Camilleri (Ed.), *Healing the inner-city child: Creative arts therapies with at-risk youth* (pp. 212–228). London: Jessica Kingsley.

Haen, C. (2011). Boys and therapy: The need for creative reformulation. In C. Haen (Ed.), *Engaging boys in treatment: Creative approaches to the therapy process* (pp. 3–40). New York, NY: Routledge.

Haen, C. (2014). Examining roles in children's group therapy: Applying a dramaturgical role instrument to group process. *The Arts in Psychotherapy, 41*(5), 554–562.

Haen, C. (2015a). Advancing a dramaturgical theory of group process. *Drama Therapy Review, 1*(2), 219–235.

Haen, C. (2015b). Fostering change when safety is fleeting: Expressive therapy groups for adolescents with complex trauma. In N. B. Webb (Ed.), *Play therapy with children and adolescents in crisis* (4th ed., pp. 239–256). New York, NY: Guilford.

Haen, C., & Weil, M. (2010). Group therapy on the edge: Adolescence, creativity, and group work. *Group, 34*(1), 37–52.

Himelstein, S. (2017). High-risk adolescents. In C. Haen & S. Aronson (Eds.), *Handbook of child and adolescent group therapy: A practitioner's reference* (pp. 441–452). New York, NY: Routledge.

Hoff, A. L., Swan, A. J., Mercado, R. J., Kagan, E. R., Crawford, E. A., & Kendall, P. C. (2017). Psychological therapy with children and adolescents: Theory and practice. In A. J. Consoli, L. E. Beutler & B. Bongar (Eds.), *Comprehensive textbook of psychotherapy: Theory and practice* (2nd ed., 267–283). New York, NY: Oxford University Press.

Hurster, T. (2017). Ethically informed group practice. In C. Haen & S. Aronson (Eds.), *Handbook of child and adolescent group therapy: A practitioner's reference* (pp. 66–78). New York, NY: Routledge.

Jensen, F. E., & Nutt, A. E. (2014). *The teenage brain: A neuroscientist's survival guide to raising adolescents and young adults.* New York, NY: HarperCollins.

Kaduson, H. (2016). Play therapy across the life span: Infants, children, adolescents, and adults. In K. J. O'Connor, C. E. Schaeffer & L. D. Braverman (Eds.), *Handbook of play therapy* (2nd ed., pp. 327–341). Hoboken, NJ: Wiley.

Karkou, V., & Joseph, J. (2017). The moving and movement identities of adolescents: Lessons from dance movement psychotherapy in a mainstream secondary school. In R. MacDonald, D. J. Hargreaves & D. Miell (Eds.), *Handbook of musical identities* (pp. 232–244). Oxford: Oxford University Press.

Kline, W. H. (2009). How do adolescents leave psychotherapy? *Journal of Infant, Child & Adolescent Psychotherapy, 8*(3–4), 169–180.

La Greca, A. M., & Lai, B. S. (2014). The role of peer relationships in youth psychopathology. In J. Ehrenreich-May & B. C. Chu (Eds.), *Transdiagnostic treatments for children and adolescents: Principles and practice* (pp. 111–137). New York, NY: Guilford.

Landy, R. J. (2008). *The couch and the stage: Integrating words and action in psychotherapy.* Lanham, MD: Jason Aronson.

Lee, F. S., Heimer, H., Giedd, J. N., Lein, E. S., Šestan, N., Weinberger, D. R., & Casey, B. J. (2014, October 31). Adolescent mental health—Opportunity and obligation: Emerging neuroscience offers hope for treatments. *Science, 346*(6209), 547–549.

Long, K., & McKechnie, B. (2008). No time to say hello, good-bye: Drama therapy with children on an inpatient psychiatric unit. In S. Brooke (Ed.), *The use of the creative therapies with survivors of domestic violence* (pp. 199–222). Springfield, IL: Charles C. Thomas.

MacLeod, L. (2016). Act before you think: Using instinct not intellect in groups. *Social Work with Groups, 39*(2–3), 208–220.

Malberg, N. T., & Midgley, N. (2017). A mentalization-based approach to working with adolescents in groups. In C. Haen & S. Aronson (Eds.), *Handbook of child and adolescent group therapy: A practitioner's reference* (pp. 148–159). New York, NY: Routledge.

Malekoff, A. (2014). *Group work with adolescents: Principles and practice* (3rd ed.). New York, NY: Guilford.

Malekoff, A. (2017). Strengths-based group work with children and adolescents. In C. D. Garvin, L. M. Gutiérrez & M. J. Galinsky (Eds.), *Handbook of social work with groups* (2nd ed., pp. 255–270). New York, NY: Guilford.

Manassis, K. (2012). *Problem solving in child and adolescent psychotherapy: A skills-based, collaborative approach.* New York, NY: Guilford.

McFerran, K. (2010). *Adolescents, music and music therapy: Methods and techniques for clinicians, educators and students.* London Jessica Kingsley.

McGrath, E. (2017). The role of music and rhythm in the development, integration and repair of the self. In E. Prendiville & J. Howard (Eds.), *Creative psychotherapy: Applying the principles of neurobiology to play and expressive arts-based practice* (pp. 21–37). New York, NY: Routledge.

Moon, B. (1998). *The dynamics of art as therapy with adolescents.* Springfield, IL: Charles C. Thomas.

Nitsun, M. (2014). *Beyond the anti-group: Survival and transformation.* New York, NY: Routledge.

Ogden, P. (2017). Play, creativity, and movement vocabulary. In T. Marks-Tarlow, M. Solomon & D. J. Siegel (Eds.), *Play and creativity in psychotherapy* (pp. 92–109). New York, NY: Norton.

Ormont, L. R. (1990). The craft of bridging. *International Journal of Group Psychotherapy, 40*(1), 3–17.

Panagiotopoulou, E. (2018). Dance therapy and the public school: The development of social and emotional skills of high school students in Greece. *The Arts in Psychotherapy, 59*, 25–33.

Phillips, A. (2011). The pleasures of working with adolescents. *Psychodynamic Practice: Individuals, Groups and Organizations, 17*(2), 187–197.

Pojman, A. P. (2017). Groups in private practice. In C. Haen & S. Aronson (Eds.), *Handbook of child and adolescent group therapy: A practitioner's reference* (pp. 217–228). New York, NY: Routledge.

Prendiville, E., & Howard, J. (2017). Neurobiologically informed psychotherapy. In E. Prendiville & J. Howard (Eds.), *Creative psychotherapy: Applying the principles of neurobiology to play and expressive arts-based practice* (pp. 21–37). New York, NY: Routledge.

Rachman, A. W. (1989). Identity group psychotherapy with adolescents: A reformulation. In F. J. Cramer Azima & L. H. Richmond (Eds.), *Adolescent group psychotherapy* (pp. 21–41). New York, NY: International Universities Press.

Riley, S. (2001). *Group process made visible: Group art therapy.* Philadelphia, PA: Brunner-Routledge.

Riviere, S. (2005). Play therapy techniques to engage adolescents. In L. Gallo-Lopez & C. E. Schaefer (Eds.), *Play therapy with adolescents* (pp. 121–142). Lanham, MD: Jason Aronson.

Rofofsky, M., Kalyanam, A., Berwald, A., & Krishnakumar, A. (2017). LGBTQ adolescents. In C. Haen & S. Aronson (Eds.), *Handbook of child and adolescent group therapy: A practitioner's reference* (pp. 453–463). New York, NY: Routledge.

Rutan, J. S., & Shay, J. J. (2017). Group therapy: Theory and practice. In A. J. Consoli, L. E. Beutler & B. Bongar (Eds.), *Comprehensive textbook of psychotherapy: Theory and practice* (2nd ed., 223–238). New York, NY: Oxford University Press.

Sawyer, K. (2007). *Group genius: The creative power of collaboration.* New York, NY: Basic Books.

Sawyer, R. K. (2018). An interdisciplinary study of group creativity. In R. J. Sternberg & J. C. Kaufman (Eds.), *The nature of human creativity* (pp. 280–290). Cambridge: Cambridge University Press.

Scrine, E., & McFerran, K. (2018). The role of a music therapist exploring gender and power with young people: Articulating an emerging anti-oppressive practice. *The Arts in Psychotherapy, 59*, 54–64.

Shatkin, J. P. (2017). *Born to be wild: Why teens take risks, and how we can help keep them safe.* New York, NY: TarcherPerigree.

Shechtman, Z. (2014). Counseling and therapy groups with children and adolescents. In J. DeLucia-Waack, C. R. Kalodner & M. T. Riva (Eds.), *Handbook of group counseling and psychotherapy* (2nd ed., pp. 585–596). Thousand Oaks, CA: Sage.

Shechtman, Z. (2017). Bridging the gap between research and practice: How research can guide group leaders. In C. Haen & S. Aronson (Eds.), *Handbook of child and adolescent group therapy: A practitioner's reference* (pp. 52–65). New York, NY: Routledge.

Shechtman, Z., & Gluk, O. (2005). An investigation of therapeutic factors in children's groups. *Group Dynamics: Theory, Research, and Practice, 9*(2), 127–134.

Shechtman, Z., & Leichtentritt, J. (2010). The association of process with outcomes in child group therapy. *Psychotherapy Research, 20*(1), 8–21.

Siegel, D. J. (2010). *The mindful therapist: A clinician's guide to mindsight and neural integration.* New York, NY: Norton.

Siegel, D. J. (2012). *The developing mind: How relationships and the brain interact to shape who we are* (2nd ed.). New York, NY: Norton.

Sloan, E., Hall, K., Moulding, R., Bryce, S., Mildred, H., & Staiger, P. K. (2017). Emotion regulation as a transdiagnostic treatment construct across anxiety, depression, substance, eating and borderline personality disorders: A systematic review. *Clinical Psychology Review, 57,* 141–163.

Stark, M. (2017). The therapeutic use of optimal stress: Precipitating disruption to trigger recovery. In M. Solomon & D. J. Siegel (Eds.), *How people change: Relationships and neuroplasticity in psychotherapy* (pp. 185–219). New York, NY: Norton.

Steinberg, L. (2014). *Age of opportunity: Lessons from the new science of adolescence.* Boston, MA: Houghton Mifflin Harcourt.

Stern, D. N. (2010a). The issue of vitality. *Nordic Journal of Music Therapy, 19,* 88–102.

Stern, D. N. (2010b). *The present moment in psychotherapy and everyday life.* New York, NY: Norton.

Straus, M. B. (2017). *Treating trauma in adolescents: Development, attachment, and the therapeutic relationship.* New York, NY: Guilford.

Taylor, A., & Abell, S. C. (2005). The use of poetry in play therapy with adolescents. In L. Gallo-Lopez & C. E. Schaefer (Eds.), *Play therapy with adolescents* (pp. 143–158). Lanham, MD: Jason Aronson.

Twenge, J. M. (2017, September). Have smartphones destroyed a generation? *The Atlantic.* Retrieved from www.theatlantic.com/magazine/archive/2017/09/has-the-smartphone-destroyed-a-generation/534198/

Verkuyten, M., & Fleischmann, F. (2017). Ethnic identity among immigrant and minority youth. In A. Rutland, D. Nesdale & C. Spears Brown (Eds.), *The Wiley handbook of group processes in children and adolescents* (pp. 23–46). Chichester: Wiley.

Waller, D. (2015). *Group interactive art therapy: Its use in training and treatment* (2nd ed.). New York, NY: Routledge.

Weber, A. M., & Haen, C. (2016). Attachment-informed drama therapy with adolescents. In C. Holmwood & S. Jennings (Eds.), *International handbook of dramatherapy* (pp. 218–229). London: Jessica Kingsley.

Weisz, J. R. (2015). Promoting youth self-regulation through psychotherapy: Redesigning treatments to fit complex youths in clinical care. In G. Oettingen & P. W. Gollwitzer (Eds.), *Self-regulation in adolescence* (pp. 332–356). New York, NY: Cambridge University Press.

Weitkamp, K., Klein, E., Hoffmann, H., Wiegand-Grefe, S., & Midgley, N. (2017). Therapy expectations of adolescents with depression entering psychodynamic psychotherapy: A qualitative study. *Journal of Infant, Child, and Adolescent Psychotherapy, 16*(1), 93–105.

Wiener, D. J. (2017). From action to insight: Uses of post-enactment processing in the action therapies. *Drama Therapy Review, 3*(2), 181–194.

Wilson, J. (2017). *Creativity in times of constraint: A practitioner's companion in mental health and social care.* London: Karnac.

Yalom, I. D., & Leszcz, M. (2005). *The theory and practice of group psychotherapy* (5th ed.). New York, NY: Basic Books.

2
Creative Arts-Based Approaches to Adolescent Group Therapy
The State of the Art

CRAIG HAEN

Research on treatment with young people has become more rigorous, specific, and developmentally sensitive within the past two decades (Hoff et al., 2017). However, there continues to be a disconnect between researchers and clinical practitioners, so that therapists often do not incorporate the findings from research studies into practice decisions, nor does the body of research adequately speak to the contexts in which therapists are working (Haen, 2017), a phenomenon known as the *research–practice gap*. There also remains far more research on adults than on young people, despite the fact that half of all mental illnesses have their onset by age 14 (Harvey, 2014).

The enduring disparities in the research landscape are not surprising. Young people are widely considered a vulnerable population whose ability to provide informed consent is questionable (Freeman & Mathison, 2009); therefore, institutional review boards scrutinize projects involving adolescents more carefully. Further, the developmental fluctuations characteristic of adolescence complicate research with this age group, as teens are in a state of ongoing and often rapid change, with physical and neuromaturation occurring at a pace comparable only to that seen during infancy (Kazak et al., 2010). In general, there are more factors that are "free to vary" with adolescents, including family dynamics and characteristics (Steele & Roberts, 2003), and developmental risk histories (Augustyniak, Brooks, Rinaldo, Bogner, & Hodges, 2009). The presence of many uncontrolled variables makes the establishment of effective control groups challenging and increases the possibility that comorbidity, the occurrence of more than one disorder, will be overlooked (Kazdin & Weisz, 1998). Likewise, studies that homogenize children and adolescents into one group are insufficient, as different interventions may be necessary based on the young person's developmental stage.

Explaining the importance of clinicians being able to read and evaluate research as part of committed, ethical treatment, Cruz and Koch (2015) wrote:

> Clinical practice is a complex endeavor that requires the therapist to hypothesize based on both knowledge and comparative data. Clients benefit when the therapist is broadly informed and engaged in reading research. In a complementary way, clinicians are best positioned from their daily work with a range

of clients to pose questions and problems to researchers about how to improve care that are worthy of research.

(p. 12)

This chapter seeks to promote the kind of dialogue between therapists and researchers that these authors suggest by summarizing studies relevant to the practice of group work with teens, as well as capturing the current state of research on creative arts-based group work more generally. In doing so, I aim to also address the scarcity of focus on group process within the creative arts therapies literature, a lack that is surprising given how often these modalities are conducted in groups (Pavlicevic, 2016). The ultimate goal is for readers to walk away with a sense of the body of research that exists and how they can utilize this information to make better 'on-the-ground' decisions.

Studying Group Therapy

Just by virtue of having multiple interacting people in a room, group therapy is complex by nature. How groups evolve, and how the interactions between group leaders, group members, and the group as a whole inform one another, does not lend itself readily to linear models of understanding (Gold & Kivlighan, 2018). Doel (2006) characterized therapy groups as "not so much a series of steps and stages as a sense of emerging 'groupness,' the erratic development of shared meanings and understandings" (p. 23).

For this reason, Piper, Ogrodniczuk, Joyce, and Weideman (2010) speculated that "the study of the process of group psychotherapy will never be a readily controlled deterministic science" (p. 157). The connections between relationship factors, techniques, and outcome represent layered phenomena that shift as a function of time, dosage, group membership, and individual patient factors (Barber, 2009). Nevertheless, researchers believe that there is an order that can be divined from this chaos, and that by seeking to clarify group process, leaders can increasingly attend to factors that might facilitate change for patients.

As Leszcz (2018) recently noted, there are three roads to therapists practicing in an evidence-informed way. They can either: 1) only use treatments that are considered evidence-supported (ESTs), 2) engage in the ongoing tracking of treatment outcomes, known as *practice-based evidence*, by using data from measures of client change and adjusting in response, or 3) incorporate evidence from studies and practice guidelines in order to enhance their own clinical judgment. Although this chapter will primarily focus on the third route, the other two will be considered within the context of adolescent group therapy.

The Trouble With Evidence-Supported Treatment

The EST movement has prompted a wide range of studies intended to demonstrate that certain therapy models are effective in addressing specific problems. Though research on cognitive behavior therapy (CBT) groups is still the most common (Burlingame & Jensen, 2017), there has been an increase in outcome studies in the creative arts therapies in recent years that speak to their effectiveness with adolescents who present with a variety of diagnoses (e.g., Cortina & Fazel, 2015; Geipel, Koenig, Hillecke, Resch, & Kaess, 2018; Greenbaum & Javdani, 2017; Kim, Kim, & Ki, 2014; Shuman, Kennedy, DeWitt, Edelblute, & Wamboldt, 2016; SmithBattle, Chantamit-o-pas, Freed, McLaughlin, & Schneider, 2017). However, the volume and level of this research does not approach the threshold for EST consideration.

By necessity, empirical outcome studies for specific disorders seek to reduce 'noise' from the data. As such, they tend to focus on patients with simple diagnostic pictures and on easily replicable therapy procedures, and communicate their findings in terms of aggregate trends. Because of these features, this type of research can only offer general predictions about what types of patients will benefit from a specific approach (Midgley, Hayes, & Cooper, 2017) and whether it will work when implemented by the generic therapist (Lebow & Jenkins, 2018). Outcome studies often struggle to capture the complexity of what happens in psychotherapy—because, in their need to reduce noise, they involve controllable conditions that don't readily map onto what treatment or patients look like in clinics, agencies, and hospitals—and they are likely to be influenced by researcher bias (Harvey, 2014; Midgley et al., 2017). The body of research establishing ESTs has promoted a focus on symptom alleviation through manualized treatments. Because there are so many variable factors in the lives of adolescents, their primary treatment needs can shift, which leads to flux in the treatment—something sequential treatment models are not designed to respond to (Weisz, Bearman, Santucci, & Jensen-Doss, 2016).

As I have pointed out elsewhere (Haen, 2017), the EST movement has served to build silos among practitioners of different disciplines, moving the field away from a collaborative atmosphere in which knowledge and approaches from one modality might be applied to another. There appears to be significant disagreement across leading international organizations about which treatments for adolescents have enough research to be considered evidence-supported (Gálvez-Lara et al., 2018). Likewise, more researchers are beginning to call the utility of ESTs into question.

In a recent study, Barlow and colleagues (2017) compared the effectiveness of a transdiagnostic, emotion-focused cognitive–behavioral intervention intended to treat patients with a range of disorders against four ESTs developed for specific anxiety disorders. Participants were 223 adults in an outpatient treatment center over the course of four years. Not only did the ESTs show no benefit over the transdiagnostic treatment at termination nor six months later, but the dropout rate was higher among those receiving ESTs. All told, these findings and the concerns presented earlier suggest the need to look to other developmentally responsive forms of therapy in treating adolescents, and to other types of research for guiding principles.

Group Therapy Process Research

While outcome studies remain the most dominant model of group psychotherapy research, there is a growing body of process studies that aim to understand how change happens within groups, as well as to identify structural and methodological components that may serve to make groups more or less effective (Greene, 2016). Group therapy process research involves intensive examination of the trajectory of a course of treatment, from the micro-moments during a single session to the gradual unfolding of dynamics and relationships over time. These studies may be either quantitative or qualitative in approach, or reflect a combination of both, as each methodology can capture different elements of the complex picture that is group treatment.

Midgley (2004) suggested that process research "allows one to study what *actually* happens in therapy, rather than what people *say* happens" (p. 101). It represents a way of addressing the research–practice gap by linking the wisdom and experience of clinical work with the logic and precision of science (Greene, 2016). While the next section will offer data about the effectiveness of adolescent treatment and group therapy generally, the majority of the chapter will focus on findings from process research. These studies provide guiding evidence related to patient and therapist factors likely to lead to better outcomes, as well as identifying structural components of group that indicate where leaders should direct their focus.

Yes, but . . . Is It Effective?

While the question of which treatment methods are most effective for different disorders is a narrow one whose answers don't offer much to therapists treating a range of patients, this doesn't mean that outcome studies are unimportant. In fact, perhaps the most fundamental question to be answered is: do young people benefit from therapy? In a recent meta-analysis of 50 years of outcome studies on child/adolescent treatment, Weisz and his colleagues (2017) calculated an *effect size* (a measure of the magnitude of treatment effect) of .46, which had a modest decline to .36 about 11 months after treatment. (Notably, this number was lower than in previous meta-analyses, where findings have varied between .54 and .88.) This finding, which did not vary significantly by patient ethnicity or between children and adolescents, suggests that psychotherapy has an overall moderate to medium effect for young people that sustains itself over time, with the greatest impact being on anxiety and the least impact on depression.

Put another way, Weisz et al.'s (2017) results show that "the probability that a randomly selected youth in the treatment condition would be better off after treatment than a randomly selected youth in the control condition was 63%—only moderately better than chance at 50%" (p. 96). As Harvey (2014) advocated, there is "substantial room for improvement" in these numbers, since "even under optimal conditions, treatment failure is alarmingly common" (pp. 20–21). Approximately 30–40% of child and adolescent patients fail to respond to CBT intervention, the most well-studied form of treatment, in clinical trials (Shirk, Jungbluth & Karver, 2012). Likewise, dropout rates are high among teens referred for therapy (Henriksen, 2017). However, little research has focused on understanding what distinguishes this large population of outliers from their more responsive peers, or on gaining a clear sense of what leads teens to leave treatment.

Creative Arts Therapies

While there are no meta-analyses that address the direct question of the effectiveness of creative arts therapies in the treatment of adolescents, there are systematic reviews (e.g., Martin et al., 2018; Dunphy, Mullane, & Jacobsson, 2014) related to adult work, and some meta-analyses of specific arts modalities with children and adolescents (e.g., Gold, Voracek, & Wigram, 2004; Travagin, Margola, & Revenson, 2015). Recently, Cheng (2015) conducted a systematic review covering 33 research studies of art, dance/movement, drama, and music therapies (29 of which were offered in groups) involving more than 4,454 children, adolescents, and young adults (ages 3–24). The author noted the effectiveness of these approaches when used for "curative, remedial, rehabilitative, and preventative purposes" (p. 77), concluding that "these cost effective methods not only mitigate mental health expenditure burdens, but more importantly enhance individual and societal wellness. Their contributions significantly support the movement toward evidence-based, inter-disciplinary development in the health humanities, and particularly in mental care issues" (p. 78). As Cheng noted, arts-based approaches are increasingly being integrated into or used to extend the reach of ESTs with young people. Taken together, these studies show that there is growing research support for the effectiveness of creative arts-based group approaches across a range of diagnoses, making them promising mental health practices.

While Weisz and colleagues' (2017) meta-analysis did not show a difference in outcomes by race or gender, the researchers also noted this may be because White youth were overrepresented within the studies they surveyed. According to Hayes (2017), preliminary data from other research suggest that young people from minority racial groups tend to derive less benefit from therapy than their White peers. However, Lin and Bratton (2015) found the opposite to be true in a meta-analysis of child-centered play therapy. They speculated that the use of action approaches in play therapy decreases the privileging of verbal communication, which may make it more accessible for young people across racial groups. Though their study focused on younger children, the idea that experiential approaches transcend cultural boundaries is not unfamiliar. Arts-based therapies offer a similar emphasis on action and, therefore, may lend themselves to the same inclusivity. However, there are currently no studies that test this theory.

Group Therapy

Is there a difference in the impact of group therapy compared to individual treatment? It appears that they are equivalently effective modalities. Burlingame et al. (2016) summarized that "when identical treatments, patients, and doses are compared, individual and group formats produce statistically indistinguishable outcomes" (p. 457). This equivalency holds true for adolescents. Hoag and Burlingame (1997) calculated an effect size of .61 in their meta-analysis of child and adolescent group therapy studies. Their finding is comparable to the effect sizes for individual therapy as well as those generated in similar meta-analyses of adult groups. Subsequent meta-analytic and narrative reviews have similarly concluded that group therapy is an effective modality for young people (Gerrity & DeLucia-Waack, 2007; Prout & Prout, 1998). There are, however, data to suggest that people with chronic or multiple problems are *more* likely to improve from group therapy (Lebow & Jenkins, 2018).

While groups have demonstrated effectiveness in adolescent treatment, it should be noted that there are exceptions. Studies have found that "get-tough" approaches such as Scared Straight and boot-camp style interventions are not only ineffective but also can exacerbate symptoms in high-risk teens (Lilienfeld, 2007). Findings about the effectiveness of treatment also vary widely depending on the clinician, an issue that will be reviewed in the next section.

Progress Feedback

It has been shown that group therapists have difficulty not only in identifying patients who are failing to make treatment progress or are deteriorating during the course of therapy, but also in accurately assessing group members' perceptions of their relationships within group (Chapman et al., 2012; Compare, Tasca, Lo Coco, & Kivlighan, 2016). Sheppard (2017) is one author who has advocated for the importance of gathering practice-based evidence in the form of routine outcome monitoring. As Marmarosh (2018) noted, such feedback-gathering allows therapists to better understand how members experienced sessions, particularly within group where reactions are varied and often unspoken. But does the feedback that comes from these data make treatment more beneficial for group members? This is a question that researchers have just started to explore in greater depth, and the results are mixed. Some new research suggests that group leaders can improve outcomes within two sessions when alerted that particular members' perception of the quality of relationships in group is deteriorating (Burlingame et al., 2018).

However, other studies found that therapists' receiving ongoing feedback about members' symptoms had no significant impact on outcomes (Davidsen et al., 2017; Koementas-de Vos, Nugter, Engelsbel, & De Jong, 2018), perhaps because, given the complexity of groups, leaders are uncertain how to best make use of the information (for example, through individual versus group-as-whole interventions; Gold & Kivlighan, 2018). In the only two studies to date that have examined this question in the treatment of young people, Shechtman (Shechtman & Sarig, 2016; Shechtman & Tutian, 2017) found no immediate benefits of receiving feedback to either treatment effectiveness or bonding with the group leader or other members. However, it may be that practice-based evidence can have more distal rather than immediate benefits, serving instead to improve group leader proficiency in the long term.

What Makes for Effective Adolescent Therapists?

According to research, psychotherapists vary widely in their effectiveness, with the most successful ones averaging 50% better outcomes and 50% fewer dropouts than the average practitioner (Meichenbaum & Lilienfeld, 2018). In fact, the skills of therapists themselves—rather than theoretical orientation, techniques used, or adherence to treatment manuals—seem to have the greatest bearing on whether patients improve (Wampold, Baldwin, Grosse Holtforth, & Imel, 2017). This phenomenon is particularly relevant to adolescent groups, where bonding with the leader is predictive of outcomes, in contrast to adult groups, where bonding with other members has greater value (Shechtman, 2017).

Hattie (2008), an educational researcher, analyzed an immense number of meta-analyses of teacher effectiveness, identifying hundreds of factors that contribute to academic achievement and generating an effect size for each. Since the publication of his book, Hattie expanded his database to include over 1,200 meta-analyses (Killian, 2017). One of the strongest teacher factors in the updated study (with an effect size of .9) was *teacher credibility*, which was divided into three components: *trusting relationships* between teacher and students, *competence* (the sense that the teacher was expert in the material, knew how to help students learn it, and could manage student behavior), and *passion*. These traits are likely to extend to therapists as well. As Edgette (2010) wrote, "Establishing credibility with adolescent clients is more important for the relationship than establishing rapport" (p. 208).

While there are few group therapy studies that measure the impact of group leader factors on outcomes for young people, recent research on school-based groups with high-risk 5th graders is instructive. In this study, Lochman, Dishion, Boxmeyer, Powell, and Qu (2017) video recorded and coded 938 sessions of Coping Power, a group approach to addressing anger issues in children and adolescents. They found the most effective leaders to be ones who functioned like an authoritative parent by balancing reasonable expectations with warmth and responsiveness, thereby cultivating stronger relationships. At the heart of this balance, they found, was the therapist's ability to regulate their emotional response to group members' limit-testing and acting-out behaviors.

Hayes and Vinca (2017) echoed this, asserting that the leader's presence, which they found to be one of the most important qualities of an effective therapist, rested on an "inward attention" (p. 92) in which they use themselves as an instrument to better understand patients. They explained: "Clients necessarily evoke reactions in therapists—emotional, cognitive, behavioral, and visceral—and attending to these reactions can provide important information about the client and the nature of the work at hand" (p. 93). Because teenagers are masters at inducing feelings in others and because they often communicate through the reactions they evoke, this kind of inner monitoring can be especially important for adolescent group leaders.

Adolescents can be articulate informants about the kinds of therapists they seek. Henriksen (2017) conducted interviews with 21 former individual therapy patients whose treatments were identified as successful by their clinicians. Generally, these teens valued therapists who fostered a secure relationship and a collaborative atmosphere in which they could notice their strengths and challenges as well as their conflicted feelings about change. Some contrasted their therapy experience with past treatments that they deemed unsuccessful, characterized by therapists having a more distant style of engagement.

Pingitore and Ferszt (2017) engaged eight female adolescents who had participated in a hospital outpatient psychotherapy group in semi-structured interviews. When asked about recommendations for group leaders, these girls discussed the importance of the comfort and privacy of the physical space, of cohesion and a small group size, and the leader being authentic, friendly, upbeat, and positive, noting how she set the tone for their own mood states. They also noted the importance of her use of redirection in helping the group feel contained and safe.

Research also suggests that therapists who have a healthy level of self-doubt, that is, questions about how effective they might be with a given patient or how to approach that patient's treatment, coupled with a positive self-concept, may be more effective (Nissen-Lie et al., 2017). These findings align with a recent study of the clinical processes of experienced integrative therapists (Oddli & McCleod, 2017), which found that these clinicians tended to adopt a flexible, improvised yet sequential approach in which various techniques were tried out and evaluated in the moment, based on how patients responded to them. This balancing of improvisation with systematic observation parallels research on creativity, which characterizes creative endeavors as involving a similar balance of flexibility and focused thinking (Boot, Baas, van Gaal, Cools, & De Dreu, 2017).

It is perhaps for this reason that Farber (2017), based on his experience training non-creative arts therapists, suggested that clinicians' personal involvement in the arts can help to enhance their clinical effectiveness by better attuning them to deeper layers of communication within patients. He wrote:

> Therapy manuals drive up the mean effectiveness of a random sample of therapists, but at the expense of constricting the effectiveness of those who would have performed higher than the mean had they not adhered to the manual. Great interpersonal competence is likely one significant discriminant between average therapists and excellent ones, but the ability to listen and respond to more than the manifest content of the words—to listen for narrative shifts, pauses, tonal variations, emotional coloring, plot lines, minor characters, and false notes, and to intervene flexibly with knowledge of such shifts and the non-linearity of change (all things that artists and other creative individuals do so well)—is arguably another variable that separates the good from the great therapist.
>
> (p. 219)

Does Experience Make for a Better Therapist?

In a large-scale, longitudinal study of therapist development over time, Goldberg et al. (2016) found that, while a large minority of therapists got better with greater experience, on average therapists were slightly less effective as they continued to practice. Fonagy (2018) suggested that this may be accounted for by the way that veteran therapists tend to apply past experience as a shortcut to understanding the patient in front of them, rather than engaging fully with discovering what makes each person uniquely constructed. However, he speculated that group therapy may help to mitigate this effect as groups offer a "whole population of naïve observers" in the room, which leads to greater *epistemic trust*, or the ability to experience knowledge that is communicated interpersonally as authentic and personally relevant to oneself (Fonagy, Campbell, & Bateman, 2017). Likewise, as groups develop, it is common for members to help to facilitate the personal work of others in the group (Stone, 2016)—another way that groups may buffer therapist competency.

Cohesion and Climate

Summarizing their extensive research on the topic, Wampold et al. (2017) concluded that "one characteristic of effective therapists is that they are able to form alliances across a range of patients" (p. 44). It is now well established that the *therapeutic alliance*, or the strength of connection between therapist and patient, has a large bearing on whether a treatment works (Lebow & Jenkins, 2018), a finding that extends to adolescent outcomes (Owen, Miller, Seidel, & Chow, 2016) and serves as a potential early predictor of dropout in individual therapy (O'Keeffe et al., 2017). In group therapy, where members have relationships with the therapist but also with other members and the group-as-a-whole, the alliance is most closely related to *cohesion* and *group climate*. Both will be reviewed here as common factors whose promotion by the leader have a significant bearing on how groups proceed.

Though definitions have varied widely, cohesion is most often defined as "the positive bond between the member and the group" (Burlingame & Jensen, 2017, p. S198), characterized by a consensus about and a commitment to group goals, or more broadly, "the sum of all the forces that are exerted on members to remain in the group" (Toseland, Jones, & Gellis, 2004, p. 17). Cohesion has been found to have a medium effect on outcomes, though the strength of this relationship can vary by leader approach, size and focus of the group, and number of sessions (Burlingame & Jensen, 2017). Noting its essentiality, Leszcz (2018) framed cohesion as "the platform upon which all other therapeutic factors operate" (Leszcz, 2018, p. 287).

Cohesion is often linked conceptually to group climate, a term that refers to the emotional atmosphere in the group. A positive climate is marked by features of high engagement, low avoidance, and an ability to manage conflict (Bakali, Baldwin, & Lorentzen, 2009). Group cohesion and positive climate do not develop in and of themselves, but instead through intentional leadership tasks (Shechtman, 2017), including experiential activities that engage members in shared experience and the use of interventions such as bridging and subgrouping that encourage empathy and mentalization (see Haen & Webb, Chapter 1, this volume).

Kivlighan and Tarrant's (2001) research supports the idea that the leader's prime job in working with adolescents, even in structured group approaches, is to focus on creating a safe atmosphere, which correlated with increased engagement in the group climate. Active engagement in turn connected to members perceiving the group as more beneficial. Similarly, a group leader focus on structure had a significant relationship with decreased conflict and distance in the group climate, which related to members perceiving a positive relationship with the therapist (which, consequently, had a direct bearing on group attendance rates). This leader focus on fostering a therapeutic group climate superseded attempting to form alliances with individual members, which the authors found negatively impacted outcomes.

However, as Greene (2017) pointed out, cohesion is not a uniformly positive force. It can also lead to negative outcomes such as increased dependence and conformity, which, when taken to an extreme, can contribute to groupthink. Similarly, recent research that looks more closely at individual differences suggests that increased cohesion is not better for everyone. Several studies have captured the importance of attachment as a moderating variable. *Moderators* are baseline characteristics that do not change during treatment but serve to influence the direction or magnitude of the relationship between treatment and outcome (Kazdin, 2007). These characteristics might be patient or therapist factors, or they may be related to structural components of the treatment package. For example, patient age, therapist theoretical orientation, session length, and group size are all moderating variables that significantly predict the magnitude of the relationship between group cohesion and patient outcome (Burlingame, Strauss, & Joyce, 2013).

Evidence-Based Practice

Beyond knowing which treatments are considered evidence-supported and tracking patient outcomes, the next way therapists can utilize research is to engage in evidence-based practice (Leszcz, 2018). This is the point where clinical intuition and skill meet with research findings. Evidence-based therapists, rather than adopting a treatment package whole, can make use of research that identifies *common factors*. These components of therapy are shared elements across approaches that help to make treatment more effective. Research on common factors often contributes to the articulation of practice guidelines. Burlingame and Jensen (2017) wrote, "Group psychotherapy seems to be most effective when group leaders take advantage of the unique interactive properties of groups and incorporate group process principles into treatment rather than treating it as simultaneously delivered individual treatment" (p. S201). In recent years, there has been increased study of structural features of groups that, when attended to, can enhance creative arts-based groups with adolescents. Several of these features will be reviewed in this section.

Attachment Style

In her recent review of lessons from a career spent studying child and adolescent groups, Shechtman (2017) highlighted the importance of attachment style (of group members as well as therapists) to both outcomes and ruptures in group process, findings that are aligned with increased research on adult groups (Marmarosh, 2017). Attachment style is both a predictor of outcomes and a moderating variable that impacts cohesion, climate, and levels of self-disclosure (Burlingame et al., 2013). Studies suggest that group members with high attachment anxiety benefit from groups where cohesion increases over time, whereas cohesion has less impact for those with an attachment avoidant style (Gallagher, Tasca, Ritchie, Balfour, & Bissada, 2014). Likewise, adolescents with avoidant attachment can be destructive to group process if overrepresented in a group (Shechtman, 2017), which suggests the importance of attending to group composition. Ultimately, as Rosenthal (1987) wrote, there are some potential members who are "unready for the frustrations of group living" (p. 114).

Group Composition

It is widely understood that the patient make-up of a group has a direct influence on what the process will look like, but few studies have examined factors that are important for leaders to consider in making decisions about group composition (Shechtman, 2015). Composition is usually framed in terms of the degree of heterogeneity versus homogeneity of a range of concrete patient factors such as age, gender, and diagnosis, to other less obvious factors including interpersonal style, capacity for engagement, group experience, and developmental level (Leszcz, 2018). While it has been suggested that groups that are more specific in focus (e.g., grief groups) generally benefit from greater homogeneity among members while more open groups need greater variety (Kealy, Ogrodniczuk, Piper, & Sierra-Hernandez, 2016), some youth issues call for balance.

For example, Shechtman (2015, 2017) found that the presence of nonaggressive young people can help mitigate *deviancy training*, or the positive reinforcement of delinquent behaviors, in groups targeted to addressing anger. Likewise, Kivlighan, Lo Coco, Gullo, Pazzagli, and Mazzeschi (2017) discovered that a diversity of attachment styles helped to reduce interpersonal conflict within groups. For example, adding a member who was high in attachment avoidance to a group that was low in avoidance helped to increase positive bonding. The researchers speculated that the group-as-a-whole could tolerate and perhaps counteract the avoidant member's attempts at distancing themselves from others.

Gender

Gender composition is another important question; namely, whether to have single or mixed-gender groups. There are a range of opinions in the literature about the benefits and drawbacks to each. In some ways, the answer will be dictated by the group focus. Garcia, Bacio, Tomlinson, Ladd, and Anderson (2015) conducted one of the few studies to examine gender as a variable in adolescent groups. In examining the influence of member interactions on group satisfaction, engagement, and endorsement of healthy behavior in an adolescent substance abuse program, the authors found that the presence of a higher proportion of girls in groups was connected to increased outcomes for both girls and boys. In other words, girls showed higher benefits from being in all-female groups, while boys showed greater benefit from mixed-gender groups. The researchers hypothesized that single-gender groups allow girls to feel greater connection and perhaps to take more assertive roles in participation, while mixed-gender groups allow boys to overcome masculinity norms the prohibit emotional communication and affiliation. These findings have been supported by Shechtman (2017), who found higher rates of verbal self-disclosure in girls, and have been mirrored by research on adult groups (Burlingame et al., 2013).

Age

Given the rapid pace of developmental changes during the teen years, older adolescents are typically quite different from their younger peers in a number of ways, and the issues they face are often distinct. Many developmental theorists divide this stage into early (11–14 years), middle (14–17 years), and late (17+ years) phases and attribute different tasks to each of these stages (Music, 2017). While heterogeneity in interpersonal style can increase vitality within groups, too wide a range of ages and developmental levels is likely to negatively affect the group.

Group Size

Research on adult groups suggests an ideal size of five to nine members (Burlingame & Jensen, 2017), though there is little research on adolescent groups that addresses the same question. The general recommendation is for five to ten members, with seven to nine considered ideal (Berg, Landreth, & Fall, 2018; Finneran, Nitza, & Patterson, 2017). In arts-based groups, group size will depend in part upon how many teens can be accommodated in the room where sessions will take place while still allowing ample space for movement and use of materials.

In an interesting study, Kivlighan, London, and Miles (2012) sought to understand how group size and leadership structure related to adolescent group member perception of treatment benefits and relationship with the leader. They found that adolescents reported greater benefit from co-led groups than from groups with a single leader. In singly led groups, as group size increased so did avoidance and a negative perception of the group. This effect was mitigated in co-led groups by the presence of a second leader. As the group got larger, members still reported positive feelings toward the group and decreased avoidance. The results suggest that a co-leader can help to attend to more group members and pick up on material that a single leader might miss when the group is bigger.

The presence of two leaders, regardless of their gender, can evoke associations and projections related to parents. This construction allows for a modeling of shared power dynamics, collaboration, and the appearance and resolution of conflict, something that might be particularly useful for group members who have witnessed conflict within their families (Davies, 2015). In addition, it provides a model of coupling for adolescents, who are often entering into their first romantic relationships.

Active Engagement

Meta-analytic results have connected a young person's level of engagement in treatment to how much benefit they derive from therapy (Hayes, 2017). This finding has been echoed in adolescent group therapy research (Shechtman and Leichtentritt, 2010), as well as in creative arts-based groups. Orkibi, Azoulay, Regev, and Snir (2017) found that a member's active engagement in role play during psychodrama groups had a positive relationship to leader perceptions of the therapeutic alliance, as well as the likelihood that the group member would demonstrate less resistance and greater productive behaviors within sessions. In a nuanced study that teased out how one group member's perceptions interact with those of the whole group, Gillis, Kivlighan, and Russell (2016) found a positive correlation between active engagement and outcomes for older adolescents and young adults, but only when the individual group member's perception of the group as actively engaged matched the perception of the majority of the rest of the group. In other words, high engagement produced better outcomes only when the young person was on the same page with how the other members were also viewing the level of engagement in the group.

Existing research supports what group therapists have long understood: that facilitating active engagement in group and creative processes leads to increased change for teens. As a caveat, it is important to note that there are a variety of ways in which group members actively engage in sessions, befitting their personalities and challenges. Quieter members do show benefits and dominant members do deteriorate during groups, depending on the quality of the interactions (Haen, 2015; Pingitore & Ferszt, 2017).

Engaging Parents

While engaging adolescents is important, Shechtman (2017) reminded that young people "do not live in a vacuum" (p. 63). Group leaders should also seek to engage parents, where possible, both to establish trust and to support gains made in the group. Parents may serve as important informants about treatment progress (Weisz et al., 2017), and depending on the problem area, they may also be engaged as consultants, additional clients, or collaborators (Brennan, Murphy, & Flessner, 2017). Teens are often well-served by having their parent participate in a corresponding support group.

How Much Does Technique Matter?

This book is centered on the idea that creative arts-based approaches can help to make for groups that are both appealing to adolescents and helpful in producing change. The evidence presented here indeed suggests that who the therapist is, and the kinds of relationships they can create, have a much stronger bearing on outcomes. However, since these outcomes also depend on active engagement of teens in the process, which supports the development of cohesion and group climate, techniques that reduce anxiety and resistance pave the way for change to happen.

It has been suggested by numerous authors that creative arts-based approaches may have particular efficacy in group therapy by promoting cohesion (Kymissis, Christenson, Swanson & Orlowski, 1996), fostering empathy and insight (Veach & Gladding, 2007), allowing for increased emotional expression without flooding (Chapman, 2014), and creating conditions that allow members to engage interpersonally in the here-and-now (Aigen, 1997). There is also evidence to suggest that these groups provide an ideal venue for the stimulation and enhancement of emotional regulation (Gruber & Oepen, 2018; Moneta & Rousseau, 2008). The following section will consider the arts within the context of evidence-based practice.

Creative Arts: Unique Change Agents or Different Path to the Same Destination?

The creative arts therapies, by necessity, involve a triadic relationship between the therapist, the group members, and the artistic process, so that members experience connections not just with other people, but also with the art they and other members are creating (Rusch & Imus, 2017). Does the involvement of creative and experiential processes mean that creative arts-based approaches involve different mechanisms of change, or are they simply a different means of enacting the same change processes that happen in other types of therapy? This question is reflective of a debate among practitioners of whether artistic creation allows for material to surface that can then be addressed clinically or whether the arts themselves are the healing element (Cruz & Feder, 2013). A similar question has been asked in play therapy as reported by Shelby, Ellingsen, and Schaefer (2016): "whether play therapy is merely a vehicle facilitating change, or whether it is the play itself that holds unique curative value" (p. 565).

Early process research studies in the field reflected a desire to identify process components specific to creative arts therapy groups. These studies included comparisons of therapeutic factors between creative arts therapy and verbal therapy groups (e.g., Goldberg, McNiel & Binder, 1988; Strauss, 2004); examination of helping and hindering factors in arts-based groups (Dokter, 2010); consideration of whether art made during session can provide reliable indicators of group dynamics (Rubin & Rosenblum, 1977); and examination of the relationship between verbal and art making processes in groups (Skaife, 2011). Ultimately, the results of these studies are mixed, with some finding no differences in therapeutic factors, while others were limited by methodology challenges or a lack of ability to generalize the findings in a meaningful way. Nevertheless, there have been subsequent bodies of research in each creative arts therapy modality that have attempted to identify unique mechanisms of change. There have also been recent attempts to synthesize change processes among the various arts modalities in order to create a shared language (Havsteen-Franklin, Jovanovic, Reed, Charles, & Lucas, 2017).

While representative studies of therapeutic factors will be reviewed below, one important approach to understanding the impact of any clinical process is to engage the patients as informants. Such studies of adolescent treatment are rare, particularly in the creative arts therapies. However, there are some notable exceptions. Forenza (2017) conducted retrospective interviews with adults who had participated in a teen theater program in which they devised and performed a variety of scenes for other teens related to timely topics. Of interest to clinicians, all ten participants in this study highlighted the way that their engagement in the artistic process fostered strong connections to their castmates and left them with a sense of being needed and valued, thereby enhancing social support. The ability of the arts to forge resonant interpersonal connections extends to the clinical realm. Trevarthen and Panksepp (2017) asserted, "Group music therapy, dance therapy and drama therapy recruit the spirit of collaboration among performers, strengthening different ways of being, different personalities and different talents" (p. 47).

Diamond and Lev-Wiesel (2016) conducted a retrospective study in which they interviewed 20 adults about their experience participating in an expressive therapies group as children or adolescents. Many of the themes derived from these interviews reflect elements common to verbal group therapy. However, participants also reported that making art in the group helped promote spontaneity and a sense of creative freedom that was lacking in their lives outside of treatment. Their reports have been echoed by a recent mixed-method study (Lange, Leonhart, Gruber, & Koch, 2018) that found a link between artistic creation and enhancement of self-efficacy and well-being in adults.

Gabel and Robb (2017) conducted a meta-synthesis of over 100 writings on group art therapy to ascertain five therapeutic factors that are distinct from those Yalom established for verbal therapy groups (Yalom & Leszcz, 2005). In order of prominence within the literature, these were: *symbolic expression, relational aesthetics* (the aforementioned triangular relationship between the leader, the members, and the art), *embodiment, pleasure and play,* and *ritual.* Koch (2017) aimed to identify specific factors applicable to all of the creative arts therapies, embedding them within a theoretical model of *embodied aesthetics.* Three of the items, *hedonism* (art for pleasure and play), *meaning making* (art for symbolizing, communicating, and being seen), and *transitional support* (art for adapting to change, which contains elements of ritual) map onto Gabel and Robb's (2017) factors. Two others, *aesthetics* (art for beauty, which serves an integrative function) and *productivity* (art for resilience, self-efficacy, and leaving something behind), are distinct.

These initial efforts toward establishing specific change factors within the creative arts therapies suggest that, while arts-based approaches share elements in common with other therapies, there are also unique ingredients connected to artistic processes. Evidence-based group practice means understanding how to draw on the effective structural elements of group therapy while also using creative arts-based approaches for the potent ways they might support treatment goals. For example, stigma surrounding mental illness can be a significant barrier to willingness to attend treatment for teens (Brennan et al., 2017), particularly in the case of group therapy (Shechtman, Vogel, Strass, & Heath, 2018), perhaps because of increased visibility. However, use of the arts can de-pathologize therapy, something reflected by participants in Diamond and Lev-Wiesel's (2017) study, who reported that they counteracted negative feelings about receiving treatment by thinking of the group as an art class or telling their friends that it was fun.

As alternative forms of expression, the arts also offer a means of working through material that adolescents would otherwise be reluctant to verbally disclose. Findings from three empirical studies conducted by Goncalo, Vincent, and Krause (2015) suggest that engaging in creative tasks can lift the sense of physical burden from keeping a secret. Important for clinical work, the researchers found that this effect carried through without participants revealing the secret they were keeping. Finally, by engaging the body, the arts may deepen the group process, allowing for stronger interpersonal connections between members. Embodiment has been seen to allow for greater attention to the present moment and facilitation of regulation, both of which allow the group to work with more emotionally sensitive material (Kimmel & Gockel, 2017).

Conclusion

Research tells us that overall, psychotherapy for youth has modest outcomes, with groups being as effective as individual treatment. While there is less research on the creative arts therapies than other more prominent forms of treatment, there is a growing evidence base that attests to its efficacy. Because the therapeutic relationship has greater impact on treatment outcome than the method practiced, it is important that group leaders working with teens establish a presence that balances warmth with expectations. Leaders should direct their efforts toward creating a therapeutic group climate that is appreciative of all members and their unique strengths, while facilitating bonding between members and active engagement in the process, both of which help to increase cohesion. Leaders who can self-regulate, attune to members' uniqueness, utilize their presence, and remain self-reflective are likely to forge alliances with a greater number of teens.

Attention to structural issues, including group composition and the degree of heterogeneity of attachment styles, age, and gender, as well as attempts to engage parents in treatment, are important. Understanding the specific ingredients of the arts and how these can be catalysts for change, applying them in a flexible way, and monitoring impact while adjusting as needed will help to strengthen treatment effectiveness. This chapter aimed to present a current snapshot of the state of the art regarding creative arts-based approaches in group work with adolescents. The chapters to follow will present a range of practice principles drawn from each of the creative arts therapy modalities, as well as present ways the arts have been used to target common issues with which adolescents struggle.

References

Aigen, K. (1997). Here we are in music: One year with an adolescent creative music therapy group. *Nordoff-Robbins Music Therapy Monograph Series*, Vol. 2. St. Louis, MO: MMB Music.

Augustyniak, K. M., Brooks, M., Rinaldo, V. J., Bogner, R., & Hodges, S. (2006). Emotional regulation: Considerations for school-based group interventions. *The Journal for Specialists in Group Work*, 34(4), 326–350.

Bakali, J. V., Baldwin, S. A., & Lorentzen, S. (2009). Modeling group process constructs at three stages in group psychotherapy. *Psychotherapy Research*, 19(3), 332–343.

Barber, J. P. (2009). Presidential address: Toward a working through of some core conflicts in psychotherapy research. *Psychotherapy Research*, 19(1), 1–12.

Barlow, D. H., Farchione, T. J., Bullis, J. R., Gallagher, M. W., Murray-Latin, H., Sauer-Zavala, S., ... Cassiello-Robbins, C. (2017). The unified protocol for transdiagnostic treatment of emotional disorders compared with diagnosis-specific protocols for anxiety disorders: A randomized clinical trial. *JAMA Psychiatry*, 74(9), 875–884.

Berg, R. C., Landreth, G. L., & Fall, K. A. (2018). Group counseling with adolescents. In *Group counseling: Concepts and procedures* (2nd ed., pp. 181–190). New York, NY: Routledge.

Boot, N., Baas, M., van Gaal, S., Cools, R., & De Dreu, C. K. W. (2017). Creative cognition and dopaminergic modulation of fronto-striatal networks: Integrative review and research agenda. *Neuroscience and Biobehavioral Reviews*, 78, 13–23.

Brennan, E., Murphy, Y. E., & Flessner, C. A. (2017). Examining developmental considerations of evidence-based practices for youth. In C. A. Flessner & J. C. Piacentini (Eds.), *Clinical handbook of psychological disorder in children and adolescents: A step-by-step treatment manual* (pp. 8–28). New York, NY: Guilford.

Burlingame, G. M., & Jensen, J. L. (2017). Small group process and outcome research highlights: A 25-year perspective. *International Journal of Group Psychotherapy*, 67(Suppl1), S194–S218.

Burlingame, G. M., Seebeck, J. D., Janis, R. A., Whitcomb, K. E., Barkowski, S., Rosendahl, J., & Straus, B. (2016). Outcome differences between individual and group formats when identical and nonidentical treatments, patients, and doses are compared: A 25-year meta-analytic perspective. *Psychotherapy*, 53(4), 446–461.

Burlingame, G. M., Strauss, B., & Joyce, A. (2013). Change mechanisms and effectiveness of small group treatments. In M. J. Lambert (Ed.), *Bergin and Garfield's handbook of psychotherapy and behavior change* (6th ed., pp. 640–689). New York, NY: Wiley.

Burlingame, G. M., Whitcomb, K. E., Woodland, S. C., Olsen, J. A., Beecher, M., & Gleave, R. (2018). The effects of relationship and progress feedback in group psychotherapy using the Group Questionnaire and Outcome Questionnaire-45: A randomized clinical trial. *Psychotherapy, 55*(2), 116–131.

Chapman, C. L., Burlingame, G. M., Gleave, R., Rees, F., Beecher, M., & Porter, G. S. (2012). Clinical prediction in group psychotherapy. *Psychotherapy Research, 22*(6), 673–681.

Chapman, L. (2014). *Neurobiologically informed trauma therapy with children and adolescents: Understanding mechanisms of change.* New York, NY: Norton.

Cheng, F. K. (2015). Effects of expressive arts based interventions on adolescent mental health. In R. Wolfe (Ed.), *Psychological health and needs research development* (pp. 57–90). New York, NY: Nova Science.

Compare, A., Tasca, G. A., Lo Coco, G., & Kivlighan, Jr., D. M. (2016). Congruence of group therapist and group member alliance judgments in emotionally focused group therapy for binge eating disorder. *Psychotherapy, 53*(2), 163–173.

Cortina, M. A., & Fazel, M. (2015). The Art Room: An evaluation of a targeted school-based group intervention for students with emotional and behavioural difficulties. *The Arts in Psychotherapy, 42*, 35–40.

Cruz, R. F., & Feder, B. (2013). *Feders' the art and science of evaluation in the arts therapies* (2nd ed.). Springfield, IL: Charles C. Thomas.

Cruz, R. F., & Koch, S. F. (2015). Reading and evaluating quantitative research in body psychotherapy. *International Body Psychotherapy Journal, 14*(1), 10–19.

Davidsen, A. H., Poulsen, S., Lindschou, J., Winkel, P., Tróndarson, M. F., Waaddegaard, M., & Lau, M. (2017). Feedback in group psychotherapy for eating disorders: A randomized clinical trial. *Journal of Consulting and Clinical Psychology, 85*(5), 484–494.

Davies, A. (2015). Co-therapy and working with others. In A. Davies, E. Richards & N. Barwick (Eds.), *Group music therapy: A group analytic approach* (pp. 139–148). New York, NY: Routledge.

Diamond, S., & Lev-Wiesel, R. (2016). Recollections of being in child expressive arts group therapy: A qualitative study of adult former clients' conceptions of their therapy as children. *International Journal of Group Psychotherapy, 66*(3), 401–421.

Diamond, S., & Lev-Wiesel, R. (2017). The title 'therapy' and what do you do with it as a child? Recollections of being in child expressive arts group therapy. *Clinical Child Psychology and Psychiatry, 22*(1), 152–164.

Doel, M. (2006). *Using groupwork.* New York, NY: Routledge.

Dokter, D. (2010). Helping and hindering processes in creative arts therapy group practice. *Group, 34*(1), 67–83.

Dunphy, K., Mullane, S., & Jacobsson, M. (2014). The effectiveness of expressive arts therapies: A review of the literature. *Psychotherapy and Counselling Journal of Australia, 2*(1). Retrieved from http://pacja.org.au/?p=1439

Edgette, J. S. (2010). Avoiding the trap of trying too hard: Appreciating the influence of natural law in adolescent therapy. In M. Kerman (Ed.), *Clinical pearls of wisdom: 21 leading therapists offer their key insights* (pp. 207–218). New York, NY: Norton.

Farber, B. A. (2017). Gaining therapeutic wisdom and skills from creative others (writers, actors, musicians, and dancers). In L. G. Castonguay & C. E. Hill (Eds.), *How and why are some therapists better than others?: Understanding therapist effects* (pp. 215–231). Washington, DC: American Psychological Association.

Finneran, K. R., Nitza, A., & Patterson, K. W. (2017). Planning for groups. In C. Haen & S. Aronson (Eds.), *Handbook of child and adolescent group therapy: A practitioner's reference* (pp. 9–19). New York, NY: Routledge.

Fonagy, P. (February 26, 2018). The technique of mentalization-based treatment for severe personality disorder. Special institute presented at the American Group Psychotherapy Association annual meeting, Houston, TX.

Fonagy, P., Campbell, C., & Bateman, A. (2017). Mentalizing, attachment, and epistemic trust in group therapy. *International Journal of Group Psychotherapy, 67*(2), 176–201.

Forenza, B. (2017). Empowering processes of a countywide arts intervention for high school youth. *Journal of Youth Development, 12*(2), 21–40.

Freeman, M., & Mathison, S. (2009). *Researching children's experiences.* New York, NY: Guilford.

Gabel, A., & Robb, B. (2017). (Re)considering psychological constructs: A thematic synthesis defining five therapeutic factors in group art therapy. *The Arts in Psychotherapy, 55,* 126–135.

Gallagher, M. E., Tasca, G. A., Ritchie, K., Balfour, L., & Bissada, H. (2014). Attachment anxiety moderates the relationship between growth in group cohesion and treatment outcomes in group psychodynamic interpersonal psychotherapy for women with binge eating disorder. *Group Dynamics: Theory, Research, and Practice, 18*(1), 38–52.

Gálvez-Lara, M., Corpas, J., Moreno, E., Venceslá, J. F., Sánchez-Raya, A., & Moriana, J. A. (2018). Psychological treatments for mental disorders in children and adolescents: A review of the evidence of leading international organizations. *Clinical Child and Family Psychology Review, 21*(3), 366–387.

Garcia, T. A., Bacio, G. A., Tomlinson, K., Ladd, B. O., & Anderson, K. G. (2015). Effects of sex composition on group processes in alcohol prevention groups for teens. *Experimental and Clinical Psychopharmacology, 23*(4), 275–283.

Geipel, J., Koenig, J., Hillecke, T. K., Resch, F., & Kaess, M. (2018). Music-based interventions to reduce internalizing symptoms in children and adolescents: A meta-analysis. *Journal of Affective Disorders, 225,* 647–656.

Gerrity, D. A., & DeLucia-Waack, J. L. (2007). Effectiveness of groups in the schools. *The Journal for Specialists in Group Work, 32*(1), 97–106.

Gillis, H. L., Jr., Kivlighan, D. M., Jr., & Russell, K. C. (2016). Between-client and within-client engagement and outcome in a residential wilderness treatment group: An actor partner interdependence analysis. *Psychotherapy, 53*(4), 413–423.

Gold, C., Voracek, M., & Wigram, T. (2004). Effects of music therapy for children and adolescents with psychopathology: A meta-analysis. *The Journal of Child Psychology and Psychiatry, 45*(6), 1054–1063.

Gold, P. B., & Kivlighan, D., Jr. (2018). It's complicated: Using group member process-feedback to improve group therapist effectiveness. *Psychotherapy, 55*(2), 164–169.

Goldberg, F. S., McNiel, D. E., & Binder, R. L. (1988). Therapeutic factors in two forms of inpatient group psychotherapy: Music therapy and verbal therapy. *Group, 12*(3), 145–156.

Goldberg, S. B., Rousmaniere, T., Miller, S. D., Whipple, J., Nielsen, S. L., Hoyt, W. T., & Wampold, B. E. (2016). Do psychotherapists improve with time and experience? A longitudinal analysis of outcomes in a clinical setting. *Journal of Counseling Psychology, 63*(1), 1–11.

Goncalo, J. A., Vincent, L. C., & Krause, V. (2015). Liberating consequences of creative work: How a creative outlet lifts the physical burden of secrecy. *Journal of Experimental Social Psychology, 59,* 32–39.

Greenbaum, C. A., & Javdani, S. (2017). Expressive writing intervention promotes resilience among juvenile justice-involved youth. *Children & Youth Services Review, 73,* 220–229.

Greene, L. (2016). A qualitative assessment of the quantitative group psychotherapy research: Past, present, and future. *Group, 40*(1), 23–28.

Greene, L. (2017). Group psychotherapy research studies that therapists might actually read: My top 10 list. *International Journal of Group Psychotherapy, 67*(1), 1–23.

Gruber, H., & Oepen, R. (2018). Emotion regulation strategies and effects in art-making: A narrative synthesis. *The Arts in Psychotherapy, 59,* 65–74.

Haen, C. (2015). Advancing a dramaturgical theory of group process. *Drama Therapy Review, 1*(2), 219–235.

Haen, C. (2017). An integrative perspective on group therapy. In C. Haen & S. Aronson (Eds.), *Handbook of child and adolescent group therapy: A practitioner's reference* (pp. 193–202). New York, NY: Routledge.

Harvey, A. G. (2014). Transdiagnostic mechanisms and treatments for youth with psychiatric disorders: An opportunity to catapult progress? In J. Ehrenreich-May & B. C. Chu (Eds.), *Transdiagnostic treatments for children and adolescents: Principles and practice* (pp. 15–31). New York, NY: Guilford.

Hattie, J. (2008). *Visible learning: A synthesis of over 800 meta-analyses relating to achievement*. New York, NY: Routledge.

Havsteen-Franklin, D., Jovanovic, N., Reed, M., Charles, M., & Lucas, C. (2017). Developing a shared language within arts psychotherapies: A personal construct psychology approach to understanding clinical change. *The Arts in Psychotherapy, 55*, 103–110.

Hayes, J. (2017). What leads to change?: I. Common factors in child therapy. In N. Midgley, J. Hayes & M. Cooper (Eds.), *Essential research findings in child and adolescent counselling and psychotherapy* (pp. 119–147). London: Sage.

Hayes, J. A., & Vinca, M. (2017). Therapist presence, absence, and extraordinary presence. In L. G. Castonguay & C. E. Hill (Eds.), *Why are some therapists better than others? Understanding therapist effects* (pp. 85–99). Washington, DC: American Psychological Association.

Henriksen, A. K. (2017). Helpful aspects at the beginning of successful outpatient treatment: Retrospective views of adolescents and their therapists. *Journal of Psychotherapy Integration, 27*(4), 508–525.

Hoag, M. J., & Burlingame, G. M. (1997). Evaluating the effectiveness of child and adolescent group treatment: A meta-analytic review. *Journal of Clinical Child Psychology, 26*(3), 234–246.

Hoff, A. L., Swan, A. J., Mercado, R. J., Kagan, E. R., Crawford, E. A., & Kendall, P. C. (2017). Psychological therapy with children and adolescents: Theory and practice. In A. J. Consoli, L. E. Beutler & B. Bongar (Eds.), *Comprehensive textbook of psychotherapy: Theory and practice* (2nd ed., pp. 267–283). New York, NY: Oxford University Press.

Kazak, A. E., Hoagwood, K., Weisz, J. R., Hood, K., Kratochwill, T. R., Vargas, L. A., & Banez, G. A. (2010). A meta-systems approach to evidence-based practice for children and adolescents. *American Psychologist, 65*(2), 85–97.

Kazdin, A. E. (2007). Mediators and mechanisms of change in psychotherapy research. *Annual Review of Clinical Psychology, 3*, 1–27.

Kazdin, A. E., & Weisz, J. R. (1998). Identifying and developing empirically supported child and adolescent treatments. *Journal of Consulting and Clinical Psychology, 66*(1), 19–36.

Kealy, D., Ogrodniczuk, J. S., Piper, W. E., & Sierra-Hernandez, C. A. (2016). When it is not a good fit: Clinical errors in patient selection and group composition in group psychotherapy. *Psychotherapy, 53*(3), 308–313.

Killian, S. (2017, January 18). Hattie effect size 2016 update. *The Australian Society for Evidence-Based Teaching.* Retrieved from www.evidencebasedteaching.org.au/hattie-effect-size-2016-update/

Kim, S., Kim, G., & Ki, J. (2014). Effects of group art therapy combined with breath meditation on the subjective well-being of depressed and anxious adolescents. *The Arts in Psychotherapy, 41*(5), 519–526.

Kimmell, A., & Gockel, A. (2017). Embodied connections: Engaging the body in group work. *Qualitative Social Work, 17*(2), 268–285.

Kivlighan, Jr., D. M., Lo Coco, G., Gullo, S., Pazzagli, C., & Mazzeschi, C. (2017). Attachment anxiety and attachment avoidance: Members' attachment fit with their group and group relationships. *International Journal of Group Psychotherapy, 67*(2), 223–239.

Kivlighan, Jr., D. M., London, K., & Miles, J. R. (2012). Are two heads better than one? The relationship between number of group leaders and group members, and group climate and group member benefit from therapy. *Group Dynamics: Theory, Research, and Practice, 16*(1), 1–13.

Kivlighan, Jr., D. M., & Tarrant, J. M. (2001). Does group climate mediate the group leadership-group member outcome relationship?: A test of Yalom's hypotheses about leadership priorities. *Group Dynamics: Theory, Research, and Practice, 5*(3), 220–234.

Koch, S. (2017). Arts and health: Active factors and a theory framework of embodied aesthetics. *The Arts in Psychotherapy, 54*, 85–91.

Koementas-de Vos, M. M. W., Nugter, M. A., Engelsbel, F., & De Jong, K. (2018). Does progress feedback enhance the outcome of group psychotherapy? *Psychotherapy, 55*(2), 151–163.

Kymissis, P., Christenson, E., Swanson, A. J., & Orlowski, B. (1996). Group treatment of adolescent inpatients: A pilot study using a structured therapy approach. *Journal of Child & Adolescent Group Therapy, 6*(1), 45–52.

Lange, G., Leonhart, R., Gruber, H., & Koch, S. C. (2018). The effect of active creation on psychological health: A feasibility study on (therapeutic) mechanisms. *Behavioral Sciences, 8*(2), 25. Retrieved from www.mdpi.com/2076-328X/8/2/25

Lebow, J. L., & Jenkins, P. H. (2018). *Research for the psychotherapist: From science to practice* (2nd ed.). New York, NY: Routledge.

Leszcz, M. (2018). The evidence-based group psychotherapist. *Psychoanalytic Inquiry, 38*(4), 285–298.

Lilienfeld, S. O. (2007). Psychological treatments that cause harm. *Perspectives on Psychological Science, 2,* 53–70.

Lin, Y.-W., & Bratton, S. (2015). A meta-analytic review of child-centered play therapy approaches. *Journal of Counseling and Development, 93*(1), 45–58.

Lochman, J. E., Dishion, T. J., Boxmeyer, C. L., Powell, N. P., & Qu, L. (2017). Variation in response to evidence-based group preventive intervention for disruptive behavior problems: A view from 938 Coping Power sessions. *Journal of Abnormal Child Psychology, 45*(7), 1271–1284.

Marmarosh, C. L. (Ed.). (2017). Attachment in group therapy [Special issue]. *International Journal of Group Psychotherapy, 67*(2).

Marmarosh, C. L. (2018). Introduction to special issue: Feedback in group psychotherapy. *Psychotherapy, 55*(2), 101–104.

Martin, L., Oepen, R., Bauer, K., Nottensteiner, A., Merheim, K., Gruber, H., & Koch, S. C. (2018). Creative arts interventions for stress management and prevention—A systematic review. *Behavioral Sciences, 8*(2), 28. Retrieved from www.mdpi.com/2076-328X/8/2/28

Meichenbaum, D., & Lilienfeld, S. (2018). How to spot hype in the field of psychotherapy: A 19-item checklist. *Professional Psychology: Research and Practice, 49*(1), 22–30.

Midgley, N. (2004). Sailing between Scylla and Charybdis: Incorporating qualitative approaches into child psychotherapy research. *Journal of Child Psychotherapy, 30*(1), 89–111.

Midgley, N., Hayes, J., & Cooper, M. (2017). Introduction: What can child therapists learn from research? In Authors (Eds.), *Essential research findings in child and adolescent counselling and psychotherapy* (pp. 1–13). London: Sage.

Moneta, I., & Rousseau, C. (2008). Emotional expression and regulation in a school-based drama workshop for immigrant adolescents with behavioral and learning difficulties. *The Arts in Psychotherapy, 35*(5), 329–340.

Music, G. (2017). *Nurturing natures: Attachment and children's emotional, sociocultural and brain development* (2nd ed.). New York, NY: Psychology Press.

Nissen-Lie, H. A., Rønnestad, M. H., Høglend, P. A., Havik, O. E., Solbakken, O. A., Stiles, T. C., & Monsen, J. T. (2017). Love yourself as a person, doubt yourself as a therapist? *Clinical Psychology & Psychotherapy, 24,* 48–60.

O'Keeffe, S., Martin, P., Goodyer, I. M., Wilkinson, P., Impact Consortium, & Midgley, N. (2017). Predicting dropout in adolescents receiving therapy for depression. *Psychotherapy Research, 28*(5), 708–721.

Oddli, H. W., & McCleod, J. (2017). Knowing-in-relation: How experienced therapists integrate different sources of knowledge in actual clinical practice. *Journal of Psychotherapy Integration, 27*(1), 107–119.

Orkibi, H., Azoulay, G., Regev, D., & Snir, S. (2017). Adolescents' dramatic engagement predicts their in-session productive behaviors: A psychodrama change process study. *The Arts in Psychotherapy, 55,* 46–53.

Owen, J., Miller, S. D., Seidel, J., & Chow, D. (2016). The working alliance in treatment of military adolescents. *Journal of Consulting and Clinical Psychology, 84*(3), 200–210.

Pavlicevic, M. (2016). Group music therapy reconsidered: Of musics, contexts, and discourses. In J. Edwards (Ed.), *The Oxford handbook of music therapy* (pp. 669–683). Oxford: Oxford University Press.

Pingitore, F., & Ferszt, G. G. (2017). "The voice" and perspectives of adolescents participating in a short-term psychotherapy group. *International Journal of Group Psychotherapy, 67*(3), 360–382.

Piper, W. E., Ogrodniczuk, J. S., Joyce, A. S., & Weideman, R. (2010). *Short-term group therapies for complicated grief: Two research-based models.* Washington, DC: American Psychological Association.

Prout, S. M., & Prout, H. T. (1998). A meta-analysis of school-based studies of counseling and psychotherapy: An update. *Journal of School Psychology, 36*(2), 121–136.

Rosenthal, L. (1987). *Resolving resistance in group psychotherapy.* Northvale, NJ: Jason Aronson.

Rubin, J. A., & Rosenblum, N. (1977). Group art and group dynamics: An experimental study. *Art Psychotherapy, 4*(3–4), 185–193.

Rusch, D. C., & Imus, S. (2017). The same kid in yet another hood—Deep game design as creative arts therapy? In D. C. Rusch, *Making deep games: Designing games with meaning and purpose* (pp. 167–192). Boca Raton, FL: CRC Press.

Shechtman, Z. (2015). Group composition in children's groups: A clinical demonstration. *Group, 39*(1), 25–38.

Shechtman, Z. (2017). Bridging the gap between research and practice: How research can guide group leaders. In C. Haen & S. Aronson (Eds.), *Handbook of child and adolescent group therapy: A practitioner's reference* (pp. 52–65). New York, NY: Routledge.

Shechtman, Z., & Leichtentritt, J. (2010). The association of process with outcomes in child group therapy. *Psychotherapy Research, 20*(1), 8–21.

Shechtman, Z., & Sarig, O. (2016). The effect of client progress feedback on child/adolescent's group-counseling outcomes. *The Journal for Specialists in Group Work, 41*(4), 334–349.

Shechtman, Z., & Tutian, R. (2017). Feedback to semi-professional counselors in treating child aggression. *Psychotherapy Research, 27*(3), 338–349.

Shechtman, Z., Vogel, D. L., Strass, H. A., & Heath, P. J. (2018). Stigma in help-seeking: The case of adolescents. *British Journal of Guidance & Counselling, 46*(1), 104–119.

Shelby, J., Ellingsen, R., & Schaefer, C. E. (2016). Play therapy research: Issues for 21st century progress. In K. J. O'Connor, C. E. Schaeffer & L. D. Braverman (Eds.), *Handbook of play therapy* (2nd ed., pp. 563–581). Hoboken, NJ: Wiley.

Sheppard, T. (2017). Evaluation and practice-based evidence. In C. Haen & S. Aronson (Eds.), *Handbook of child and adolescent group therapy: A practitioner's reference* (pp. 40–51). New York, NY: Routledge.

Shirk, S., Jungbluth, N., & Karver, M. (2012). Change processes and active components. In P. C. Kendall (Ed.), *Child and adolescent therapy: Cognitive-behavioral procedures* (4th ed., pp. 379–397). New York, NY: Guilford.

Shuman, J., Kennedy, H., DeWitt, P., Edelblute, A., & Wamboldt, M. Z. (2016). Group music therapy impacts mood states of adolescents in a psychiatric hospital setting. *The Arts in Psychotherapy, 49*, 50–56.

Skaife, S. (2011). Maps and mess: Group members' experience of the relationship between art and talk in an art therapy group. In A. Gilroy (Ed.), *Art therapy research in practice* (pp. 251–267). Oxford: Peter Lang.

SmithBattle, L., Chantamit-o-pas, C., Freed, P., McLaughlin, D., & Schneider, J. K. (2017). Moms growing together: Piloting action methods and expressive arts in a therapeutic group for teen mothers. *Journal of Child and Adolescent Psychiatric Nursing, 30*(2), 72–79.

Steele, R. G., & Roberts, M. C. (2003). Therapy and intervention research with children and adolescents. In M. C. Roberts & S. S. Ilardi (Ed.), *Handbook of research methods in clinical psychology* (pp. 307–328). Malden, MA: Blackwell.

Stone, M. H. (2016). The role of group members in facilitating treatment. *Universal Journal of Psychology, 4*(6), 270–276.

Strauss, B. (2004). Naturalistic studies within different group treatment formats. *International Journal of Group Psychotherapy, 54*(2), 253–259.

Toseland, R. W., Jones, L. V., & Gellis, Z. D. (2004). Group dynamics. In C. D. Garvin, L. M. Gutierrez & M. J. Galinsky (Eds.), *Handbook of social work with groups* (pp. 13–31). New York, NY: Guilford.

Travagin, G., Margola, D., & Revenson, T. A. (2015). How effective are expressive writing interventions for adolescents? A meta-analytic review. *Child Psychology Review, 36*, 42–55.

Trevarthen, C., & Panksepp, J. (2017). In tune with feeling: Musical play with emotions of creativity, inspiring neuroaffective development and self-confidence for learning in company. In

S. Hart (Ed.), *Inclusion, play and empathy: Neuroaffective development in children's groups* (pp. 29–54). London: Jessica Kingsley.

Veach, L. J., & Gladding, S. T. (2007). Using creative group techniques in high schools. *The Journal for Specialists in Group Work, 32*(1), 71–81.

Wampold, B. E., Baldwin, S. A., Grosse Holtforth, M., & Imel, Z. E. (2017). What characterizes effective therapists? In L. G. Castonguay & C. E. Hill (Eds.), *How and why are some therapists better than others?: Understanding therapist effects* (pp. 37–53). Washington, DC: American Psychological Association.

Weisz, J., Bearman, S. K., Santucci, L. C., & Jensen-Doss, A. (2016). Initial test of a principle-guided approach to transdiagnostic psychotherapy with children and adolescents. *Journal of Clinical Child & Adolescent Psychology, 46*(1), 44–58.

Weisz, J. R., Kuppens, S., Ng, M. Y., Eckshtain, D., Ugueto, A. M., Vaughn-Coaxum, R . . . Fordwood, S. R. (2017). What five decades of research tells us about the effects of youth psychological therapy: A multilevel meta-analysis and implications for science and practice. *American Psychologist, 72*(2), 79–117.

Yalom, I. D., & Leszcz, M. (2005). *The theory and practice of group psychotherapy* (5th ed.). New York, NY: Basic Books.

3

A Neuroscience Perspective on Creative Arts Therapies and Adolescent Groups

TERRY MARKS-TARLOW AND CRAIG HAEN

During the Middle Ages, many religious paintings of Madonna and child depicted the child as a miniature adult. These paintings look odd, with head and body proportions bearing little relationship to actual youngsters. It appears that the artists didn't examine real children when creating their masterpieces, but instead drew upon idealized forms from imagination. This may be because the very concept of childhood didn't exist during the Middle Ages (Aries, 1962). With the infant and toddler mortality rate so high, and with no clear indication of who would live and who would die, it may have been too risky to pour attention onto young children. Not until the Renaissance, with the development of three-dimensional perspective, did artists start rendering children and babies in correct proportions.

As creative arts therapists already know, art communicates powerfully about broader social trends. An interesting parallel exists within the field of psychology. During the early twentieth century, when psychoanalysis arose, the concept of childhood definitely existed, yet an empirically based developmental perspective was part of neither theory nor practice. Instead, early analysts such as Sigmund Freud and Klein (1932/1975) hypothesized about development by abstracting backwards from work with adults. Because their theories were not based on direct observation, they misattributed cognitive processes and defensive operations to children whose prefrontal cortexes had not yet matured enough for such high levels of abstraction.

Mahler (Mahler, Pine, & Bergman, 1975) was among the first psychoanalysts to draw upon actual experience with children and their caretakers. Bowlby (1969) was another analyst highly influenced by empirical observation of mothers and their offspring, including those of other mammals. Bowlby introduced attachment theory as a developmental framework, and this perspective has proven unusually valuable. Whereas securely attached children are likely to have good self-esteem and lasting relationships, contributing to successful futures, insecurely attached children tend to encounter problems that last into adulthood, including with school, forming relationships, and developing emotional and even physical symptoms. Those with disorganized attachment are most vulnerable to future psychiatric and medical conditions (Puig, Englund, Simpson, & Collins, 2013; Zeanah, 2012). With Bowlby's development of attachment theory, all preconceptions and abstract ideas had been set aside. The emotional needs of real children were placed front and center, including implications for ideal parenting and optimal therapeutic healing.

The 1990s are considered the 'decade of the brain,' bringing an understanding of stages of childhood to new levels. Neuropsychologist Schore (1994, 2012) extended Bowlby's findings, translating concepts into the language of brain and autonomic nervous system circuitry. Schore's modern attachment theory goes by the name *regulation theory*. Along with including neural aspects, he shifted Bowlby's emphasis from a behavioral focus to a central concern with emotion, which is mediated primarily by *subcortical* (beneath the cortex) and *cortical* (conscious thinking, reasoning, symbolizing, and self-awareness) structures of the *limbic* (emotional processing) *system* at the center of healthy development and relationships. Schore's regulation theory is both evolutionary and developmental, identifying neural underpinnings of healthy or unhealthy minds, brains, and bodies as they arise from attuned or misattuned early relationships.

This chapter aims to educate clinicians about the nature and distinct features of the adolescent brain, as well as to suggest ways that neuroscientific understanding can help to articulate the benefits of creative arts-based groups in working with teens. Adolescence is a time of great transition that prepares young people for adulthood, yet ushers in a period characterized by emotional dysregulation and unpredictability, particularly in social situations (Guyer, Silk, & Nelson, 2016; Victor & Hariri, 2017). A good understanding of any adolescent's early developmental history, plus genetic background, can be crucial in discerning whether symptoms are likely to be transient or part of a broader syndrome. By adding a conception of what is going on in the brain and autonomic nervous system, therapists are better equipped to sort out age- and stage-related factors from purely idiosyncratic ones.

Puberty Versus Adolescence

Puberty was once considered the end-point of brain maturation, but now we understand that the *prefrontal cortex* (forwardmost part of the brain, behind the eyes and forehead) doesn't finish developing until young adults reach their mid- to late 20s (Gogtay et al., 2004)—well past the end of puberty. The concepts of puberty and adolescence, though loosely connected, are often confused with one another. Puberty is a biological concept related to sexual maturation. During puberty, a tide of gonadal hormones sweeps through the body, changing the voice, initiating the growth of pubic and facial hair, and readying the sexual organs for procreation. All these changes are physical, linear, discrete, and time-limited, reaching their peak between 15 and 16 years of age (van Duijvenvoorde, Peters, Braams, & Corne, 2016).

By contrast, adolescence extends over a much longer period, representing the nonlinear transition between childhood and adulthood that may be best thought of as ending when the young person achieves self-sufficiency (Kilford, Garrett, & Blakemore, 2016). Adolescence is an emergent time of life characterized by many emotional, social, and behavioral changes, which are highly unique to each child and variable across culture. While hormones are important in affecting adolescent behavior, they don't determine it. In fact, there are no simple, one-to-one correlations between the flow of gonadal hormones and prototypical adolescent behavior (Spear, 2000).

The idea that adolescent development extends well into the 20s has tremendous implications across multiple domains. As an example, the courts in many American states frequently have responded to teenagers who commit murder as if they are identical to fully mature adults. When this has occurred, the fact that executive areas of teenage brains remain underdeveloped was not taken into account, either in determining punishment or in considering chances for rehabilitation or recidivism (Cohen, Bonnie, Taylor-Thompson, & Casey, 2015).

Psychotherapy is another realm in which an understanding of the adolescent brain can guide both clinicians and parents, especially in determining what is developmentally appropriate and normative versus problematic and pathological. Most people with mental health problems differ from those without by virtue of frequency and intensity of symptoms (Harvey, 2014). Indeed, in adolescence, the distinction between a 'normal' teen presentation and that which indicates mental health problems is often quite thin (Brennan, Murphy, & Flessner, 2017). This chapter brings both the evolutionary and developmental perspectives of interpersonal neurobiology to an examination of the adolescent brain. We begin with a description of adolescent behavior and concomitant brain processes, and conclude with implications for group psychotherapy, with a special emphasis on the importance of the creative arts.

The Animal Brain

Only recently, with the advent of fMRI technology, among other methods, have researchers been able to study the adolescent brain in context. Until then, animal studies of the juvenile period of rodents and other non-human primates had yielded a wealth of information about neurochemical and cellular changes that occur as a function of age. Given the absence of psychological stresses unique to humans, some people question the validity of animal models for studying adolescence. Yet, it turns out that a host of mammals, such as rodents and other non-human primates, exhibit behaviors very similar to human adolescents. Examples include increased attraction to peers and social interactions (Primus & Kellogg, 1989), as well as enhanced novelty seeking and risk-taking behaviors (Adriani, Chiatrotti, & Laviola, 1998). An important set of findings gleaned from rodent studies involves distinct changes within the limbic and *prefrontal* (executive functions, personality, social processing, moral reasoning) regions of the brain during adolescence.

Beginning with Darwin (1872) and continuing through Ekman (2003), interest in the neurobiology of emotion has led researchers to examine discrete emotional circuits in the brains of animals. Panksepp (2004; Davis & Panksepp, 2018; Panksepp & Biven, 2012), considered the 'father' of affective neuroscience, identified seven emotional/motivational circuits common to all mammals: SEEKING, FEAR, RAGE, LUST, CARE, PANIC/GRIEF, and PLAY (capitalized to emphasize their universality). Each has distinct neural architecture to link sensory, motivational, and behavioral areas of the brain. Yet overlap exists in the neurochemical cocktail of excitatory and inhibitory transmitters released into synaptic gaps between neighboring neurons. *Glutamate*, the most widespread excitatory neurotransmitter, works in tandem with *GABA*, its chemical precursor and most widespread inhibitory neurotransmitter.

We humans love to pride ourselves on our differences from other animals, as the only species with multiple languages, books for our young, and computers that interconnect our social and political existences across the globe. It is easy to privilege the power of symbolic thinking. Yet the more we grasp about the centrality of emotion, the more we realize that to have a rational mind, we need a solid emotional foundation. It is the affective core we share with other mammals that lends us the capacity for compassion, the passion to play artfully, and the courage to help others. Meanwhile, the teenage brain is especially sensitized to emotion (Burnett, Sebastian, Cohen Kadosh, & Blakemore, 2011), so it is important for clinicians to put this into proper context.

Beginning in the 1960s, MacLean (1990) introduced his concept of the *triune brain*, the idea that the brain consists of three structures: the reptilian brain, the limbic brain, and the neocortex.

- The *reptilian brain* is the oldest of the three layers, serving as the foundation as relates to reflex and survival needs. The reptilian brain controls the body's vital functions, such as heart rate, breathing, temperature, and balance. Its main structures, the brain stem and cerebellum, lie deep within the subcortical part of the brain.
- Next is the *limbic brain*, which MacLean believed first emerged in mammals. By recording memories of behaviors that produce agreeable or disagreeable social experiences, the limbic layer introduces emotion and motivation connected to modulate basic needs. The main limbic structures include the *hypothalamus* (involved in sleep and emotional activity; coordinates the autonomic nervous system; regulates hormonal activity of the pituitary relevant to body temperature, thirst, hunger, and other homeostatic systems), the *amygdala* (processes emotional experiences; encodes memories for safety, danger, fear, and other strong emotions), and the *hippocampus* (encodes autobiographical and semantic memories).
- In humans, the reptilian and mammalian brains are both topped by the *neocortex*, which consists of two large cerebral hemispheres (right and left) permitting the more conscious experiences of self-reflection, planning, imagination, language, abstract thought, and symbolic representation. Whereas the subcortical layer of the human brain is the origin of impulse and emotion, the cortical layer helps Homo sapiens develop self-control, largely through cortical inhibition of subcortical impulses and feelings. By standing back and reflecting, the cortex allows us to slow everything down, to think about what is happening, to be mindful about what we are feeling, and to consciously decide what action to take in response. Our mature, cortical capacity to make decisions is what allows adults to override the natural impulses that drive children, adolescents, and animals.

MacLean's triune brain (Figure 3.1) and Panksepp's emotional/motivational circuits go hand in hand. Contemporary neuroscience has revealed that the first four circuits previously listed—SEEKING, FEAR, RAGE, and LUST—also characterize the reptilian brain, while the last three circuits—CARE, PANIC/GRIEF, and PLAY—are unique to the social brain of mammals. The SEEKING circuit (also called the reward

Triune Brain

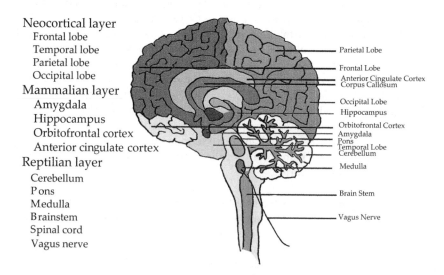

Neocortical layer
  Frontal lobe
  Temporal lobe
  Parietal lobe
  Occipital lobe
Mammalian layer
  Amygdala
  Hippocampus
  Orbitofrontal cortex
  Anterior cingulate cortex
Reptilian layer
  Cerebellum
  Pons
  Medulla
  Brainstem
  Spinal cord
  Vagus nerve

Parietal Lobe
Frontal Lobe
Anterior Cingulate Cortex
Corpus Callosum
Occipital Lobe
Hippocampus
Orbitofrontal Cortex
Amygdala
Pons
Temporal Lobe
Cerebellum
Medulla
Brain Stem
Vagus Nerve

Figure 3.1

circuit) energizes humans, mammals, and reptiles to go out into the world and get their needs met. This circuit, enervated by the neurotransmitter *dopamine*, plays a large role in the emotional sensitivity of teenagers as well as in the underlying incentives that drive the adolescent brain.

Each circuit extends downward into lower subcortical centers in the brain stem as well as upward into higher, uniquely human cortical areas. In people, the neocortex is necessary for emotional experience to reach full awareness, yet this higher part of the brain cannot generate feeling states. Overlap also exists in how the circuits function, with blended emotions such as guilt or righteous indignation being a mixture of different emotional circuits blended with cognitive elements. Meanwhile, the subcortical origin of all feelings means that animals probably do experience emotion, but from a fully immersed vantage point, without reflective awareness.

The CARE circuit is considered part of the social brain because of its importance in attachment dynamics that drive mammalian parents to care for their young, strangers to empathize with one another, and members of one species at times to care for members of another. From a neural perspective, human empathy consists of two interrelated circuits (Decety & Ickes, 2009); one, online from birth, is purely emotional, consisting of affective resonance. Affective resonance is why babies so easily cry when they hear other babies crying, why joy, fear, and humor are so contagious, and why depression and trauma are difficult for loved ones to bear. While mammals share affective resonance, human empathy's other neural pathway is purely cognitive. It consists of two aspects: 1) *theory of mind*, the ability to put ourselves in the shoes of another and see the world through their eyes, and 2) the ability to differentiate self from other (even if we share the same feelings, we are not exactly in the same circumstances as others). Within all psychotherapists, the affective dimension of empathy supplies great meaning in helping even strangers with their problems, while the cognitive dimension protects us from burnout and compassion fatigue (see Marks-Tarlow, 2012).

The Adolescent Brain

During adolescence, the brain undergoes a process that can be likened to a software upgrade on a computer, in which circuitry is consolidated, networks are reorganized, and processes are rendered more efficient and specialized (Giedd, 2015). Sercombe and Paus (2009) provided a helpful metaphor when they suggested thinking of the brain as an unchartered region like the Australian outback. The first people to arrive to this region forge their own pathways, and subsequent travelers follow those paths but then diverge in a number of directions. Over time, the most heavily used paths become easier to travel and eventually are paved to make efficient roads; the lesser-used ones grow over and their remnants fade with time. The child brain is represented by that set of multiple pathways, which are blazed by the millions of pieces of information that children take in, while the adult brain is represented by modern society, which has a reliable highway system that gets travelers to their destination more directly and efficiently. The adolescent brain serves as the transition between those two states.

During early puberty, an overproduction of axons and synapses occurs that is followed by a period of rapid *pruning* (or elimination of circuits) during later adolescence (Crews, He, & Hodge, 2007). Synaptic networks are reorganized, and their connections rendered stronger and more efficient through a process known as *myelination*, which involves an increase in white matter volume and a corresponding decrease in gray matter (Kilford et al., 2016). As different areas of the brain develop more quickly than others, there is a gap between the advancement of emotional responsiveness and motivation (subcortical processes) and the point when cognitive control mechanisms (cortical processes) come fully online. It is this gap, as will be discussed later, that is implicated in many of the risky and seemingly mind-boggling decisions that teenagers make.

Because the brain is in a state of development during adolescence, the common view is that teens are a 'work in progress' and that their inconsistency is attributable to their learning to use their new neural systems, a phenomenon that Abigail Baird aptly referred to as "neural gawkiness" (Dobbs, 2011, para. 19). During this period, the brain is particularly open to growth and change, a quality referred to as *neuroplasticity*. Steinberg (2016) defined plasticity as "the capacity of the brain to change in response to experience" (p. 345), and this openness to modification allows for important growth, as well as making adolescents particularly vulnerable to stress and the onset of mental illness (Tottenham & Galván, 2016).

Subcortical structures that mediate exaggerated emotional sensitivity and enhanced evaluation of incentives get reorganized during adolescence. So, it is no wonder this stage of life renders them so vulnerable to the onset of affective, eating, and addictive disorders. Fortunately, most teenagers successfully navigate the transition from depending upon caregivers for food, shelter, protection, and financial support to supplying these things for themselves by becoming self-sufficient, contributing members of society. Unfortunately, some struggle to make this transition, and a small number never succeed. Amid so many physical and behavioral changes, the peak age of onset for many psychiatric disorders, including depression, anxiety, personality disorders, and psychoses, is adolescence (Giedd, 2015). Paus, Keshavan, and Giedd (2008) suggested that the pathophysiology of these disorders arises from aberrations of maturational changes that naturally occur within the adolescent brain.

As humans age, brain development is generally characterized by a shifting balance of decreased plasticity and increased stability (Fett, Gromann, Giampietro, Shergill, & Krabbendam, 2014). Preliminary evidence suggests that greater plasticity during adolescence is related to greater intelligence (Blakemore, 2018). The notion of experience as a catalyst highlights the importance of therapy processes rooted in the experiential domain, particularly during this window when the brain remains especially adaptable.

The Developmental Importance of Play and the Arts

Out of all mammals, the human's brain has the most open wiring. This circuitry allows for postnatal experience and learning to shape how each brain will become wired through culture and upbringing. For this reason, human babies are born with highly immature brains that require a more extended childhood than any other animal. As mentioned, two main sets of social instincts separate the open wiring of the mammalian brain from the closed wiring of the reptilian brain upon which it sits: care of the young and the tendency to play. PANIC/GRIEF is a third circuit of the mammalian brain that signals separation distress. When fear, panic, or grief is highly active, all play stops, while in the context of relational and emotional safety play can proceed.

Hand in hand with brain plasticity, another great development in the evolution of human knowing was curiosity. Instead of merely responding to the press of innate survival needs, as reptiles do, through play mammals became proactive, adventurous, and inquisitive. In most species, the urge to play occurs within a critical window during the juvenile period (Beatty, Dodge, Dodge, White, & Panksepp, 1982). Human play resembles that of other mammals in also having a critical window for normal development. As with many other mammalian species, rough-and-tumble play during the early childhood years appears especially related to cognitive capacities to settle down and focus attention. This led Panksepp (2018) to suggest that early education should begin each day on the playground. He saw running, romping, and grappling as preventative measures against increasing diagnoses of attention deficit/hyperactivity disorder amid a backdrop of decreasing interest in and funding for physical education.

Across all descriptive levels, neurobiological, psychological, sociological, and anthropological investigations have identified a host of affective, cognitive, social, and motor capacities that accompany children's play (for a summary, see Marks-Tarlow, 2010). These include:

- Brain growth
- Self-regulation of behavior and emotions

- Development of imagination and symbolic representation
- Meaning making
- Development of language and narrative
- Meta-communication (communication about communication)
- Creativity and divergent thinking
- Self-transformation
- Social competence
- Gender identification
- Community membership
- Cultural awareness and creation

Humans differ from other species, which typically cease playing outside of their critical developmental window. People often continue playing right into adulthood, which includes our lifelong attraction to sports and the arts. Play is so important because it enhances positive feelings, provides passion for life and intrinsic motivation, and allows novel experiences (Marks-Tarlow, Solomon, & Siegel, 2018). Not just children, but also adolescents and even adults experiment with new ways to think, act, and be through play (Dissanayake, 2017). This is what makes the creative arts therapies and play therapy such vital modalities.

Along with its extension throughout the lifespan, human play differs from that of other species in another significant aspect. Beyond the rough-and-tumble variety common to other mammals, human play also diverges into symbolic realms and imaginative landscapes. As play becomes increasingly symbolic, social, and imaginative, it moves from implicit, preconscious, and nonverbal roots to include more explicit, conscious, and verbal elements. While still facilitated by safe attachment and primary caretaker involvement, children's play develops in opposite directions simultaneously: toward greater autonomy as well as toward fuller coordination with others.

Marks-Tarlow (2010, 2012) suggested that children learn how to operate intuitively in an internally grounded fashion, from the inside-out, through ample opportunities for free play during the early years. When mammals are meant to play but do not, whatever the reason, consequences can be severe. Brown, a psychiatrist at Stanford, stumbled into a professional focus on play after unearthing a chilling example (Brown & Eberle, 2018). As a psychiatric resident in 1969, Brown worked within prison settings, conducting clinical interviews on 26 young incarcerated murderers in hopes of finding common threads. At first, he was puzzled by the diverse backgrounds of these felons. They came from such different social classes, ethnicities, levels of trauma and deprivation, as well as varying opportunities in life. Then he came across a single factor these violent men appeared to have in common: the absence of play during childhood. Perhaps because of its necessity for normal development, play in psychotherapy is especially powerful at all ages.

Playing during psychotherapy is not engagement in frivolous activity (Marks-Tarlow, 2015a, 2015b); rather, it can provide safety in the context of what can be otherwise intolerable emotions. Playing helps to expand intersubjective space by relaxing defenses and allowing for safe exploration of even darker places when necessary (Haen, 2015). This potential is familiar to yoga teachers, who frequently guide students to approach the *asanas*, or poses, playfully as a means of creating more space inside the mind, body, and spirit. The more present we are in our bodies, the more we lengthen out, relax in, and breathe through our movements, the more freedom we gain to create additional possibilities. Within the enterprise of psychotherapy, then, play grants more freedom of being, feeling, doing, moving, and relating in the context of a trusting bond.

The interpersonal neurobiology of attachment illustrates how the self grows, unfolds, and builds new structure through play. Freedom to play without inhibition or constriction is a key ingredient for joy, interest, passion, and vitality later in life. Within all juvenile animals, the mixing of pleasure and pain through play also expands emotional tolerance (Pellis & Pellis, 2010). For this reason, children often play in ways that serve to draw them toward the edges of their regulatory boundaries (Marks-Tarlow, 2012). Young children love to throw themselves into disequilibrium by spinning, jumping, climbing, and hurling their bodies right to the edges of what they can tolerate emotionally. Adolescents take these urges to play and explore new edges to unprecedented levels.

Impulsivity and Risk Taking

One hallmark of adolescence is a love of new experiences and especially risky ones. Teens feel driven in hot pursuit of novelty, often with a very present-centered state of mind that lacks consideration for future outcomes or negative consequences of their actions. Based on the 2005 National Youth Risk Behavior Survey, Casey, Jones, and Hare (2008) reported that adolescents engage in behaviors that increase the likelihood of their death or illness in multiple ways: by binge drinking, driving a vehicle while intoxicated, not wearing seat belts, carrying weapons, using illegal substances, and engaging in unprotected casual sex that results either in unintended pregnancies or sexually transmitted diseases.

Clearly, such risky behavior leaves them extremely vulnerable. In fact, the risk of injury or death is higher during adolescence than in childhood or adulthood, with suicide being the second leading cause of death among young people (Heron, 2017). To understand what is happening in the brain corresponding to such riskiness, it is first important to distinguish between two different concepts: *risk* and *impulse*. Casey and colleagues (2008) noted that adolescent behavior is often described as both impulsive and risky nearly synonymously, yet these behaviors rely on different cognitive as well as neural processes. This means that risk and impulse are distinct, with differing developmental trajectories.

The opposite of impulse is impulse control, which involves the capacity to suppress inappropriate thoughts and actions. Impulse control, or the ability to delay gratification in favor of goal-directed behavior, is a cornerstone of cognitive and behavioral development. Consider Mischel's classic "marshmallow experiments" (e.g., Mischel, Shoda, & Rodriguez, 1989; Mischel, 2014). A group of 4-year-old children were offered opportunities to either indulge in a smaller treat right away, such as one marshmallow, or resist immediate gratification to receive a bigger treat later in time, such as two marshmallows. This same group was tracked longitudinally. By the time they reached adolescence, subjects who could delay gratification at age 4 had developed greater social and emotional competence by adolescence.

Not only did they do better academically, but they also excelled at self-regulation. Experiments such as these suggest that goal-directed behavior requiring control of impulses to optimize outcomes matures steadily across childhood and adolescence.

A review of the literature suggests that impulsivity diminishes with age and is associated with protracted development of the prefrontal cortex (Casey, Galván, & Hare, 2005; Chein, Albert, O'Brien, Uckert, & Steinberg, 2010). It is important to know that brain development moves both from bottom to top (subcortical to cortical structures) and back to front (posterior to anterior). The highest, most frontal area of the brain—the prefrontal cortex—is the last to develop, only coming into full maturation between the ages of 26 and 28 years, and generally reaching full maturity for females more quickly than for males. The prefrontal cortex coordinates and adjusts complex behavior. It contains several subareas, each with distinct functions. Some relate to executive functioning, such as focusing and organizing attention, decision making, planning, prioritizing competing and simultaneous information, and task accomplishment. Others relate to personality and social processing of self and other, including theory of mind, empathy, and moral judgment.

A recently discovered area receiving a great deal of attention is the *default mode network*, which generally includes the medial prefrontal cortex, posterior cingulate cortex, inferior parietal lobule, lateral temporal cortex, hippocampal formation, and precuneus (Chan & Siegel, 2018). The default mode network is the most active part of the brain and uses the most metabolic energy. Although initially thought to represent internal resting states apart from external tasks, researchers now understand its significance to self-referential and social processing. This is the part of the brain we use for daydreaming, rumination, and associative acts of creativity. It is also an area highly affected by mindfulness practices. In general, the midline or *medial* areas of the prefrontal cortex are part of the cortical level of limbic circuitry that are emotionally toned for social and emotional information. The *lateral* areas of the prefrontal cortex farthest from the midline, such as the *dorsolateral cortex*, are non-limbic and more related to strictly cognitive processing and intellectual tasks.

In contrast to the gradual, linear increase in impulse control associated with age, there is a nonlinear increase in sensation seeking associated with late adolescence (Casey et al., 2005). What this means is that risk taking increases in late adolescence, peaking at around age 19, and because it is higher during adolescence than in either childhood or adulthood, when graphed it appears like an inverted U. Unlike impulsivity, which relates to slower prefrontal cortical development, differences in risk taking appear to relate more to subcortical limbic processing connected to affective information and evaluation of incentives. In a recent large-scale study of 5,000 participants across 11 countries, Steinberg and colleagues (2017) found that these trends appear across cultures, as does a steady increase in self-regulation skills from pre-adolescence to young adulthood. Of note, the findings also suggested that while adolescence is generally a time for greater propensity toward risk taking, how and to what degree these behaviors are expressed is influenced in part by one's culture.

fMRI studies (e.g., Ernst et al., 2005) reveal two important subcortical structures that become more highly activated in adolescents as they face risky choices or process emotional information: the *amygdala* and *nucleus accumbens*. Both structures, online at birth, undergo deep transformation during puberty, accompanying the influx of adrenal and gonadal hormones. The amygdala, which represents the first line of emotional and social processing, is central in the neuroception of safety versus danger, including the experience of fear (Porges, 2011). The nucleus accumbens, which lies in the basal ganglia within the brain stem, represents the first line of processing incentives by the reward or SEEKING system. (Panksepp believed the term 'reward system' a misnomer, because this circuitry is not involved with actually enjoying the reward once we've found what we're looking for.)

As mentioned previously, the SEEKING system is energized by the dopamine neurotransmitter and is deeply connected with attachment dynamics. This includes the absolute joy of connection during infancy, beginning around 3 months, as part of interactive regulation of emotions and arousal. When all goes well with the attachment process, the SEEKING system makes a gradual and smooth transition between interactive regulation by caregivers and autoregulation through self-soothing and self-stimulating behaviors. If, for whatever reason, there are problematic early attachment dynamics, and especially in cases of relational trauma (see Schore, 2012) where the primary caregiver is abusive, neglectful, or otherwise not fully available, the infant may be forced into autoregulation too early in life. If this happens, the SEEKING system is in danger of getting co-opted by autoregulatory strategies such as addiction. All the same underlying mechanisms and subcortical structures come into play, whether the addiction involves food, drugs, sex, or alcohol (see Katehakis, 2016).

The subcortical part of the adolescent brain story also explains something else that would otherwise be puzzling. If the impulsivity, poor judgment, and risky behavior so characteristic of adolescents were purely a function of an immature prefrontal cortex (which suggests irrationality, a feeling of invulnerability, and an inability to perceive risks), then young children would also be high-risk takers. But this is not the case, for as mentioned, risk taking peaks during adolescence (Steinberg et al., 2017). What is more, research reveals that unlike small children, adolescents do have the cognitive ability to anticipate and understand the potential risks of behaviors in which they engage (Steinberg, 2015). These findings underscore the difference between intellectual understanding in a 'cold context' (decisions made in isolation or preemptively) and emotional response in the 'hot context' of embodied existence, such as in the presence of peers, in the moments of sexual engagement, or while under the influence of substances (Blakemore, 2018; Victor & Hariri, 2017). The latter necessitates both reflection and emotion regulation, involving different underlying brain systems, and often requires quick decision making (Zelazo & Doebel, 2015).

To understand what is happening in the brain, it is important to consider both cortical as well as subcortical levels. The brain is highly complex and rarely reduces down to a single thing. The combination of levels also reveals how the developmental mechanisms that underlie impulsivity are fundamentally different from those that underlie risk taking. The most prominent explanatory framework is the *dual systems model*, which attributes the increase in risk-taking behaviors in adolescence to a developmental mismatch between the rapidly developing reward system in the limbic and paralimbic regions and the more gradual neuromaturation of the cognitive control system localized in the lateral prefrontal and parietal cortices and synaptically connected parts of the anterior cingulate (Steinberg, 2015).

This asynchrony is thought to underlie teens' propensity for seeking sensation and novelty, their increased sensitivity to rewards, and their difficulty applying internal brakes to reflect on risky choices before acting on them.

While a useful heuristic, this model has been criticized (e.g., by Casey, Galván, & Somerville, 2016; Victor & Hariri, 2017) for oversimplifying neural processes and not sufficiently capturing how these two brain systems interact or how behavior is dependent on context (for example, with whom the teen is interacting). Likewise, Blakemore (2018) recently noted individual variability in these patterns, with some adolescents having both their amygdala and nucleus accumbens reach full maturity before their prefrontal cortex, while other teen brains showed acceleration in only one of these limbic regions, or neither. But as a parsimonious explanation, the dual systems model offers important ways for clinicians, parents, and teens to understand the often-confounding choices adolescents make from a non-pathologizing stance.

Given the incredible vulnerability to disease and even death that enhanced riskiness confers on adolescents, is there any evolutionary advantage to this state of affairs? Here is where an evolutionary perspective complements a developmental eye so well. Spear (2000) speculated that novelty seeking and willingness to take risks help the adolescent separate from their home territory. Given that this occurs exactly at the peak of puberty, the willingness to leave one's own village in search of adventure and sexual liaisons, in combination with increased emotional sensitivity supporting the neuroception of danger, appears to maximize successes of mating by mixing and spreading one's genes far and wide. This may be how the precise combination of novelty seeking, emotional reactivity, and elevated risk taking observed across so many different species of animals can confer evolutionary advantages.

It is now well established that adolescents are far more likely to take increased risks in the presence of peers, or even under conditions in which they believe peers are observing them. Less emphasized are findings that reflect the potentially positive influence peers can have, such as the ability to influence increased prosocial behavior, especially when that behavior is accompanied by positive peer feedback (Guyer et al., 2016). Likewise, Telzer and colleagues (Telzer, Fuligni, Lieberman, Miernicki, & Galván, 2015) found teen risk taking to be moderated by the amount and quality of existing peer support, with those adolescents who reported more peer conflict or exclusion also tending to take greater risks.

Significance of Emotional Dysregulation

Within all mammals, the detection, expression, and regulation of emotion is a specialty of the right hemisphere (McGilchrist, 2009; Schore, 1994), whose circuitry is lateralized to reach deep into the body's internal systems through the interface between limbic and autonomic nervous systems. Whereas the central nervous system consists of the brain and spinal cord, the peripheral nervous system consists of the *somatic nervous system*, which controls the striated muscles of the body, and the *autonomic nervous system* (ANS), which controls the smooth muscles of the internal organs. Along with the *enteric* division, which helps us to digest food, the ANS includes two branches. The *sympathetic* division up-regulates emotional arousal to deal with fight-or-flight or intense joy. The *parasympathetic* division down-regulates arousal to bring the body back to rest and relaxation.

Within humans, whether in teenagers, younger children, or adults, most symptoms that cause concern and bring people to psychotherapy involve problems with emotional arousal. But adolescents are especially prone to emotional dysregulation, informed by their increased sensitivity to social threat and peer rejection. As the ability to *mentalize*, or to understand the mental and emotional states of others, is under development during this developmental period, there is a tendency for teens to misperceive threat, engaging in "faulty neuroception" (Flores, 2017, p. 212). As such, adolescents tend to show greater brain activity than adults in areas related to social cognition when engaging in self-reflection, suggesting that how they see themselves is highly informed by how they believe others see them (Guyer et al., 2016).

It is important for clinicians and parents to understand the neurobiology of emotion. Emotional experience carries two dimensions: *intensity* (high or low arousal) and *valence* (negative or positive emotional experience). Adolescents tend to experience greater extremes of both positive and negative emotions in response to social situations. Also, their joyful feelings tend not to last as long as they do in adults, which leads to heightened stress (Burnett et al., 2011; Tottenham & Galván, 2016). When dealing with the dark and dramatic turns of the teenage repertoire, it is helpful to remember that everyone, not just teenagers, needs the full range of emotional experience. What is more, even negative emotions pass relatively quickly when given full expression. Finally, most emotional problems involve difficulties tolerating the intensity and not the valence of felt emotions.

What Group Therapy Offers

The neurobiology of adolescence suggests targets for intervention that groups are uniquely suited to address. Namely, groups can capitalize on social influence and novel experiences while fostering self-regulatory skills. When working clinically with adolescents, it is important to redirect the SEEKING circuit by helping teens experience inherent rewards within the search for self-understanding and growth. Given that creativity is a sophisticated form of play, and play is inherently growth-promoting and intrinsically rewarding—not to mention the most complex sophisticated mammalian circuit—creative arts-based groups may be particularly potent in supporting teenagers through this emotional time period and developing the skills to ease their developmental transition to adulthood.

As adolescents experience a shift from the importance of caregivers as primary attachment figures to a broadening of the attachment network to include peers, they are often caught in a dance between wanting to retain the security of the parent relationship for support and seeing that relationship as a threat to their need to establish independence and social connections (Allen & Tan, 2016). The drive toward connection with peers, the power of peer influence, and the opportunity to have these connections facilitated by an adult render group therapy a developmentally responsive form of intervention for teens.

As numerous authors (Badenoch & Cox, 2015; Flores, 2017; Goldstein, 2018; Grossmark, 2017; Mark-Goldstein & Ogden, 2015) have asserted, a prime value of group therapy comes from how it evokes past relational experiences from one's family-of-origin or other important groups, and how these often-traumatic experiences can be held, understood, and repaired within the group itself. During group, when interactions mirror past interpersonal experiences as encoded in implicit as opposed to explicit memory, related emotions and behaviors tend to surface automatically (Livingston & Scott, 2017). By slowing down the process and bringing implicit reactions to conscious awareness and reflection, the group helps to regulate affect in real time, while habitual responses can be modified in the face of powerful new experiences. Leszcz (2017) succinctly wrote, "Group therapy can be viewed as a neural exercise in the co-construction of regulatory capacity" (p. 283). These regulatory moments have the possibility of fostering new neural connections within the brain, stimulating growth that accompanies the emergence of new behavior patterns (Kinley & Reyno, 2016).

As Schermer (2016) noted, knowledge of neuroscience cannot yet provide specific best practices, but can increase the therapist's attunement to underlying individual and group processes. Knowledge of neuroscience also underscores the importance of therapist intuition by providing "a conceptual map that can supplement the intuitive maps inwardly available to the therapist" (p. 181). This sort of 'bottom-up' understanding relates to the importance of emotions and novel experiences for adolescents when it comes to effecting learning and change. Yet, there remains a propensity of 'top-down' approaches to adolescent treatment that largely target cognition and fear extinction. Recent neuroscience literature notes that heightened emotional reactivity and diminished fear extinction characteristic of the teen years make these approaches less effective for adolescents (Fett et al., 2014; Guyer et al., 2016; Lee et al., 2014). Instead, modalities that provide prosocial forms of risk taking in the context of novel stimuli, regulatory activities, and opportunities for reflection may show the greatest promise (Suleiman & Dahl, 2017). In the following section, we highlight the value of creative arts-based groups through a neuroscience lens.

What Arts-Based Groups Offer

While the arts are ubiquitous among young people, they have not yet been given proper attention by developmental researchers. Goldstein, Lerner, and Winner (2017) asserted that the arts represent an important area for study. Embedded within their praxis are abilities important to development, including self-control, executive function, attention, engagement, motivation, emotion regulation, and understanding of others. Dissanayake (2017) also noted their developmental significance by locating the origin of the arts within the attachment relationship, emerging out of the patterned interactions of children and their caregivers.

Whereas the reptilian layer matures in the womb, the mammalian and cortical levels of the brain mature after birth through interaction with primary caregivers and other experiences in the environment. The first two years of a baby's life provide the emotional foundation upon which cognitive development occurs. Right-brain to right-brain communication between parents and child enables primary care-givers to sense and respond to their infant's emotional needs (see Schore, 2003a, 2003b). Creative arts-based therapies can similarly serve as an important form of interactive regulation. Interactive regulation takes place through empathically based communication, occurring through nonverbal, subcortical channels that use paralinguistic features like facial expression, tone and rhythm of voice, posture, and movements. Precisely because the expressive arts employ body-based, nonverbal techniques, they quickly shoot under defenses to reach preverbal levels of develop-ment. In this way, creative arts therapies can help uncover and heal early relational wounds, as well as channel negative emotion, contain high arousal, and provide a safe way to take emotional risks.

For adolescents, whose regulatory systems are still maturing and who may there-fore find it particularly difficult to remain present through the interpersonal friction that can come from interacting with others, groups also offer the opportunity to see another group member engaged in a rupture and repair sequence. These moments may register for teens more fully from the slightly more distanced but nevertheless emotionally resonant position of witness. Witnessing provides a sense of the others' emotional experience through what has been termed *embodied simulation*. Gallese (2017) described this process as such:

> When perceiving others expressing disgust, or experiencing touch or pain, some of the same brain areas are activated as when we subjectively experience the same emotion or sensation. We do not fully experience their qualitative content, which remains largely opaque to us, however, embodied simulation enables us to experience others as experiencing emotions or sensations we know from the inside.
>
> (p. 44)

Embodied simulation is closely linked to the discovery of *mirror neurons*, or the finding that when one watches another engaged in intentional action, the same areas of the brain activated in the person who is being observed are stimulated in the viewer (Gallese & Goldman, 1998).

In arts-based methods, in which group members observe others performing intentional actions, whether through the creation of a piece of art, engagement in a movement sequence, the taking on of a role, or the playing of a musical phrase, the firing of mirror neurons and the "jointly-evoked sensory and emotional reac-tions" (Gallese, 2017, p. 45) are facilitative of empathic connections. While it is not uncommon for teens to engage in criticism and judgmental behavior toward peers during the verbal process of psychotherapy groups, there is often a respect that emerges during the action sequences of arts-based approaches that helps to create connection through attunement (Haen, 2015). Linking the arts to the play that is so vital for human development, Brown and Vaughan (2009) eloquently observed, "Art is part of a deep, preverbal communication that binds people together. It is literally a communion" (p. 62).

Likewise, experiential approaches rooted in the arts and play allow for forms of mobilization of the body that, in contrast to typical manifestations related to aggression and defense, allow for a "neuroception of safety even with heightened arousal" (Kestly, 2014, p. 35). This ability to create safety may be particularly apt for those young people who would otherwise find therapy groups—with their emphasis on being with and seeing others—especially threatening, such as teens with complex trauma (Haen, 2015). More generally, the arts lend themselves to embodiment in a way that teens sitting in a circle and talking during verbal group therapy simply does not. As such, it is possible to both observe and explicitly work with "the sensations, gestures, tensions, movement patterns" that underlie feelings, thoughts and behaviors as they are "happening live" (Mark-Goldstein & Ogden, 2015, p. 124).

Recently, researchers have established an intriguing correlation between levels of patient–therapist bodily synchrony during individual sessions and both ratings of the strength of the therapeutic relationship and treatment outcomes (Ramseyer & Tschacher, 2011; Tschacher & Pfammatter, 2016/2017). Likewise, depressed patients may have lower levels of nonverbal synchrony, perhaps reflecting their heightened focus on self or a loss of hope in the possibility of connection (Paulick et al., 2018). In societal groups, synchronized activities, such as moving or singing together, have been found to increase group cohesion and cooperation (Wiltermuth & Heath, 2009), as well as to enhance sense of belonging (Welch, Himonides, Suanders, Papageorgi, & Sarazin, 2014). Creative arts-based groups often use shared movement, communal singing, group mirroring, and other forms of synchronized action as a means of bringing members into shared affective space. As a complement to the sense of universality that operates as a therapeutic factor within verbal groups, these facilitated forms of connection likely help to establish an implicit sense of 'we' among adolescents—who often feel isolated or that their problems and feelings are unique.

This sense of 'we' might alter an adolescent's construction of self. As group members become engaged in arts-based work, they also begin to see themselves as artists, a role that can empower teens and help them develop agency. Likewise, adolescents frequently experience a shift in their sense of who they are in relationship to others, transcending differences in ways that have ramifications beyond the group room. For example, studies on the impact of group membership suggest that humans are neurologically primed to empathize with those they associate with their in-group, particularly regarding race and culture (Eres & Molenberghs, 2013). Likewise, children as young as 6 years old, regardless of their race, demonstrate implicit bias toward White individuals (Stevens & Abernethy, 2018).

However, preliminary data suggest that the affective, cognitive, and regulatory components of empathy can be modified, and racial and cultural bias reduced, through experiences in which one identifies, even temporarily, as a member of a group composed of diverse others (Van Bavel, Packer, & Cunningham, 2008). This is particularly true in the context of emotional experiences (Stevens & Abernethy, 2018). Evidence suggests that these findings reliably apply to relationships across gender as well (Martin et al., 2017). In other words, factors such as race and gender that often mark a division between 'us' and 'them' can be transformed through shared group experiences.

Conclusion

Despite all that is known about the adolescent brain and how that knowledge can inform what motivates and produces change for teenagers, there remain outdated approaches to group therapy that privilege verbalization as the hallmark of adolescent treatment progress and that view action as connected to pathology (e.g., Sharp & Ahmed, 2016). Creative arts-based group therapy provides an alternative approach that redirects the SEEKING system using novel stimuli and attuned forms of interactive regulation. An arts approach allows for embodiment that fosters cohesion and connection. Creative arts-based groups also provide safe distance for witnessing and reflection. As one adolescent member, summarizing his group experience, so aptly stated: "We came (to group), we made (art), we bonded, and we grew."

References

Adriani, W., Chiatrotti, F., & Laviola, G. (1998). Elevated novelty seeking and peculiar d-amphetamine sensitization in peri-adolescent mice compared with adult mice. *Behavioral Neuroscience, 112*(5), 1152–1166.

Allen, J. P., & Tan, J. S. (2016). The multiple faces of attachment in adolescence. In J. Cassidy & P. R. Shaver (Eds.), *Handbook of attachment: Theory, research, and clinical applications* (3rd ed., pp. 399–415). New York, NY: Guilford.

Aries, P. (1962). *Centuries of childhood* (R. Baldick, Trans.). New York, NY: Knopf.

Badenoch, B., & Cox, P. (2015). Integrating interpersonal neurobiology with group psychotherapy. In S. P. Gantt & B. Badenoch (Eds.), *The interpersonal neurobiology of group psychotherapy and group process* (pp. 1–23). London: Karnac.

Beatty, W. W., Dodge, A. M., Dodge, L. J., White, K. A., & Panksepp, J. (1982). Psychomotor stimulants, social deprivation and play in juvenile rats. *Pharmacology, Biochemistry & Behavior, 16*(3), 417–422.

Blakemore, S. J. (2018). *Inventing ourselves: The secret life of the teenage brain*. New York, NY: Public Affairs.

Bowlby, J. (1969). *Attachment* (Vol. 1). New York, NY: Basic Books.

Brennan, E., Murphy, Y. E., & Flessner, C. A. (2017). Examining developmental considerations of evidence-based practices for youth. In C. A. Flessner & J. C. Piacentini (Eds.), *Clinical handbook of psychological disorder in children and adolescents: A step-by-step treatment manual* (pp. 8–28). New York, NY: Guilford.

Brown, S., & Eberle, M. (2018). A closer look at play. In T. Marks-Tarlow, M. Solomon & D. J. Siegel (Eds.), *Play and creativity in psychotherapy* (pp. 21–38). New York, NY: Norton.

Brown, S., & Vaughan, C. (2009). *Play: How it shapes the brain, opens the imagination, and invigorates the soul*. New York, NY: Avery.

Burnett, S., Sebastian, C., Cohen Kadosh, K., & Blakemore, S. J. (2011). The social brain in adolescence: Evidence from functional magnetic resonance imaging and behavioural studies. *Neuroscience and Biobehavioral Reviews, 35*, 1654–1664.

Casey, B. J., Galván, A., & Hare, T. A. (2005). Changes in cerebral functional organization during cognitive development. *Current Opinion in Neurobiology, 15*(2), 239–244.

Casey, B. J., Galván, A., & Somerville, L. H. (2016). Beyond simple models of adolescence to an integrated circuit-based account: A commentary. *Developmental Cognitive Neuroscience, 17*, 128–130.

Casey, B. J., Jones, R. M., & Hare, T. (2008). The adolescent brain. *Annals of the New York Academy of Sciences, 1124*, 111–126.

Chan, A., & Siegel, D. J. (2018). Play and the default mode: Interpersonal neurobiology, self, and creativity. In T. Marks-Tarlow, M. Solomon & D. J. Siegel (Eds.), *Play and creativity in psychotherapy* (pp. 39–63). New York, NY: Norton.

Chein, J., Albert, D., O'Brien, L., Uckert, K., & Steinberg, L. (2010). Peers increase adolescent risk taking by enhancing activity in the brain's reward circuitry. *Developmental Science, 14*(2), F1-F10.

Cohen, A., Bonnie, R., Taylor-Thompson, K., & Casey, B. J. (2015). *When does a juvenile become an adult? Implications for law and policy. Temple Law Review,* 88, 769.

Crews, F., He, J., & Hodge, C. (2007). Adolescent cortical development: A critical period of vulnerability for addiction. *Pharmacology, Biochemistry & Behavior,* 86(2), 189–199.

Darwin, C. (1872). *The expression of emotion in animals and man.* London: Methuen.

Davis, K. L., & Panksepp, J. (2018). *The emotional foundations of personality: A neurobiological and evolutionary approach.* New York, NY: Norton.

Decety, J., & Ickes, W. (2009). *The social neuroscience of empathy.* Cambridge, MA: MIT Press.

Dissanayake, E. (2017). Ethology, interpersonal neurobiology, and play: Insights into the evolutionary origin of the arts. *American Journal of Play,* 9(2), 143–168.

Dobbs, D. (2011, November). Beautiful brains. *National Geographic.* Retrieved from www.nationalgeographic.com/magazine/2011/10/beautiful-brains/

Ekman, P. (Ed.). (2003). *Emotions inside out: 130 years after Darwin's "The Expression of the Emotions in Man and Animals"* (1st ed.). New York, NY: New York Academy of Sciences.

Eres, R., & Molenberghs, P. (2013). The influence of group membership on the neural correlates involved in empathy. *Frontiers in Human Neuroscience,* 7, 1–6.

Ernst, M., Nelson, E. E., Jazbec, S., McClure, E. B., Monk, C. S., Leibenluft, E., . . . Pine, D. S. (2005). Amygdala and nucleus accumbens in responses to receipt and omission of gains in adults and adolescents. *Neuroimage,* 25(4), 1279–1291.

Fett, A. J., Gromann, P. M., Giampietro, V., Shergill, S. S., & Krabbendam, L. (2014). Default distrust? An fMRI investigation of the neural development of trust and cooperation. *SCAN,* 9, 395–402.

Flores, P. J. (2017). Group psychotherapy as a neural exercise: Bridging polyvagal theory and attachment theory. *International Journal of Group Psychotherapy,* 67(2), 202–222.

Gallese, V. (2017). Visions of the body: Embodied simulation and aesthetic experience. *Aisthesis,* 1(1), 41–50.

Gallese, V., & Goldman, A. (1998). Mirror neurons and the simulation theory of mind-reading. *Trends in Cognitive Sciences,* 2(12), 493–501.

Giedd, J. N. (2015). Commentary: Adolescent neuroscience of addiction: A new era. *Developmental Cognitive Neuroscience,* 16, 192–193.

Gogtay, N., Giedd, J. N., Lusk, L., Hayashi, K. M., Greenstein, D., Vaituzis, A. C., . . . & Rapoport, J. L. (2004). Dynamic mapping of human cortical development during childhood through early adulthood. *Proceedings of the National Academy of Sciences of the United States of America,* 101(21), 8174–8179.

Goldstein, B. (2018). Cultivating curiosity, creativity, confidence, and self-awareness through mindful group therapy for children and adolescents. In T. Marks-Tarlow, M. Solomon & D. J. Siegel (Eds.), *Play and creativity in psychotherapy* (pp. 338–358). New York, NY: Norton.

Goldstein, T. R., Lerner, M. D., & Winner, E. (2017). The arts as a venue for developmental science: Realizing a latent opportunity. *Child Development,* 88(5), 1505–1512.

Grossmark, R. (2017). Narrating the unsayable: Enactment, repair, and creative multiplicity in group psychotherapy. *International Journal of Group Psychotherapy,* 67(1), 27–46.

Guyer, A. E., Silk, J. S., & Nelson, E. E. (2016). The neurobiology of the emotional adolescent: From the inside out. *Neuroscience and Biobehavioral Reviews,* 70, 74–85.

Haen, C. (2015). Expressive therapy groups with chronically traumatized adolescents: Fostering change when safety is fleeting. In N. B. Webb (Ed.), *Play therapy with children and adolescents in crisis* (4th ed., pp. 239–256). New York, NY: Guilford.

Harvey, A. G. (2014). Transdiagnostic mechanisms and treatments for youth with psychiatric disorders: An opportunity to catapult progress? In J. Ehrenreich-May & B. C. Chu (Eds.), *Transdiagnostic treatments for children and adolescents: Principles and practice* (pp. 15–31). New York, NY: Guilford.

Heron, M. (2017, November 27). Deaths: Leading causes for 2015. *National Vital Statistics Reports,* 66(5). Retrieved from www.cdc.gov/nchs/data/nvsr/nvsr66/nvsr66_05.pdf

Katehakis, A. (2016). *Sex addiction as affect dysregulation: A neurobiologically informed holistic treatment.* New York, NY: Norton.

Kestly, T. A. (2014). *The interpersonal neurobiology of play: Brain-building interventions for emotional well-being*. New York, NY: Norton.

Kilford, E. J., Garrett, E., & Blakemore, S.-J. (2016). The development of social cognition in adolescence: An integrated perspective. *Neuroscience and Biobehavioral Reviews, 70*, 106–120.

Kinley, J. L., & Reyno, S. M. (2016). Dynamic relational group psychotherapy: A neurobiologically informed model of change. *International Journal of Group Psychotherapy, 66*(2), 161–178.

Klein, M. (1975). *The psychoanalysis of children* (rev. ed., A. Strachey, Trans.). London: Hogarth. (Original work published 1932)

Lee, F. S., Heimer, H., Giedd, J. N., Lein, E. S., Šestan, N., Weinberger, D. R., & Casey, B. J. (2014, October 31). Adolescent mental health—Opportunity and obligation: Emerging neuroscience offers hope for treatments. *Science, 346*(6209), 547–549.

Leszcz, M. (2017). Commentary: How understanding attachment enhances group therapist effectiveness. *International Journal of Group Psychotherapy, 67*(2), 280–287.

Livingston, M., & Scott, C. A. (2017). Sustained empathic focus and the creation of a "we space" revisited in the light of recent findings in neurobiology. *International Journal of Group Psychotherapy, 67*(4), 479–499.

MacLean, P. (1990). *The triune brain in evolution: Role in paleocerebral functioning*. New York, NY: Springer.

Mahler, M., Pine, F., & Bergman, A. (1975). *The psychological birth of the human infant: Symbiosis and individuation*. New York, NY: Basic Books.

Mark-Goldstein, B., & Ogden, P. (2015). Sensorimotor psychotherapy as a foundation for group psychotherapy with younger clients. In S. P. Gantt & B. Badenoch (Eds.), *The interpersonal neurobiology of group psychotherapy and group process* (pp. 123–145). London: Karnac.

Marks-Tarlow, T. (2010). The fractal self at play. *American Journal of Play, 3*(1), 31–62.

Marks-Tarlow, T. (2012). *Clinical intuition in psychotherapy: The neurobiology of embodied response*. New York, NY: Norton.

Marks-Tarlow, T. (2015a). Games therapists play: Hide and seek in the therapeutic dialogue. In J. Johnson, S. Eberle, T. Hendricks & D. Kuschner (Eds.), *Handbook of the study of play* (Vol. 2, pp. 271–286). New York, NY: Rowman & Littlefield.

Marks-Tarlow, T. (2015b). From emergency to emergence: The deep structure of play in psychotherapy. *Psychoanalytic Dialogues, 25*(1), 108–123.

Marks-Tarlow, T., Solomon, M., & Siegel, D. J. (Eds.). (2018). *Play and creativity in psychotherapy*. New York, NY: Norton.

Martin, C. L., Fabes, R. A., Hanish, L. D., Gaertner, B., Miller, C. F., Foster, S., & Updegraff, K. A. (2017). Using an intergroup contact approach to improve gender relationships: A case study of a classroom-based intervention. In A. Rutland, D. Nesdale & C. Spears Brown (Eds.), *The Wiley handbook of group processes in children and adolescents* (pp. 437–454). Chichester: Wiley.

McGilchrist, I. (2009). *The master and his emissary: The divided brain and the making of the Western world*. New Haven, CT: Yale University Press.

Mischel, W. (2014). *The marshmallow test: Why self-control is the engine of success*. New York, NY: Little, Brown.

Mischel, W., Shoda, Y., & Rodriquez, M. (1989). Delay of gratification in children. *Science, 244*(4907), 933–938.

Panksepp, J. (2004). *Affective neuroscience: The foundations of human and animal emotions*. Oxford: Oxford University Press.

Panksepp, J. (2018). PLAY and the construction of creativity, cleverness, and reversal of ADD in our social brains. In T. Marks-Tarlow, M. Solomon & D. J. Siegel (Eds.), *Play and creativity in psychotherapy* (pp. 242–270). New York, NY: Norton.

Panksepp, J., & Biven, L. (2012). *The archaeology of mind: Neuroevolutionary origins of human emotions*. New York, NY: Norton.

Paulick, J., Rubel, J. A., Deisenhofer, A.-K., Schwartz, B., Thielemann, D., Altmann, U., . . . Lutz, W. (2018). Diagnostic features of nonverbal synchrony in psychotherapy: Comparing depression and anxiety. *Cognitive Therapy and Research, 42*(5), 539–551.

Paus, T., Keshavan, M., & Giedd, J. N. (2008). Why do many psychiatric disorders emerge during adolescence? *Neuroscience, 9,* 947–957.

Pellis, S., & Pellis, V. (2010). *The playful brain: Venturing to the limits of neuroscience.* Oxford: Oneworld.

Porges, S. (2011). *The polyvagal theory: Neurophysiological foundations of emotions, attachment, communication, and self-regulation.* New York, NY: Norton.

Primus, R. J., & Kellogg, C. K. (1989). Pubertal-related changes influence the development of environment-related social interaction in the male rat. *Developmental Psychobiology, 11*(6), 633–643.

Puig, J., Englund, M. M., Simpson, J. A., & Collins, W. A. (2013). Predicting adult physical illness from infant attachment: A prospective longitudinal study. *Health Psychology, 32*(4), 409–417.

Ramseyer, F., & Tschacher, W. (2011). Nonverbal synchrony in psychotherapy: Coordinated body movement reflects relationship quality and outcome. *Journal of Consulting and Clinical Psychology, 79*(3), 284–295.

Schermer, V. L. (2016). Commentary on: Kinley, J. L. and Reyno, S. M. Dynamic Relational Group Psychotherapy: A neurobiologically informed model of change. *International Journal of Group Psychotherapy, 66*(2), 179–185.

Schore, A. (1994). *Affect regulation and the origin of the self.* New York, NY: Erlbaum.

Schore, A. (2003a). *Affect dysregulation and disorders of the self.* New York, NY: Norton.

Schore, A. (2003b). *Affect dysregulation and the repair of the self.* New York, NY: Norton.

Schore, A. (2012). *The science of the art of psychotherapy.* New York, NY: Norton.

Sercombe, H., & Paus, T. (2009). The "teen brain" research: An introduction and implications for practitioners. *Youth & Policy, 103,* 25–37.

Sharp, W., & Ahmed, K. (2016). Talk and action: Iatrogenic effects and the research-practitioner balance. *Group, 40*(4), 291–301.

Spear, L. P. (2000). The adolescent brain and age-related behavioral manifestations. *Neuroscience & Biobehavioral Reviews, 24*(4), 417–463.

Steinberg, L. (2015). The neural underpinnings of adolescent risk-taking: The roles of reward-seeking, impulse control, and peers. In G. Oettingen & P. W. Gollwitzer (Eds.), *Self-regulation in adolescence* (pp. 173–192). New York, NY: Cambridge University Press.

Steinberg, L. (2016). Commentary on special issue on the adolescent brain: Redefining adolescence. *Neuroscience and Biobehavioral Reviews, 70,* 343–346.

Steinberg, L., Icenogle, G., Shulman, E. P., Breiner, K., Chein, J., Bacchini, D., . . . Takash, H. M. S. (2017). Around the world, adolescence is a time of heightened sensation seeking and immature self-regulation. *Developmental Science, 21*(2), e12532.

Stevens, F. L., & Abernethy, A. D. (2018). Neuroscience and racism: The power of groups for overcoming implicit bias. *International Journal of Group Psychotherapy, 68*(4), 561–584.

Suleiman, A. B., & Dahl, R. E. (2017). Leveraging neuroscience to inform adolescent health: The need for an innovative transdisciplinary developmental science of adolescence. *Journal of Adolescent Health, 60*(3), 240–248.

Telzer, E. H., Fuligni, A. J., Lieberman, M. D., Miernicki, M. E., & Galván, A. (2015). The quality of adolescents' peer relationships modulates neural sensitivity to risk taking. *SCAN, 10*(3), 389–398.

Tottenham, N., & Galván, A. (2016). Stress and the adolescent brain: Amygdala-prefrontal cortex circuitry and ventral striatum as developmental targets. *Neuroscience & Biobehavioral Reviews, 70,* 217–227.

Tschacher, W., & Pfammatter, M. (2016/2017). Embodiment in psychotherapy—A necessary complement to the canon of common factors? *European Psychotherapy, 13,* 9–25.

Van Bavel, J. J., Packer, D. J., & Cunningham, W. A. (2008). The neural substrates of in-group bias: A functional magnetic resonance imaging investigation. *Psychological Science, 19*(11), 1131–1139.

van Duijvenvoorde, A. C. K., Peters, S., Braams, B. R., & Corne, E. A. (2016). What motivates adolescents? Neural responses to rewards and their influence on adolescents' risk taking, learning, and cognitive control. *Neuroscience and Biobehavioral Reviews, 70,* 135–147.

Victor, E. C., & Hariri, A. R. (2017). A neuroscience perspective on sexual risk behavior in adolescence and emerging adulthood. *Development and Psychopathology, 28*(2), 471–487.

Welch, G. F., Himonides, E., Suanders, J., Papageorgi, I., & Sarazin, M. (2014). Singing and social inclusion. *Frontiers in Psychology, 5*, Article 803.

Wiltermuth, S. S., & Heath, C. (2009). Synchrony and cooperation. *Psychological Science, 20*(1), 1–5.

Zeanah, C. H. (2009). *Handbook of infant mental health* (3rd ed.). New York, NY: Guilford.

Zelazo, P. D., & Doebel, S. (2015). The role of reflection in promoting adolescent self-regulation. In G. Oettingen & P. W. Gollwitzer (Eds.), *Self-regulation in adolescence* (pp. 212–239). New York, NY: Cambridge University Press.

Section 2
Creative Arts Therapies in Action

4

Adolescent Group Art Therapy[1]

DENISE WOLF

Thomas Edison famously said, "I failed my way to success" (57 Greatest Thomas Edison Quotes, n.d.). This chapter will present both successes and "therapy fails." "Fails," particularly in adolescent work, are most instructive because they offer opportunities for growth and connection. Utilizing the art process takes advantage of multiple ways to give and receive information other than relying solely on words. Art making adds visual, tactile, and kinesthetic pathways to exchange information (Rubin, 2010). Along with an exploration of historical and structural foundations, real-world applications of theory will be shared through clinical vignettes from over 15 years of facilitating group art therapy with adolescents.

Therapeutic Space and Group Dynamics

Therapeutic space has been understood as a crucial part of psychotherapy since its inception. In group work, the holding space is created by the group itself, and the group becomes the real/not real space, much like the art (Winnicott, 1971). This is a space where new behaviors and responses are acknowledged, tested, practiced, and can be explored, honed, or sampled for reaction and response (Geyer, 2017). It is the work of the facilitators to create and maintain this space, as well as to teach group members how to use it. This awareness of roles can be enacted through practicing and responding vis-à-vis the art process. Group interactions and dynamics parallel those of families, and often group becomes a new type of family (Rubin, 2005).

An important developmental task of adolescence is the creation of identity, as both an individual and also a member of a newly formed family of peers (Erikson, 1950/1993). Because the implicit conflict of forming and maintaining two seemingly opposing identities can create anxiety for adolescent group members, one important leadership focus is on reducing anxiety that may be a barrier to joining or engaging in group. Rubin's (2005) Framework for Freedom is a therapeutic approach to art making that provides both structure and the ability to make choices within that structure. Her approach can be adapted to adolescent art therapy groups as a flexible and transparent structure that contributes to the reduction of initial anxiety. Gabel and Robb (2017), in identifying the mechanisms of change in group art therapy, highlighted the importance of ritual, specifically presented through the preparation and routine use of materials or the provision of a consistent group structure.

Wood, Bruner, and Ross (1976) identified learning as a tiered process that builds on skills and knowledge, resulting in more meaningful and richer understanding for the learner. Albert (2010) noted that the creating of specific steps for structuring art tasks is often overlooked in art therapy practice. She described the technique of *frontloading*, or introducing "ideas to facilitate specific understanding before expressive art making" (p. 92). This approach is supported by Rubin (2005), who asserted that use of a "warm up" activity is essential for adolescents, to reduce self-consciousness and to access personal creativity. A frontloaded, sequenced approach to art therapy allows group members to experience the attainment of advanced skills and concepts, as well as benefit from increased therapeutic gains. This shift results in a heightened capacity to work toward the creation of powerful symbols and metaphors. Within the structure of both the overall group and the specific art task, clients ultimately make their own choices. It is through these choices that more in-depth symbolic content can be accessed.

For adolescents, the group can often become an experimental family as their identity and roles shift from family-of-origin to being part of the larger community (Erikson, 1950/1993; Gatta, Gallo, & Vianello, 2014; Yalom & Leszcz, 2005). Group leaders are tasked with maintaining a balance between being leader and guide in this transitional process. The group functions as a real-yet-not-real space in which interpersonal dynamics can be tried on and either accepted or discarded, much the way an adolescent may try on new clothes (Geyer, 2017; Moon, 2016; Winnicott, 1971). A therapist who is strict and authoritarian may be rejected by the group. A therapist who is too temperate in their approach may be discounted altogether. Either extreme renders the therapist ineffectual in maintaining the group as a safe place for expression and exploration.

Balance in leadership style is especially important in an adolescent art therapy group, where the therapeutic space holds the overlap of imagination, creative processes, and sensory activities (Yasenik & Gardner, 2017). It is imperative, then, that the art therapist build specific art interventions that activate group dynamics (Gabel & Robb, 2017). I have found that holding an awareness of Tuckman's model of group development is useful. To summarize, Tuckman and Jensen (1977) identified five stages of group growth: *forming, storming, norming, performing*, and *adjourning*.

Bonebright (2010) applied Tuckman's stages to modern theories of counseling. He maintained that understanding these stages is useful in describing ways group members interact, as well as in providing facilitators a way to predict the stages of growth in groups. *Forming* is the establishment of structure within a new group, including the time and day, expectations, and ground rules. Boundaries are identified and tested, and relationships among the members and with the leader are established. Group art therapy can assist members in clarifying the roles they take on in group, such as intruder, compromiser, outsider, facilitator, or disruptor (Rubin, 2010).

Storming is a stage of conflict typified by division and opposition. Members appear guarded and look to find security. In the third phase, *norming*, there is an overall acceptance of these roles and the beginning of the group's establishment of their own group-specific norms. In the final stage of the original model (Tuckman, 1965), *performing* is when meaningful therapeutic work takes place. Connections between members are maintained and flourish. Bonebright (2010) identified a fifth stage, *adjourning*. In its broadest definition, it is when the group begins to end.

These stages can be noted over the lifetime of a group, but the group may also pass through them within each session. Often, delineation between the stages is not clear. In best practice, the therapist should use a developmental framework to guide decision making (Yasenik & Gardner, 2017). A student I was supervising asked for help with group tasks for a new group she was leading at an adolescent detention center. Reportedly, the members were disengaged, fidgety, and resistant. She was looking for tasks that would hold their interest and attention. My response to her was to acknowledge the *forming* stage of the group, as well as the normative adolescent desire to "overthrow the leader." I suggested she attempt to connect to adolescent culture by generating art tasks around favorite musical artists, redesigning packaging for bestselling snack foods, or even fully joining the resistance by asking them to create an image of where else they would rather be. I also reminded her that this was a normative stage of both group and adolescent development, and her role wasn't so much to find the "perfect" art task but rather to provide the overall structure of the group so that therapeutic work could take place.

The following vignettes will illustrate these principles through a retelling of clinical failures and successes that led to growth and learning for the group leader. By offering some of my own therapy fails, I hope to underscore the importance of acknowledging the developmental stage of the group as well as predictable group dynamics. Further, I wish for the reader to see fails as an opportunity for therapist and group growth through the therapist modeling vulnerability and reconciliation.

Failure! Papermaking

The following vignette took place within a residential treatment facility serving urban youth with mental health diagnoses where I was the on-site school art therapist.

There was a lot of screaming and yelling and crying, and that was just from me! I had been working for three months with a cohesive classroom of co-ed 15- and 16-year-old urban youth, identified by their primary teacher for art therapy to engage in a service learning project. They were fundraising for their selected charity, the Make-A-Wish Foundation. Together, we had made over one hundred peppermint wreaths and sold them to the community, keeping in mind the budget and projected donation amount. The project culminated in a field trip to the regional Make-A-Wish office, where we presented them with a rather rag-tag stack of one- and five-dollar bills, with the occasional ten . . . a total donation of $250. Although we had been in contact with the regional manager, he failed to hide his surprise at the appearance of my group. "S" proudly presented him the monies, as he openly gawked at the large, Old English font, script tattoo on her neck that read, "Thug Life." We returned to the school feeling successful and extremely proud. The primary teacher suggested the group continue their work in art therapy, as she had seen great improvement in her overall classroom climate: improved grades, fewer behavioral outbursts, and a marked decrease in physical altercations between students in the group.

I was excited to continue with the cohesive group. Roles and norms had been established and I felt that now we could get to the deeper therapeutic work (Tuckman & Jensen, 1977; Yalom & Leszcz, 2005). I decided they were ready to engage in the rigorous and rewarding task of papermaking. This activity has change and transformation inherent to the process, utilizes sequential steps that allow for practicing delayed gratification, and has many sensory components. I felt these were important therapeutic themes for the group to explore and to work toward attaining mastery. In preparation, I spent ten minutes before they entered the room pulling out screens, deckles, paper to be recycled, a blender, and other papermaking supplies. With what I thought was flourish and flair, I did a quick demonstration of the papermaking process: create the pulp with the shredded paper and water in a blender, set up the deckles and screens, pour the pulp, sponge off the excess water, move paper to the drying rack. I opened for questions and no one asked. They seemed eager to get started. I asked them to partner up, since I only had enough supplies for half the students to engage at one time, and set them to work.

The noise level in the room rose as they began creating their piles of torn paper to bring to me, to blend and create pulp. A line began to form at the blender, and some students had an increasingly difficult time being patient. As I poured the pulp into containers and sent the students back to their tables, I began to hear comments: "Yo, this pulp feels like dookie," "Why you touchin' dookie?" Some giggling erupted, followed by several wet splats. A group of three students began chasing each other around the room, flinging handfuls of paper pulp. One student overturned the water drainage bin. Another began to verbally aggress with her partner as water from the table seeped into her backpack. Mayhem ensued—an art therapist's sloppy, material-ridden, regressive nightmare. My gentle prompts for redirection and refocusing on the task were ineffective.

As anxiety rose in the group, I became more agitated and found myself yelling at the students. I ended the group early and had them collect their personal belongings, and promptly walked them back to class. I returned to a wet and messy art therapy room. After stewing in my anger, I began to realize that the group behaved exactly like a group of teens does without structure, goals, or cohesion. I was dreading next week's meeting with them, until I created a frame, or structure, for not only our next group meeting, but also a reworking of the overall balance between structure and autonomy within the larger context of this group. I had failed to scaffold the tasks into discrete, attainable steps and wasn't mindful of the regressive nature of the media.

Before our next meeting, I made a large vat of paper pulp and created 'papermaking stations' around the room suited for a team of two, with all the supplies laid out. I was more aware of my treatment approach and philosophy. Asking group members to work together offers opportunities for engaging in problem solving and interpersonal interaction. I called upon Rubin (2010) and defined my role as facilitator in strengthening therapeutic movement by controlling structure, media, and roles.

When the group entered the room, I was curious about their expectations for the day, as they were uncharacteristically quiet and sluggish, heads down and hoodies up. I had pulled the chairs into a circle, setting a different physical space and tone than they had been accustomed to, an attempt to signal that something different was happening. Once we were all seated, I began with an apology for my own behavior during the prior session—screaming at them, kicking them out early, and not structuring or explaining the process in a way that was useful. They accepted my apology and, surprisingly, a few of the students provided unprompted apologies of their own. Perhaps because I modeled a way to initiate repair, they followed suit. I took this opportunity to review and renew our group norms in terms of behavioral expectations. I told them I wanted to try papermaking with them again and asked what they thought might be more useful for success, offering them agency and control. They agreed. I began by showing them some examples of finished samples of handmade papers from previous students.

I then engaged them in a brain-storming session about how they think paper is made and where it comes from, activating any background knowledge and increasing motivation through offering small, attainable steps. I reviewed the steps of papermaking with them by first having them each tear a small amount of paper, so that collectively we made one blender-full of paper pulp, which I added to the vat. As a group, we all made one sheet together and I selected some of the "pulp throwers" from the previous week to assist me. It is often important as a group leader, particularly with adolescents, to align oneself with the leaders among the members of the group (Yalom & Leszcz, 2005).

I asked if they had any questions so far and cleared up some of the questions they asked about the process. I assigned them partners, based on my knowledge of group and interpersonal dynamics, alleviating some anxiety they may have had previously about finding a partner. After assigning the dyads to stations, I directed them to leave their personal belongings in the front of the room, where they would remain clean and dry. The students were given choice of the shape of their deckle (traditional frame, half sheet, or cookie cutter shapes) as well as pots of various color-dyed pulp. We spent the next three weeks successfully making paper and interacting as a group. At the close of each session, I ensured that there was not only enough time to clean up, but also to talk about techniques used, successes, obstacles, and their plan for the following meeting. The students engaged in this process with similar excitement and pride to what they seemed to experience during the service learning project.

The level of structure, expectation, and motivation, combined with opportunities for choice and autonomy, resulted in a group experience that promoted the exploration of interpersonal relationships, distress tolerance, emotional management, adherence to rules, delayed gratification, repetition for mastery, and opportunities for sensory regulation. By removing the anxiety caused by uncertainty and lack of structure, possibilities for growth and success were afforded. There is also great value in the leader recognizing and revealing her own errors to group members. Self-disclosure with adolescents is an incredibly useful tool when used with caution and clinical relevance for the benefit of the clients. We model vulnerability. We show how to make repairs. We honor the relationships, which are the basis of any therapeutic process.

Soft Sculpture Misses the Mark!

Early in my career, I was interning as a therapeutic art educator in an urban elementary school. I had to submit lesson plans incorporating art education standards, requiring some advanced planning of group art tasks. I had created a plan for a second grade class to create a soft sculpture face, utilizing stockings and poly fill. The plan was to guide the students to create a face with an identified expression using the listed materials in conjunction with a needle and thread utilizing basic stitching and knotting by "scrunching up" sections of stocking and fill and sewing around it to create facial features. This activity was selected specifically after the completion of a unit on macramé, which they had recently covered in art class. The soft sculptures were intended to provide opportunities to achieve mastery of previously learned skills as well as to work on identifying emotions and their functions.

I began with a motivating discussion about facial expressions and the function of emotions as communication to both self and others. I reviewed basic stitching and utilized assigned "table captains" for material management. Although I felt I had carefully planned and scaffolded the task, I was unprepared for how difficult this was for the students. They did not seem to have the capacity for abstract thinking required to form the facial features from a lump of poly fill or the fine motor control to use the needle. Although it seemed the group members understood the expectations, there was limited success through the class of 28 to create something that they felt resembled a face.

I could not seem to move through the room fast enough to offer support, and the group's frustration gradually increased. My desire to alleviate the students' anxiety took over and I made an announcement: this task was over, and students should collect their materials and return them to the table captains. I walked, table to table, with a trash can and assisted the students in discarding their partially formed faces and lumps of stocking and poly fill. I thought they seemed relieved. The bell rang, and the students lined up and exited a clean and chaos-free art room.

My on-site supervisor was observing and patted the seat next to him at his desk for what I thought would be a congratulatory discussion. He asked me about what message I thought I'd communicated to the children. I shared what I thought were my sage opinions about frustration tolerance, awareness of developmental levels and physiological maturation, and overall goodness of fit. He challenged me and asked if I may have unintentionally communicated to the students to throw their feelings (and parts of themselves) in the trash. I was horrified! In my effort to alleviate the immediate stress, I had accidentally failed to value their work and efforts, and may have further communicated the message that "when it gets difficult, quit."

Often therapy doesn't feel good, and guides or facilitators must be willing and able to tolerate distress, so their young clients can learn that they can as well. Rankanen (2014) wrote, "The unpleasant experiences of facing negative emotions or thoughts foster constructive therapeutic change when the experience is integrated with emerging self-reflection and insights" (p. 203). Further, distress tolerance leads to effective problem solving.

With the support of my supervisor, I retrieved the stocking lumps from the trash. The next week, when the group returned for their art therapy session, I was prepared with buttons, jewels, pompoms, glue, and needles for those who wanted another opportunity to work toward mastery, and an apology.

Holding the frame effectively requires that we also hold an awareness of what we are framing as well as acknowledging the times when we drop it. As Rubin (2005) noted, "Each new group is an adventure, and part of what makes group art therapy exciting is that it is impossible to know its path in advance" (p. 226). Working with groups requires that the facilitator balance maintaining direction with allowing the group to determine its own path. In my eagerness to plan the group, I had perhaps "overplanned." Steadfastly adhering to my intention of the creation of sewn faces blinded me to see that the members did not have skills to engage. Perhaps if I had been open to an ongoing assessment of the group's interest and ability, I could have adjusted the task before sweeping their projects into the trashcan!

The Fish Sandwich Problem

As an art therapy educator and clinical supervisor, I find that a great deal of frustration comes from working with ineffective co-leaders. Direct care staff working with adolescents with challenging behaviors may often give in to the immediate problem without much thought about the long-term consequences. I think of this as the "fish sandwich problem."

During dinner at a residential treatment facility for adolescent males, there was one client who was the leader of the group of residents and would often exhibit disruptive and aggressive behaviors if his immediate requests were not met. This night at dinner, he was requesting a fish sandwich instead of what was being served. The shift leader initially said "no," until this resident's behavior escalated into throwing chairs and threatening staff. The shift leader quickly produced a fish sandwich for him, while the other boys ate the prepared dinner of beef stew. I attempted to talk to the shift leader about shaping behaviors and setting limits. The shift leader let me know that I was leaving in an hour and he was "on the clock" until midnight. This is a failure with success avoided.

Often, we are quick to ameliorate the behavioral responses of adolescents and lose an opportunity to find deeper meaning and create circumstances for behavioral change. Working with adolescents, we must prepare ourselves to tolerate what might be initially thought of as intolerable behaviors in order to access more important therapeutic opportunities.

Finding the balance between facilitating an effective group and working with co-leaders and direct care staff is an ongoing challenge. Contrary to the point made above, where an authoritative stance does not necessarily encourage a positive response, a high level of authority and power differential can be incredibly useful. I came to understand this through my work at a juvenile prison.

After being buzzed in through two gates and a large metal door, I stood before the prison activity director. I was tasked with facilitating four back-to-back therapeutic art groups for adjudicated adolescent males. Materials were limited; no sharp objects, no strings, no wire or anything that could be fashioned into a "shank." I had planned a blackout poetry experience (see Figure 4.1 for an example) utilizing patterning to cover unwanted text,

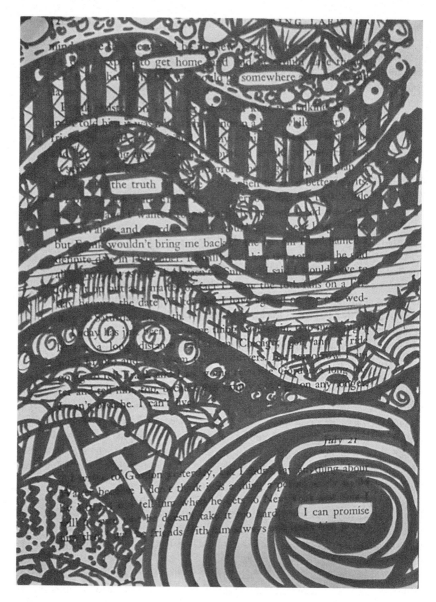

Figure 4.1

instead of complete coverage or blackout. The allure of destroying a book is strong, directly in opposition to grade school admonishments not to draw in or destroy texts.

I thought this would entice this population. Groups of 15 to 20 males were marched into the activity room by at least six muscled guards. I hadn't accounted for the possibility that guards would be present for the duration of the groups. I wondered how their presence would impact the group process. I felt slightly intimidated, fearful that I would do something wrong, and concerned that the guards would interrupt my therapeutic flow. I wondered if the group members had similar responses. The boys quietly sat down while the guards positioned themselves strategically around the room. My banter and attempts at humor fell flat. The participants appeared alert and silent, perhaps in fear of reprimand from the guards. I explained the process of creating blackout poetry, shared an example, and provided pattern sheets to prompt creative filling of the background spaces.

One client, clearly a leader of the group, told me he was awaiting a call to court and would be leaving soon, so he wasn't going to participate. I encouraged him, echoed by the guards: "Do what the lady says." He sat down and began creating, but he was shortly called to report to the on-site court room. To my surprise, before leaving he asked if he could share his poem. He had encircled every lowercase and capital "I" on the page and covered the remainder of the text with color and pattern. "I, I, I, I, i, i, I, I, i, i, i, i, i, i, I, i" he read. The presence of the guards discouraged any laughter or criticism from his peers. During all four groups that morning, at least half of the members volunteered to share their poetry. They read about sons and daughters lost to the system, family members left behind. They gave voice to struggles with addiction, neglect, and abuse. There were empathic looks and concessions of "Me too, bro." The guards held the rules of engagement. There was no taunting, no shaming.

In this setting, the power differential and threat of consequence for engaging in group-destroying behavior created the third space in art therapy: creative expression and exploration without fear of rejection. I believe, in this context, the presence of the guards made this possible. I had wondered if the clients would be loud, disruptive, or disengaged. I did not account for the role of the guards in making sure the members participated. Perhaps by their forced involvement, they realized that they liked making blackout poetry, writing their stories on top of what was already written. Maybe this sense of autonomy, the power of the art process, is what inspired the boys to share their stories.

Leadership Styles With Adolescents

"Adolescence is synonymous with transformation" (Gatta et al., 2014, p. 1). Working with a group of adolescents can present many challenges. By the nature of their physiological development, the capacity for emotional processing is not yet fully developed (Yasenik & Gardner, 2017). What may otherwise be labeled aggressive, oppositional, or resistant behaviors are all normative in adolescence (Moon, 2015). An effective group leader is one who balances maintenance of rules with non-judgmental acceptance. I have found a way to synthesize these seemingly opposite principles using humor. When group members are resistant to accept and engage with new members, I may reply, "This is not Burger King, you can't have it your way." I think of this approach as "out-crazying" the clients. This allows me to join with them while also asserting myself as the leader and gatekeeper.

I have learned to praise positive change and only validate the valid. If I offer overgeneralized praise, such as "That looks great" (if it doesn't), my adolescent clients are quick to call me out on inauthenticity. I might respond, "You're right, it's awful. My dog threw up this morning and it looked better than that." Again, this use of humor and irreverence disrupts the expected power struggle. I would be quick to follow up with client specific praise such as, "I appreciate the way you are taking your time and thinking through this task" or "Your color choice is really exciting." The key is to follow adolescent resistance, instead of perceiving it as opposition or threat. Managing the balance of humor, irreverence, and appropriate role modeling seems to generate the best responses.

When giving specific directives that help structure the art task, often size and measurements are important. More adolescents know the relative size of an M&M candy than what a quarter-inch looks like. I have found relating size to cookies and loaves of bread, textures to fruit snacks and crackers, and color saturation to packaging to be great ways to access knowledge. One of my all-time favorite responses to the ubiquitous call of "I'm done" is: "What are you, a Thanksgiving turkey?"

Just as art allows group members a simultaneous, nonverbal experience, so do other non-art activities (Rubin, 2010). In my school-based office at an adolescent residential treatment facility, I often began individual therapy sessions with a mindfulness practice. A favorite of many of my clients was the mindful use of eucalyptus stress-reduction lotion. It was not unusual to receive a random, frantic knock on my office door. "Miss, sorry but I just need some stress lotion real quick." I was happy to oblige. This appeared to me as skillful behavior, as well as an opportunity to build and maintain relationships with group members outside of session. Often, building rapport with teens can be a slow process. Engaging in non-art warm-up activities provides a safe, non-threatening way to begin. I often open new groups by asking clients to engage in look-and-find puzzles like *Where's Waldo*, or allowing different group members to select a song to mindfully listen to at the start of group.

Success, and Failure Avoided: When a Member–Leader Leaves the Group

I was facilitating a co-ed, long-term adolescent group in a residential treatment facility. One of the members, "M," had become the reluctant leader over the past year and had an impending discharge. As her discharge date approached, I observed a recurrence of earlier 'storming' behaviors within the group, such as lateness, name calling, and aggressive threats. It seemed to me that the group was aware they were losing their leader. Members were again vying for role of 'top dog.' These behaviors may have also served to mask or alleviate anxiety around change and loss.

During the second-to-last group with M, I prompted her to identify who she thought would be most effective in taking over the explicit roles she had normally filled in group such as collecting homework, passing out and collecting materials, moderating discussion, even redirecting disruptive behaviors. This moved the group forward from storming into norming, and made conscious the contributions and roles of various members. Because the new role assignments were largely facilitated by a member of the group, I did not take on the role of authoritarian. This allowed me to sidestep a power struggle with the members. My role as facilitator allowed me to question the "best fit" of some of the role assignments offered by M and guide the group toward effective growth.

The role of the group leader varies. It can be instructive, passive, participatory, instigating, or just what is needed in the moment (Rubin, 2005). Co-leadership models a dyadic relationship. Co-leadership also allows for the modeling of content and process. It's invaluable to have clear and consistent roles for leader and co-leader. Dialectical Behavioral Therapy (DBT) suggests that co-leaders act as the most effective members of the group, and that co-leaders are responsible for modeling the behavior they want to see from the members (Miller, Rathus, & Linehan, 2006). Another function of the co-leader is to address group-destroying or disruptive behaviors, unless it's useful to acknowledge the behaviors with the whole group (Rathbone & Gaul, 2017). Adolescents explore and integrate multiple roles toward the creation of an adult identity through the observation of adult behaviors surrounding them (Erikson, 1950/1993). The relationships between co-leaders can and do model real-life ones. Adolescents seem to learn the most from what we are not actively trying to teach.

Sometimes, a co-leader can be a barrier to an effective group. For example, if the co-leader is not aware of the expectations of their role, their presence in group can be detrimental. Often, I was randomly assigned co-leaders from available mental health staff, based on availability. There was no consistency in these choices, which understandably impacted the group members' ability to establish norms and trust. Additionally, I would sometimes be assigned a co-leader who was disinterested in or misinformed about the purpose of the group. I have had the experience of co-leaders prompting my clients to make "pretty" art, support staff who openly texted their friends or engaged with social media during group or who made inflammatory comments about group members or other staff, and even overtly slept during the group meeting! My mentor Ron Hays would often say, "The clients are the easy part, it's with the staff that you need to use your therapeutic skills."

In the moment, it is often challenging to address destructive group behavior from a co-leader, mental health staff, or other adult who is in a place of authority. I make every attempt to brief my co-leader prior to the beginning of group about norms and expectations for the upcoming session. If I do not have this opportunity, I may utilize the group members to "tell" the new co-leader what the norms are. This reinforces the groups' norms and welcomes the new co-leader in a way that doesn't feel intimidating. If a co-leader is disruptive or harming the group, I may ask them to leave, just as I would for a client displaying the same behaviors. Doing so protects the members and communicates to the group as a whole that my role as leader/facilitator is to protect the group integrity.

Success! Art History, Technique, and Art Making

The following vignette took place at the previously described residential treatment on-site school. I was working with a pre-existing classroom of mixed-gender adolescents, 16–18 years old, who were required to attend art therapy as part of the day treatment program.

The students were often dismissive of art therapy and were free with their expressions of "I can't draw," "How can art help me with my life?" and "This art sh*t is stupid." I developed a sequenced art therapy task, based on the life and art of Georgia O'Keeffe. We began the initial meeting with a gallery walk, where the students moved around the art room observing O'Keeffe prints of floral close-up paintings. This activity was *intended to be motivating through the activation of relevant prior knowledge as well as offering a space to compensate for missing knowledge. Next, the group engaged in a non-graded and private writing activity in response to a prompting question. They could select a question to respond to such as: Which image did you like and why? Why do you think O'Keeffe painted close-ups of flowers? How can a close-up image of a flower be similar to a self-portrait? Write down everything you know about flowers. Create a list of as many items you can think of that would make interesting close-ups.*

After allowing the students some time to answer, they were engaged in a group discussion in response to these prompts. This process was intended to encourage a direct connection with the content as well as promote interaction between members. Following this was skill building, facilitated by engaging the students in drawing the other half of a flower image (see Figure 4.2). To close the session, I asked the students to reflect on why they thought O'Keeffe didn't sign many of her paintings. One student replied, "Because they're not just for her." This began a group discussion about the nature of ownership as well as the expression of identity (both significant ideas regarding the very essence of adolescence). The students used the objective work of O'Keeffe to begin the exploration of their own identities, using the same distanced symbol of a flower as O'Keeffe did.

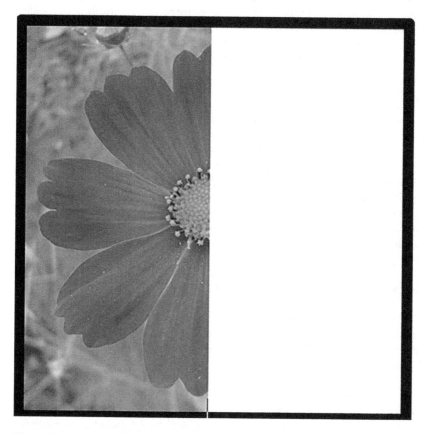

Figure 4.2

Our next session began with my asking the students to respond to O'Keeffe's statement, "I found I could say things with colors and shapes that I couldn't say any other way, things I had no words for" (Georgia Okeeffe Quotes, n.d.). This was intended to expand upon their thinking and feeling about the ability for art to communicate both to self and others. I had brought in several flower pots of mums and directed students to engage in viewing the flowers closely, as O'Keeffe might have. Although there was some laughter and comments about "stupid flowers," this sensory-rich activity engrossed the group, perhaps partially due to the fact that the flowers were alive. It placed them in the seat of O'Keeffe and offered a parallel in-vivo experience. Some group members asked why I brought the flowers in. They seemed surprised to learn that I had purchased them specifically for this activity. I was communicating through my actions that I cared about them by "going out of my way" to do something extraordinary. One student remembered aloud about a garden kept by her mother and shared a story about summers spent working alongside her in the garden. Another usually withdrawn student talked about his work with the horticultural program on campus. Although cautious at first, the group increasingly engaged in dialogue and the forming of relationships took place through the sharing of life experiences.

In a continuation of the scaffolded approach, in the next session the students were engaged in creating a wax-resist watercolor flower portrait. By brushing watercolor paint over crayon (wax), the paint would bead on top of the crayon and be absorbed by the rest of the paper. This appears as a 'magical' effect. First, the students were directed to create four small sketches of close-up views of the live flowers, prompted to completely fill and even go off the page. They then were asked to select their most "successful" sketch, giving them choice and autonomy. The wax resist and watercolor process was demonstrated. This bodily experience is visually stimulating as well as success oriented.

Finally, students were prompted to add large salt crystals to the wet watercolor, designed to create irregularities in the drying process (see Figure 4.3). The students had previously viewed visual samples of this result, to help guide their process and further reduce anxiety. The addition of the salt step asks that students give up some control, offering relief and paralleling other parts of this art process. Further, this loss of control may also mirror aspects of their own emotional lives and provide an opportunity to master those feelings. We closed this sequence with a final gallery walk of the students' completed portrait paintings and engaged in concluding discussion.

A Closer Look

"L" was a 17-year-old African American who felt she was losing at everything. She had been living in residential care for almost two years, with limited contact with her biological family. Once we began sketching, she sat close to the pot of flowers at a table by herself. When other students approached, she yelled, "Get your own flowers over there!" L was a self-identified "bad artist." With some prompting and third-hand interventions (Kramer, 1986), she began her sketches. A third-hand approach directs the art therapist to offer verbal and artistic assistance when the client becomes discouraged with the artmaking process, to help improve their ability to create symbolically significant imagery (Kramer, 1986).

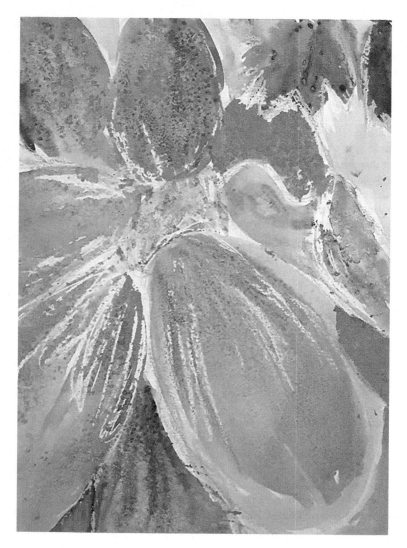

Figure 4.3

"Mmmmmm, these smell so good!" she exclaimed loudly to no one, as she repeatedly put her face deep into the blooms. After completing the four sketches, she was excited to select her "best one" and copy in onto high-quality watercolor paper.

L loved sprinkling the salt on the wet paint. "Here's salt in your wounds!" she called out joyfully. Unprompted, she went around the room to show others just how to do it. "Dang, this is bangin'," she said as she observed her paint drying, her artwork coming to life. She asked permission to leave class to show it to her favorite teachers and residential staff. L traveled through the school that day proudly holding her painting in front of her, both as shield and billboard. This structured, sequenced intervention had just enough dyscontrol to allow her to trust the process, engage, and connect with her own sense of agency.

Geyer (2017) asserted that "difference, group belonging, and dynamics of acceptance and rejection are hugely important for young people's developing sense of identity, self-worth and belonging" (p. 213). The author supports the use of a high level of structure and an orientation toward success when facilitating adolescent group art therapy, especially in a school setting. As Rankanen (2014) wrote, "Art making and observing provides perspective, a novel attitude, and clarity to personal experiences" (p. 199). Through this planned process, group members gained skills and confidence to utilize art for symbolic communication with self and others.

Art therapy groups make use of the creative process in conjunction with sensory-based activities and can foster connections among members in a way that is safe and supportive (Moon, 2016). Sketching, as opposed to drawing, was emphasized to decrease anxiety and prompt an atmosphere of acceptance, integral to effective group process (Rankanen, 2014). Rubin (2005) declared, "Art allows for more informal, non-spotlighted communication between and among group members" (p. 236). Art becomes the third space, where the concepts of identity and ownership that arose through this process can be safely examined. L's initial resistance relented, and she ultimately made a symbolic and personally meaningful connection with the content and process. She expressed joy.

A Cautionary Tale

In the style of Rubin (2005), a word of warning for the non-art therapist in using art media in their clinical work. Art therapy is a mental health profession facilitated by the art therapist (American Art Therapy Association, n.d.). The art therapist is knowledgeable about how specific media may enhance or inhibit the process of development and therefore never randomly selects materials (Chapman, 2014; Yasenik & Gardner, 2017). Instead, art therapists based their choices on understanding the inherent nature of the art media and the potential impact on the group. The non-art therapist may find that specific art media and/or processes elicit unexpected behavioral or emotional responses.

That being said, art making in mental health practices does not solely belong to art therapists. It is important to think about how art incorporated into one's practice can take advantage of the potency of both the art and the group, and how art can be used as a group warm-up to reduce anxiety (Rubin, 2010). Rubin (2005) recommended such visual starters as a scribble, a line, or selection of a photograph or magazine image to communicate mood.

For more rigorous art making, it is recommended that group leaders make use of structured tasks and media that guide participants toward a success-oriented and aesthetically pleasing outcome that promotes two of the basic tenets of group work: connection and communication. One way this can be facilitated is through a group mural making process. By asking members to work on a joint project, the therapist can observe their decision making and interaction processes (Rubin, 2005). A group mural is a structured task that promotes these, and if carefully implemented can result in an aesthetically pleasing result that is permanent. This creation process can foster a sense of agency and impact on the world, critical to adolescent development (Erikson, 1950/1993). The first step is to establish the content of the mural. The therapist can ask the group questions such as: *What do you want others to think and feel when they see this mural? What message do you want to send?*

Once a theme is identified through active group discussion, I suggest utilizing images that the participants either create or select from an open-use media site. These images can be found by searching the internet for images that are designated for reuse or licensed as 'creative commons.' The leader should take care to ensure that overall images have aesthetic value, to promote feelings of success and pride. Using a projector, the smaller images can be made larger by being projected onto the surface on which the mural will be created. Group members can work together in small groups to trace the images onto the surface. I recommend the use of paint pens to outline the images, providing clear boundaries. Colors can be established in a "paint-by-number" fashion. Participants can be guided toward success by using small brushes and small containers of paint to foster greater control of the media. Nearing completion, the participants and/or group facilitator can re-trace the outlines with the paint pen, ensuring aesthetic qualities and reinforcing boundaries.

When using art in therapy, here are some useful things to consider:

- *The inherent nature of the media.* Is it loose like paint or pastels, or structured like collage images and stencil drawing? Will the group members become frustrated with the media?
- *Structuring the tasks.* How can you help as a "third hand" (Kramer, 1986)? Can you provide some skill building so that the members can enter the task with the ability to create symbolically meaningful imagery?
- *Material management.* What materials will you need? Is there any preparation you can do ahead of time to reduce frustration and increase the time members spend engaging in art making? How will group members access the materials? Where will they be stored? What is the expectation around cleaning up?
- *Process and product.* What steps do the members need to take in their art making? What is the goal of the task? Would offering visual examples be useful?
- *Allowing resistance while maintaining the role of facilitator.* How can you use art media and process to allow for the exploration of adolescent resistance, inquiry, failure, and resultant recovery?

Summary

In facilitating art therapy groups with adolescents, the rule of improvisational acting applies: "Yes, and . . ." For leaders, this means looking for the dialectical synthesis, or what is being left out. How can the facilitator be both leader and guide, honoring structure and flexibility? We must view opposition not as resistance, but as an opportunity for engagement (see Landis & Williams, this volume). There is a saying that "for every finger you point at someone else, there are three pointing back at you." We must harness our own responsibility for our successes as well as our therapy 'fails' as ways to build and maintain relationships, move therapy forward, and grow as group clinicians.

Note

1. I extend enormous gratitude to the following people:
   - Juliet King for her initial support and encouragement as well as her ongoing clinical insight. Juliet developed the three tenets of art therapy that guide my ongoing practice (King, 2016).
   - Lynn Langan for her proofreading, editing, and clarity. Her strong attention to clear, concise language has been invaluable in not only my writing but also my overall communication style. Her assistance has continually taught me to keep growing from my failures.

References

57 Greatest Thomas Edison Quotes. (n.d.). Retrieved from https://succeedfeed.com/thomas-edison-quotes

Albert, R. (2010). Being both: An integrated model of art therapy and alternative art education. *Art Therapy: Journal of the American Art Therapy Association, 27*(2), 90–95.

American Art Therapy Association. (n.d.). *About art therapy.* Retrieved from http://arttherapy.org/about-art-therapy

Bonebright, D. A. (2010). 40 years of storming: A historical review of Tuckman's model of small group development. *Human Resource Development International, 13*(1), 111–120.

Chapman, L. (2014). *Neurobiologically informed trauma therapy with children and adolescents: Understanding mechanisms of change.* New York, NY: Norton.

Erikson, E. H. (1993). *Childhood and society* (2nd ed.). New York, NY: Norton. (Original work published 1950)

Gabel, A., & Robb, M. (2017). (Re)considering psychological constructs: A thematic synthesis defining five therapeutic factors in group art therapy. *The Arts in Psychotherapy, 55*, 125–135.

Gatta, M., Gallo, C., & Vianello, M. (2014). Art therapy groups for adolescents with personality disorders. *The Arts in Psychotherapy, 41*(1), 1–6.

Georgia O'Keeffe Quotes. (n.d.). Retrieved from www.georgiaokeeffe.net/quotes.jsp

Geyer, C. (2017). The social unconscious in action: Linking theory to group work with young adults. *Group Analysis, 50*(2), 203–216.

King, J. L. (2016). *Art therapy, trauma, and neuroscience: Theoretical and practical perspectives.* New York, NY: Routledge.

Kramer, E. (1986). The art therapist's third hand: Reflections on art, art therapy, and society at large. *American Journal of Art Therapy, 24*(3), 71–86.

Miller, A. L., Rathus, J. H., & Linehan, M. M. (2006). *Dialectical Behavior Therapy with suicidal adolescents.* New York, NY: Guilford.

Moon, B. L. (2015). *Ethical issues in art therapy.* Springfield, IL: Charles C. Thomas.

Moon, B. L. (2016). *Art-based group therapy: Theory and practice.* Springfield, IL: Charles C. Thomas.

Rankanen, M. (2014). Clients' positive and negative experiences of experiential art therapy group process. *The Arts in Psychotherapy, 41*(2), 193–204.

Rathbone, B. H., & Gaul, J. (2017). Dialectical Behavior Therapy skills groups for adolescents. In C. Haen & S. Aronson (Eds.), *Handbook of child and adolescent group therapy: A practitioner's reference* (pp. 137–147). New York, NY: Routledge.

Rubin, J. A. (2005). *Child art therapy* (25th anniversary ed.). Hoboken, NJ: Wiley.

Rubin, J. A. (2010). *Introduction to art therapy: Sources & resources.* New York, NY: Taylor & Francis.

Tuckman, B. W. (1965). Developmental sequence in small groups. *Psychological Bulletin, 63*(6), 384–399.

Tuckman, B. W., & Jensen, M. A. (1977). Stages of small-group development revisited. *Group and Organization Studies 2*(4), 419–427.

Winnicott, D. W. (1971). *Playing and reality.* London: Psychology Press.

Wood, D., Bruner, J., & Ross, G. (1976). The role of tutoring in problem solving. *Journal of Child Psychology and Psychiatry, 17*, 89–100.

Yalom, I. D., & Leszcz, M. (2005). *The theory and practice of group psychotherapy* (5th ed.). New York, NY: Basic Books.

Yasenik, L., & Gardner, K. (2017). Counseling skills in action with children, adolescents, and adults. In E. Prendiville & J. Howard (Eds.), *Creative psychotherapy: Applying the principles of neurobiology to play and expressive arts-based practice* (pp. 59–80). New York, NY: Routledge.

5

Bibliotherapy in Adolescent Groups

ZIPORA SHECHTMAN

Most of us recognize the power of therapeutic reading. We find ourselves entering the world described in the pages of a good book, or appearing in the scene of a good movie, and we become involved with the characters. We feel happy or sad, we cry with the character who suffers, we want the good ones to cope and the bad ones to be punished; we really care. We usually end up gaining new insights and ideas for ourselves as well. Just reading high-quality literature, then, is a healing process that can enrich our lives.

The term *bibliotherapy* goes back to the beginning of the twentieth century, when it was coined by Crothes (1916). The use of books for treatment purposes received special and widespread attention following World Wars I and II. With many soldiers returning from battle with post-traumatic stress disorder or symptoms, bibliotherapy was considered a cost-effective treatment. Since then, the use of bibliotherapy has expanded and is currently employed in nearly every helping profession, with every age group, and with multiple populations. Bibliotherapy is used by school counselors, social workers, mental health nurses, teachers, and librarians. A wide range of issues and problems are addressed through this approach. Many use books in character-education programs; others use them for more specific difficulties, such as death and dying, divorce, behavior problems, and aggression.

Definition and Types of Bibliotherapy

The term bibliotherapy is made up of two components: *biblio*, originating from the Greek word *biblus* (book), and *therapy*, referring to psychological help. Simply stated, bibliotherapy can be defined as the use of books to help people solve problems. Webster's Dictionary (1985) defines it as "guidance in the solution of personal problems through reading" (p. 148). Gladding (2005) provided a more comprehensive perspective, referring to a family of techniques for structuring interaction between a facilitator and a participant based on their mutual sharing of literature. Baker (1998) suggested a more clinical perception as he uses literature and poetry in the treatment of people with emotional or mental illness.

All the above definitions share one common thread: bibliotherapy requires some form of reading, but not all agree if the reading should be fiction or nonfiction (Pardeck & Pardeck, 1984), and there is a clear split regarding the emphasis placed on therapy and therapist involvement. The amount of therapy falls on a continuum, from self-help books at one extreme (in which the book is the major therapeutic agent and the involvement of a therapist is minimal) to bibliotherapy as an adjunct to therapy (in which the therapy process is the major therapeutic agent of change, with the book serving as a helping tool, and the involvement of a therapist is critical). These differences in the amount of therapy in bibliotherapy treatment have been influenced mostly by the theoretical orientation of the therapists. Indeed, this difference in theoretical orientations is responsible for the split between two major schools of bibliotherapy: "cognitive" and "affective."

Because cognitive therapists perceive learning processes as the major mechanisms of change, nonfiction written materials for educating individuals are generally the preferred form to treat people. Those can include written programs to improve functioning and to solve problems, and they are usually administered as self-help therapy, with no therapist involved or with minimal therapist contact. In contrast, affective bibliotherapy originated from psychodynamic theories that can be traced back to Sigmund Freud. This approach refers to the use of written materials to uncover repressed thoughts, feelings, and experiences. It is assumed that while the character works through a problem, readers are emotionally involved in the struggle and ultimately achieve insight into their own situation. Strong emphasis is placed on the promotion of emotional responses through identification with the experiences that the literary figures undergo. To permit such identification processes to happen, fictional literature is needed—fiction of literary merit, so that it can mirror a person's dilemma and help him or her to connect to the emotions and pain with minimal fear (Gladding, 2005). High-quality literature presenting complex psychological life events arouses deep emotions; therefore, it cannot be self-help treatment and requires the involvement of a therapist, particularly when dealing with a sensitive population like adolescents.

Studies on bibliotherapy, in general, are quite limited. One group of researchers led by Scogin (Floyd et al., 2004; Main & Scogin, 2003) evaluated the effectiveness of cognitive bibliotherapy for patients diagnosed with depression, employing the book *Feeling Good* (Burns, 1980). The general conclusion of these studies was that cognitive bibliotherapy is an effective method of treatment, particularly for issues of depression in adults (see review by McKendree-Smith, Floyd, & Scogin, 2003). One study (Ackerson, Scogin, McKendree-Smith, & Lyman, 1998) was conducted using the same book with depressed adolescents, with outcomes indicating greater treatment progress for participants compared to a no-treatment control group; however, parents didn't report noticing significant change and, more importantly, one third of the population dropped out early from treatment.

Teglasi and Rothman (2001) performed a cognitive-oriented intervention in the classroom, aimed at fostering social problem-solving skills. The stories used included content that sets models and standards for appropriate behavior, which the children could use for their increased understanding of social situations. The authors reported only partial success. Based on teacher reports of externalizing behavior, a decrease in problem behavior was found only for children who were not defined as aggressive; scores for the aggressive children actually increased following the intervention.

In a recent study (Shechtman, Baram, Danino, & Barak, 2017), self-help bibliotherapy with parents of children diagnosed with attention deficit/hyperactivity disorder (ADHD) was compared with individual coaching. Parents in the self-help condition read the book *Parent as Coach* (Danino, 2007). The therapist only monitored the reading through a few phone calls made to parents during the period of treatment. Results indicated positive results for all parents, with only a slight difference in favor of coaching. However, dropout rates were much higher in the self-help condition.

It appears that cognitive bibliotherapy may be helpful under certain conditions: patients need to be motivated, self-directed, and intelligent to utilize the book and learn from it. Most adolescents do not have such capacities; monitoring by a therapist is therefore required to help them gain the most out of their reading materials. Moreover, children connect better to fiction stories than to didactic information. Young people love stories! For some, it is the only way to connect to emotional experiences and human situations through the process of identification (Gurian, 1997). Stories are helpful in overcoming defensiveness through the creation of a safe distance, bringing the child and adolescent indirectly to the edge of sensitive issues, those that are threatening and probably too painful to face directly (Corr, 2003). Stories are also helpful in offering insight into personal problems due to the great wisdom incorporated into them (Yalom, 1998). Good literature also offers constructive solutions to human problems, from which children can learn. Finally, affective bibliotherapists believe that identifying, exploring, and reflecting on emotions are important components of the therapeutic process (Greenberg, 2002; Hill, 2005), and they are offered through the identification with the literary characters in stories.

In short, high-quality literature presents a wide range of human thoughts and emotions that readers can identify with, learn from, and apply to their own lives. Such literature goes beyond fictional stories; for example, a great deal of poetry expresses subtle and overt wisdom that clients may come to personalize and apply to their own lives. Similarly, films exhibit psychological situations, dilemmas, and conflicts that adolescents can easily identify with. In the process, the reader or listener is believed to pass through three stages: *identification* with the character and events in the story; *catharsis*, when the reader becomes emotionally involved in the story and is able to release pent-up emotions under safe conditions; and *insight* resulting from the cathartic experiences, whereby readers may become aware of their problems and of possible solutions to them.

Because the process does not rely on cognitive learning alone but rather seeks to uncover repressed or unconscious materials, the involvement of a therapist is crucial. The infinite richness of complexity, which is an advantage of affective bibliotherapy, may be overwhelming, threatening, and anxiety provoking. Moreover, books may also model undesirable behaviors. Finally, the messages conveyed to the reader may be misunderstood, misinterpreted, and even distorted, particularly when adolescents and other high-risk populations are involved.

For example, we read a poem to groups of adolescents who had suffered loss. In this poem, the character deals with a dilemma of being happy when she is expected to be sad. She feels guilty and ashamed for forgetting her father. This is a powerful poem, which presents the emotional dilemmas of mourning and allows for a cathartic experience around the sense of loss. However, some young people over-identify with the literary character and conclude that they should literally not forget and never be happy. This is, of course, not the desired conclusion, and a skillful therapist can help shape how the poem is internalized.

We once read this poem to a group of adolescent girls, one of whom was an Ethiopian immigrant to Israel. Mira's mother had died while giving birth to her on the long journey to Israel; hence, her birthday was also her mother's memorial day. Mira mentioned that she had never celebrated her own birthday; she didn't think it was appropriate and couldn't feel happy while her father was so sad. The facilitated discussion that followed clearly highlighted her distorted thoughts. A psychodrama was played out in which her mom begged her to be happy. In the next session, Mira reported to the group that she celebrated her birthday with a few friends and that it was the happiest day of her life. She also brought a cake to celebrate her birthday with the group.

For many years affective bibliotherapy was understudied empirically despite its wide use with adolescents. The few reviews published in the 1990s show mixed results. Paradeck and Paradeck (1984), in their literature review, found 24 studies supporting the positive use of fiction books in shifting the attitudes of clients, increasing client assertiveness, and changing behavior. A more recent review (Heath, Sheen, Leavy, Young, & Money, 2005) also reported mixed results. The researchers concluded that affective bibliotherapy is helpful when working with children and families dealing with loss and transition, in helping adopted children to adjust to their new families, and in enhancing interpersonal relationship, but it is not effective in improving social skills, in changing attitudes toward individuals with mental illnesses, or in decreasing test anxiety.

Shechtman (2010) conducted a series of studies comprised of children and adolescents with behavior problems and high levels of aggression. These angry and disruptive youngsters tend to be quite resistant to psychotherapy. Using bibliotherapy with them seemed appealing, as they particularly have difficulties expressing their anger and controlling their behavior. Results show more salient outcomes than the above reviews.

Shechtman (2006) evaluated the unique contribution of affective bibliotherapy to adolescents with behavior problems by comparing bibliotherapy with a treatment of the same orientation but with no use of bibliotherapy. Results pointed to more favorable outcomes for participants in the bibliotherapy condition. These young people showed greater increases in empathy, reached a more advanced stage in the change process, and had higher frequencies of insight and reported change compared to teenagers in the control group. In addition, counselors who worked with bibliotherapy reported higher satisfaction with the process.

Several studies compared outcomes of adolescents treated with bibliotherapy to those who were waitlisted for treatment. Regardless of setting (for example, mainstream classrooms [Shechtman & Birani-Nasaraladin, 2006] or special education schools [Shechtman & Nachshol, 1996]) or facilitator (for example, teachers [Shechtman & Tutian, 2015] or psychologists [Mieksner & Shechtman, 2017]), the consistency of results is striking. In all studies, young people receiving bibliotherapy showed more favorable outcomes than those who received no treatment, as reflected by self, teacher, parent, and peer measures. Moreover, results of the process measures further point to both cognitive and emotional changes in participants.

The study most relevant to this chapter was published by Betzalel and Shecht-man (2010). In their research, children and adolescents in a residential facility were randomly placed into one of two conditions: cognitive or affective bibliotherapy. Participants were evaluated on levels of anxiety and aggression, and on traumatic symptoms. Results showed more favorable outcomes on all measures for children who were treated with affective bibliotherapy.

Taken together, these research outcomes clearly point to the superiority of affec-tive bibliotherapy. It seems that guiding adolescents through a cognitive process is not sufficient to effect change in behavior. Identifying with literary characters, going through cathartic experiences, talking about their own difficulties, and exploring them on both cognitive and emotional levels has been demonstrated to be the path to behavior change.

How Does Bibliotherapy Work?

The application of affective bibliotherapy starts with the selection of literature appropriate for the group process. The criteria of selecting literature include: qual-ity, the themes offered, suitability to the change process, and appropriateness for the group members' developmental levels. The group process includes the follow-ing four stages: *reading the literature/watching the film; identifying feelings; under-standing human dynamics; self-exploration*. It is the therapist's role to navigate the therapeutic discussion of the literature, help teens make connections between the literature and their personal experiences, and guide them in exploring those expe-riences in order to gain insight and make necessary changes in behavior.

Selecting the Literature

The most important characteristic of the literature is its literary quality. Whether a story, film, poem, or picture, it has to be complex; that is, it should include emotions, an internal or interpersonal conflict, a dilemma, or a debate. It should enable ado-lescents to recognize and discuss emotions, struggles, and conflicts with which they can identify, and it should allow them to explore their own issues before a solution is offered. The type of literature that we seek for affective bibliotherapy has the power to bring out feelings that permit cathartic experiences, is rich in conflict, and doesn't explicitly say what should be changed. The poem "Joey" by Shel Silverstein (1974) is one such example. In the poem, Joey throws a stone that knocks out the sun, leads to total darkness, and eventually falls back on his toe. The poem bears several psychological messages: anger may lead to aggression; an aggressive reaction can be out of control; and the aggressive individual suffers from their own aggression, as does their social environment.

The poem presents a child who spontaneously throws a stone, but the conse-quences are dramatic. We don't know why Joey did it, and this ambiguity is good because it allows young people to project their motives for anger and aggression onto the situation. The poem doesn't judge Joey, which helps group members to identify with his pain (as the stone fell on his toe), and his sadness, sorrow, and regret in facing the outcomes of his deed. Teens can identify with those impulsive acts that they have done and the consequences that followed. They may decide that such acts are too harmful and look for change in their behavior. Although short and simple, I consider this poem to be of high quality for affective bibliotherapy.

Themes for Discussion

The literature selected for affective bibliotherapy should be within the realm of the group members' problems and represent both the difficulties they experience in life and the dynamics of their behavior. When working with young people from divorced families, the literature should present the complexity of divorce; when working with those who have experienced loss, the literature should present the difficulties of grief; when working on issues of social inclusion, it should offer characters who suffer social rejection. Generally speaking, the group members should be able to identify with the characters, so that they can perhaps also learn from their experiences.

For example, in a very recent study (Betzalel & Shechtman, 2017) conducted in two residential facilities, the authors selected stories about heroes presented in books and films. The assumption was that adolescents treated with this type of literature not only will identify with those heroes because most of them had a poor childhood but also will be encouraged by their final achievements. In this study, all children in two homes were compared in three treatment conditions: bibliotherapy using the heroes literature, bibliotherapy with no heroes, and control/no treatment.

In one session, the story of Batman was presented through the movie *Batman Begins* (Melniker, Uslan, & Nolan, 2005). This story describes the "birth" and evolution of this superhero: the tragedy of parental loss; the associated trauma, hurt, sadness, bereavement, and confusion; the self-destruction; and the journey the character undergoes to recover. Through the development of empathy to his own pain and that of others, the major character develops altruistic behavior and finds the strength to be of help to and fight for others. Batman's complex character is in a constant search for self-redemption and finds purpose and hope in moving forward. The legacy of his late father and his words of encouragement, "*Why do we fall? So we can learn to pick ourselves up,*" guides Batman throughout his life. By association, the participating adolescents who are engaged in the story are also exposed to dilemmas of right versus wrong while observing the superhero's agency and power of choice.

Results of this study (Betzalel & Shechtman, 2017) indicated positive outcomes for both types of bibliotherapy, compared to control/no-treatment adolescents. However, children in the superhero condition showed more salient and consistent outcomes. Children in this condition showed a sharper reduction in anxiety, both statistically and clinically. They showed a reduction in aggressive behavior and improved their future orientation; that is, they displayed more hope for the future than participants in bibliotherapy without superhero characters.

Hence, the results of this study (Betzalel & Shechtman, 2017) support previous research showing that bibliotherapy is an effective method in treating young people with high levels of anxiety and aggression. However, these research findings go one step further, supporting the contribution of specific content in bibliotherapy treatment, a previously unexplored component. Results clearly indicate that superhero literature is effective in treating children who experience parental absence, and is particularly effective with boys.

Adjusting the Literature to the Group Process

A group is developed in stages; therefore, the literature should be selected according to the stage of change. At the *initial stage*, the group facilitator must actively provide structure to the group sessions, with the aim of achieving the goal of forming relationships, developing a language of feelings, establishing constructive group norms, and providing a sense of security. At this stage, the book *The Soul Bird* (Snunit, 1999) is a helpful tool to develop a language of emotions. The bird represents one's emotional life and is made up of drawers, each containing a feeling. The metaphor offers a language of feelings and promotes the idea that members need to be attuned to them and experiment with them in the group, both feelings from outside the group as well as those that occur in the here-and-now.

The Working Stage

During the *working stage*, group members are focused on identifying goals and concerns and are willing to work both within and outside the group to address these concerns. Therapeutic goals may be unique to the individual or common to all members, depending on whether the group is focal or not. In both types of groups, however, the focus of treatment is both intrapsychic and interpersonal (Yalom & Leszcz, 2005). That is, the interpersonal interaction among members is used to enhance the release of emotions and to increase self-understanding and behavior change.

For example, in a group with adolescents of divorce, we read a short story called "He did not come" (Tester, 1974). In this story, Samuel is a teen from a divorced family who lives with his mother. His father often promises to see him but rarely keeps his promise. On one such day, Samuel is waiting for him long enough to become extremely disappointed. He goes out but can't really play with his friend. He acts aggressively toward his friend, toward objects, and even toward his own mother who tries to reach out to him. He is jealous of others who spend time with their parents, yet keeps saying that he doesn't care.

Despite the similar situation for members of this particular group—divorced parents—each of them dealt with different issues, under the circumstances. In this particular story, the child deals with neglect by his father. His reaction is quite defensive; he doesn't own his anger and pretends he doesn't care. Being disconnected from his own feelings, he accumulates anger and hatred. Instead of looking for resources for connection and comfort, he becomes even lonelier. The goals for those young people who identify with parental neglect would be: to identify their true emotions, express their anger, recognize the defenses they use, and find more constructive ways to deal with the situation. Other children of divorced families who don't necessarily deal with neglect can still identify common feelings of anger, frustration, and fear. They may share their own experiences, gain insight about their difficulties, and provide emotional support to each other.

In a group of early adolescents, following the reading of the above story, one boy shared his hatred for his mother who neglected him years ago. He had refused to talk to her, shut down her phone calls, and returned the presents she has sent him for his birthdays. The other group members helped him explore the situation, when at one point one girl said to him, "You may be angry at her, but you don't hate her. You may be missing her." In response to this feedback, the boy started crying and admitted to his more vulnerable feelings. Then the group suggested that they all help him write a letter to his mother. They wrote a letter in which feeling of loneliness, insult, and pain were presented. He never sent the letter, but during the next session he shared with the group his sense of relief and peace, and reported that he'd decided to talk to his mother the next time she calls. At this point he also expressed his love to the group members (Shechtman, 2007).

The Termination Stage

Termination is more than the end of treatment. It is an integral part of the therapy process and an important force for change. A successful ending of a group will have a strong impact on members' self-esteem, sense of accomplishment, and self-confidence. It may also have a long-term impact on their future interpersonal relationships, on attitudes toward groups and therapy, and on behavior. As every ending is also a new beginning, the successful end of the group may be the force for continuing personal growth in real life.

Accomplishing a successful termination process requires several sessions, as it involves a number of tasks: dealing with feelings of loss and separation; evaluating one's growth inside and outside the group; identifying areas in need of continued work; and developing plans and directions for continuing without the group. Each of these goals can rely on a piece of literature. One example for the goal of accomplishment is a poem named "I am my own Commander" (Bokek, 1994; translated from Hebrew in Shechtman, 2010). It tells about a child who reacts angrily and aggressively to any discomfort; when someone touches him even by accident, or just stares at him, or simply doesn't include him in a game, he immediately reacts. Then one day he decides that from now on he will be in charge of himself; he will decide how to react; he will become his own commander.

I use this poem frequently with highly aggressive adolescents during the termination stage. At this point they may be able to summarize their gains in regard to self-control (a major problem for highly aggressive participants or those with ADHD). They are also able to understand how the group helped them and to receive feedback from other members. The decision to take charge of one's behavior is a crucial one in the change process. It is particularly significant to adolescents striving for their freedom and independence. Adolescents often use the title of this particular poem as a metaphor for self-improvement and control.

Summary

This chapter presented bibliotherapy as an affective mode of group treatment and as an adjunct to a therapeutic process. Peseschkian (1979) has stipulated that stories of intuition and irrationality, with their playful characters and closeness to fantasy, can be used as effective mediators in therapy:

> They give the patient a basis for identification, and at the same time they are a protector for him; by associating with the story, he talks about himself, his conflicts, and his desires. Especially when there is resistance to be dealt with, the stories have proved their value. Without attaching a patient or his concepts and values, we suggest a change of positions, which at first has more the character of a game. This change of position finally allows the patient to see his own-sided concepts in relation to others, to reinterpret them and to extend the theme.
>
> (p. xv)

In his therapeutic work with adults, Peseschkian uses fictional stories of Asian origin as a tool of psychotherapy. Actually using literature adjusted to a certain culture is a great option as it increases the identification process. Many use more universal literature such as fairy tales. In general, fiction is particularly helpful in working with adolescents because of the safe distance it provides, and sometimes it is the only way to reach them.

However, fiction stories are not the only written material that can be used effectively. Poems are another rich source of therapy as they are extremely rich in human wisdom and often have the benefit of being short. I once had a chance to help a teenager who suffered from an anxiety attack. Until then, he had refused any help. When I offered stories, he agreed. At the end of the single session we had, he asked for more literary texts, which I didn't have with me at the moment. Through the stories, he experienced meaningful cathartic experiences and felt much better at the end, but any attempt to move directly to his difficulties met a wall of resistance. Usually, I try to make a connection to the client's own life, but when it seems too painful I leave it there.

Films are another alternative to bibliotherapy, which adolescents like even more. In our work with highly aggressive adolescents we use the movie *Mady*. In this movie, a terrible accident occurs following a fight between two teenagers, in which the victim remains paralyzed. The film presents the pain of the victim and the aggressor's process of remorse. Group participants learn a lot about their anger and impulsive behavior, which further helps them reappraise conflict situations and find alternative ways to respond.

In a most recent study (Haddad & Shechtman, 2017), we explored the impact of film therapy on adolescents who engage in high levels of conflict with their parents. Assuming that films will be more attractive to teenagers than talk therapy, we compared bibliotherapy and film therapy to no treatment with adolescents. Results did not show superiority of films over bibliotherapy, but both interventions produced more favorable outcomes compared to their no-treatment peers. Teenagers and parents in both treatment conditions reported a reduction in the frequency and severity of child–parent conflicts.

Regardless of the type of literature used, the common bibliotherapy format is comprised of the following steps: getting familiar with the text, identifying the character's emotions, discussing the character's behavior, connecting to the character on a personal level, and, lastly, exploring one's own behavior. This is a basic sequence, but one should not be rigid about it; the order of these components may change.

Bibliotherapy may be delivered in different modalities, including individual therapy, duo therapy, small groups, or large groups (classrooms). Group treatment, however, seems to be better for several reasons—first and foremost, for the obvious reason of cost-effectiveness; working with groups, we can reach more young people. Nevertheless, the most important reason is that group treatment is at least as effective as individual therapy (Burlingame, Strauss, & Joyce, 2013). Moreover, using bibliotherapy in group leads to a richer discussion compared to individual therapy, and so the suggestions for alternative behaviors are more meaningful because they are offered by peers rather than adults.

Finally, the supportive feedback one gets in a small group cannot be comparable to that of individual therapy. Take the following example: Arnie summarized his experience in the group as follows: "I like it here because I get to know other children in depth and befriend them, but I also feel embarrassed to need help." To this, Stan responded, "It doesn't matter as long as it helps, and everyone here can see that you are more relaxed." Arnie seemed to be relieved.

Conclusion

Research suggests that bibliotherapy in group treatment is effective with challenging youth; it is superior to no treatment, and gains seem to sustain after a few months. Moreover, bibliotherapy shows a unique contribution to outcomes compared to therapy without the use of stories, and affective group therapy produces more favorable outcomes than cognitive bibliotherapy (Betzalel & Shechtman, 2010). Taken as a whole, the research outcomes provide a strong evidence base for affective bibliotherapy treatment. Bibliotherapy can be used with all ages and in different cultures, provided that the literature is adjusted to children's age or culture and is led by a trained therapist. We are in the beginning of examining bibliotherapy as a helping technique in therapy with youth. More research is needed on the type of population that may best benefit from bibliotherapy as well as the type of literature and its content that may best assist young clients.

References

Ackerson, J., Scogin, F., McKendree-Smith, N., & Lyman, R. D. (1998). Cognitive bibliotherapy for mild and moderate adolescent depressive symptomatology. *Journal of Consulting and Clinical Psychology, 66*(4), 685–690.

Baker, J. A. (1998). *The social dictionary.* Silver Springs, MD: NASW.

Betzalel, N., & Shechtman, Z. (2010). Cognitive and affective bibliotherapy with children. *The Creative Arts in Counseling and Mental Health, 5*(4), 426–439.

Betzalel, N., & Shechtman, Z. (2017). The impact of bibliotherapy superheroes on youth who experience parental absence. *School Psychology International, 38*(5), 473–490.

Bibliotherapy. (1985). In *Webster's new twentieth century dictionary of the English language.* Cleveland, OH: Collins & World.

Burlingame, G. M., Strauss, B., & Joyce, A. (2013). Change mechanisms and effectiveness of small group treatment. In M. J. Lambert (Ed.), *Bergin and Garfield's handbook of psychotherapy and behavior change* (6th ed., pp. 640–689). New York, NY: Wiley.

Burns, D. D. (1980). *Feeling good: The new mood therapy.* New York, NY: Guilford.

Corr, C. A. (2003). Bereavement, grief, and mourning in death-related literature for children. *Omega, 48*(4), 337–363.

Crothes, S. M. (1916). A literary clinic. *Atlantic Monthly,* 118, 291–301.

Danino, M. (2007). *The parent as a coach.* Tel Aviv, Israel: Rimonim (Hebrew).

Floyd, M., Rohen, N., Shackelford, J. A. M., Hubbard, K. L., Parnell, M. B., Scogin, F., & Coates, A. (2004). Two-year follow-up of bibliotherapy and individual cognitive therapy for depressed older adults. *Behavior Modification, 30*(3), 281–294.

Gladding, S. T. (2005). *Counseling as an art: The creative arts in counseling* (4th ed.). Alexandria, VA: American Counseling Association.

Greenberg, L. S. (2002). *Emotion-focused therapy: Coaching clients to work through their feelings.* Washington, DC: American Psychological Association.

Gurian, M. (1997). *The wonder of boys.* New York, NY: Tarcher/Putman.

Haddad, L., & Shechtman, Z. (2017). School-based groups for adolescent-parent high conflict. Unpublished manuscript.

Heath, M. A., Sheen, D., Leavy, D., Young, E., & Money, K. (2005). Bibliotherapy: A resource to facilitate emotional healing and growth. *School Psychology International, 26*(5), 563–580.

Hill, C. E. (2005). *Helping skills: Facilitating exploration, insight, and action* (2nd ed.). Washington, DC: American Psychological Association.

Main, J. A., & Scogin, F. R. (2003). The effectiveness of self-administered treatments: A practice-friendly review of the research. *Journal of Clinical Psychology, 59*(2), 237–246.

McKendree-Smith, N. L., Floyd, M., & Scogin, F. R. (2003). Self-administered treatments for depression: A review. *Journal of Clinical Psychology, 59*(3), 275–288.

Melniker, B., Uslan, M. E. (Producers), & Nolan, C. (Director). (2005). *Batman begins* [Motion picture]. United States: Warner Brothers.

Mieksner, K., & Shechtman, Z. (2017). Reappraisal in group treatment of aggressive children/adolescents. Unpublished manuscript.

Pardeck, J. A., & Pardeck, J. T. (1984). *Young people with problems: A guide to bibliotherapy.* Westport, CT: Greenwood Press.

Peseschkian, N. (1979). *Oriental stories as tools in psychotherapy: The merchant and the parrot.* Berlin, Germany: Springer-Verlag.

Shechtman, Z. (2006). The contribution of bibliotherapy to counseling of aggressive boys. *Psychotherapy Research, 16*(5), 631–636.

Shechtman, Z. (2007). *Group counseling and psychotherapy with children and adolescents: Theory, research, and practice.* Mahwah, NJ: Erlbaum.

Shechtman, Z. (2010). *Treating child and adolescent aggression through bibliotherapy.* New York, NY: Springer.

Shechtman, Z., Baram, Z., Danino, M., & Barak, A. (2017). Coaching vs. self-help for parents of children with ADHD: Outcomes and processes. Unpublished manuscript.

Shechtman, Z., & Birani-Nasaraladin, D. (2006). Treating mothers of aggressive children: A research study. *International Journal of Group Psychotherapy, 56*(1), 93–112.

Shechtman, Z., & Nachshol, R. (1996). A school-based intervention to reduce aggressive behavior in maladjusted adolescents. *Journal of Applied Developmental Psychology, 17*(4), 535–353.

Shechtman, Z., & Tutian, R. (2015). Teachers treat aggressive children: An outcome study. *Teaching and Teacher Education, 58,* 28–34.

Silverstein, S. (1974). *Where the sidewalk ends.* New York, NY: Harper/Collins.

Snunit, M. (1999). *The soul bird.* New York, NY: Hyperion.

Teglasi, H., & Rothman, L. (2001). STORIES: A classroom-based program to reduce aggressive behavior. *Journal of School Psychology, 39*(1), 71–94.

Tester, S. (1974). He did not come. In *Moods and emotions* (pp. 19–20). Elgin, IL: David Cook.

Yalom, B. (Ed.) (1998). *The Yalom reader: Selections from the work of a master therapist and storyteller.* New York, NY: Basic Books.

Yalom, I. D., & Leszcz, M. (2005). *The theory and practice of group psychotherapy* (5th ed.). New York, NY: Basic Books.

6
Dance/Movement Therapy With Groups of Teens

DAWN MORNINGSTAR AND ROBYN FLAUM CRUZ

Adolescence is recognized as a time of turmoil, rapid change, and growth. Even typically developing teens, with supportive and loving families and with no major traumas, can experience adolescence as a difficult time of adjustment. Teenagers are tasked with trying to develop new, more "adult" behaviors amid rapid changes in growth, and the lack of stability within so much change can be challenging. Teens especially need opportunities to gain experience in their new and rapidly developing bodies. Dance/movement therapy (DMT) is a body-based, relational therapy that can directly address some of the developmental and psychological challenges teens face.

Through DMT, teens can creatively embody new ways of behaving and relating. Group DMT can lead adolescents to new discoveries about themselves and others. They can learn to express emotions like anger and sadness in different and often healthier ways, and they can practice social skills and learn new coping mechanisms and other skills related to increasing maturity. This chapter will look at DMT interventions designed for adolescents, and how working with the body using body-centered techniques can be emotionally healing and transformative. We begin with a brief introduction to the field of DMT and to adolescent development, including the manifestations that occur on a physical level. The appropriateness of DMT will be examined, and successful intervention examples will be presented.

Dance/Movement Therapy: An Introduction

In the 1940s, DMT began to be developed in the United States as a formal psychotherapy practice. The modern dance movement that started at the end of the nineteenth century and flourished in the twentieth so significantly influenced the origins of DMT that one can say DMT might never have developed without it. That was because the modern dance movement introduced the idea in both Europe and the United States that dance as an art form could be expressive and communicative, capable not only of entertaining but also of moving people emotionally (Cruz, 2002). While the early focus was on working within psychiatric settings, DMT has come to be used with a broad range of populations and a full array of treatment needs. A professional association, the American Dance Therapy Association, began in 1966 to support the new profession and the development of specific graduate training programs, and certification of practitioners followed. It did not take long for DMT to spread to other countries, and a strong international presence for DMT with many national associations around the globe has been firmly established for some time (Capello, 2017; Dulicai & Berger, 2005).

Various theories of growth-oriented and psychodynamic psychotherapy are used in DMT as frames of reference and are integrated into specific training in and understanding of the body, movement, and nonverbal communication. While no centrally established theory regarding the efficacy of movement in psychotherapy serves the profession (Acolin, 2016; Cruz, 2002), emerging research in neurobiology, especially related to mirror neurons, neuroplasticity, and intersubjectivity, provides key support for principles of and techniques used in the work (Berrol, 2016). In fact, a range of research findings across many related disciplines support foundational assumptions of DMT (Koch & Fischman, 2011), such as, that the body, body motion, and sensorimotor experience play a role "in the formation of concepts and abstract thinking" (p. 57).

The expanding canon of clinical research on the effects of DMT has long used meta-analysis to aggregate documented effects on anxiety, self-concept (Cruz & Sabers, 1998; Ritter & Low, 1996), body awareness, subjective well-being, body image, mood, and affect (Koch, Kunz, Lykou, & Cruz, 2014). These meta-analyses serve to establish the basis of efficacy of DMT via randomized controlled trials, while clinical trials address its effectiveness in the 'real world' for DMT practice with adolescents and adults across many populations and settings. DMT research with a focus on adolescents is somewhat rare, similar to the situation with regard to psychotherapy generally. Haen (2017), in a review of integrative approaches included in the *Handbook of Child and Adolescent Group Therapy*, noted that psychotherapy process research "remains rare, particularly in the treatment of children and adolescents" (p. 195).

Highlights of Adolescent Development in Brief

During typical adolescence, significant developmental changes, both physical and mental, occur. The major goal of this developmental period is to move from childhood to adulthood or from a state of dependence to independence or interdependence, depending on the cultural context. Adolescence can be divided into three stages: *prepuberty* (approximately ages 11–14 years), *puberty* (approximately 14–18 years), and *late adolescence* (approximately 18–24 years) (Newman & Newman, 2015). Developmentally, there are changes in all areas of functioning—physical, cognitive, and socioemotional—that come into play and carry over across these stages, creating a perfect storm of precipitous transformation. Thinking becomes much less concrete and more abstract. A teen might be more argumentative and have very different ideas than adults about how they want to accomplish a task. Teens start to have a sense of themselves as separate from their families and want to try things out independently and feel more agency. Erikson (1963) called this stage *identity versus role confusion*, reflecting the exploration teens use to establish sense of self and sense of direction in life. From a social perspective, during the teen years peers often become more important than family.

Biologically, there are rapid changes as adolescents grow in both height and weight and start to experience the effects of hormonal changes: developing secondary sexual characteristics, like breast and hip growth in females along with menstruation; and voice changes and nocturnal emissions for boys (Ginsburg & Kinsman, 2014). Due to so many rapid changes, teens can have a hard time figuring out who they are and can develop a diminished sense of self, although some studies have shown that a strong cultural identity can mitigate some self-esteem issues in teens (Swanson, Cunningham, Youngblood, & Spencer, 2009).

While the phenomenon of physical changes during adolescence is noteworthy to parents and other observers, the impact of these changes on adolescents may be underestimated. While there is a wide range in growth velocity, on average, girls will gain 10 inches and boys will gain 11 inches in height. These changes in height are accompanied by corresponding changes in bone growth and weight (Rogel, Clark, & Roemmich, 2000). Physical changes can be psychologically troublesome, especially if they occur much earlier or later for a teenager than for their peers. If a teen is gender non-conforming, transgender, or *genderqueer*, the physical changes in puberty may result in increased depression, suicidal thoughts or actions, and negative feelings about oneself (Herbert, 2011). Social pressures from peers, parents, and society at large can add significantly to that distress. During puberty, the body may not match the internal sense of self and may complicate sense of identity, as well as understanding of the identities of peers and others, creating useful opportunities for exploration through dance and movement (Thomas, 2015).

In the past 15 years strides have been made in brain studies, particularly research on the adolescent brain. For example, most researchers of adolescent brain development describe a mismatch between the *prefrontal cortex* and the *limbic system* (Mills, Goddings, Clasen, Giedd, & Blakemore, 2014). The prefrontal cortex is responsible for planning, decision making, judgment, control of impulses, regulation of emotion, understanding social interactions, and self-awareness. The limbic system is responsible for emotions, attention, and social processing. The prefrontal cortex of the brain does not develop fast enough to effectively limit the limbic system, which creates a mismatch, so teens are often observed to make bad choices, act impulsively, and overreact to emotionally laden situations (Blakemore, 2012; Giedd, 2015; Mills et al., 2014).

From a movement perspective, if development proceeds at a typical pace, teens start from a relatively integrated place physically in latency. Gross and fine motor control has been established to the extent that the body is stable with a solid trunk, differentiated limbs, and predictable, coordinated motor phrasing (Kestenberg, 1995). Due to all the rapid changes mentioned above during puberty, the body and movement become dysregulated and coordination of movements reflect that shift. A preteen can look "gangly," as the one-unit torso is more mobile and limbs are suddenly unexpectedly longer than they were even days ago. Often, body boundaries also change due to rapid physical changes. Preteens can misjudge personal space and literally run into others, looking much like a "bull in a china shop." Teens who were previously comfortable being in close physical proximity to a family member may become self-conscious and need more personal space.

In addition, movement intensity in teens can show rapid changes from high to low intensity, and these highs and lows can be more powerful than in adult or latency development (Kestenberg, 1995). High-intensity movement is the type of energy used in jumping jacks and many forms of street dance, while low intensity movement is epitomized by flopping onto a couch and staring at a smart phone or the television without moving for long periods of time. During adolescence, cycling from one intensity to another frequently happens quite quickly and can be often, giving the impression of simply not being able to "get comfortable."

Characteristics typically associated with adolescents from a behavioral perspective include defiance, secretiveness, impulsivity, taking unnecessary risks, exhibiting emotional lability, and acting self-centered while also being concerned about what peers do and think. Many develop body image and self-esteem difficulties (Sommers-Flanagan, Richardson, & Sommers-Flanagan, 2010). Thankfully, in contrast, adolescents are also receptive to learning and interested in bringing ideas and people together; thus, they can be creative and imaginative, and the approach of group DMT can be used to work within this paradoxical phase of development to maximize teens' best qualities and promote growth.

What Do DMT Groups Offer?

DMT offers a way to connect to both mind and body, providing an outlet for creativity and expression and offering a chance to experience deeper connections to others. It also provides a way to connect to symbols and metaphors, allowing participants to understand themselves in both literal and non-literal ways (Samaritter, 2009). A typical DMT group begins with a physical warm-up to prepare the group to move together. This might involve mobilizing different body parts, connecting to breath, or stretching or shaking parts of the body. A dance/movement therapist will choose how to structure the warm-up based on observing the individual group members. Observation of the body and movement is a key DMT skill that receives specific educational focus in training. Cruz (2006) described the ongoing assessment of movement in DMT as equivalent to the "listening" used by traditional verbal psychotherapists. Beginning with simple assessment of visible energy level and whole-body posture, dance/movement therapists also note subtle physical manifestations such as use of space and body parts and differences in energy flow, timing, and spatial attention. Systems of movement observation that focus on description of movement dynamics exist that are useful in this assessment, but are unfortunately beyond the scope of this chapter.

The goal of DMT groups with adolescents is a connection between the mind and the body, encouraging the group members to become more cohesive and start to attune to each other. This might happen through the introduction of rhythms, synchronizing movements by having the group follow the movement form and tempo of different group members in turn, or *mirroring*, a DMT technique involving physically reflecting the essence of a movement's shape, intensity, and timing. Once the members have begun to connect, the dance/movement therapist will introduce or clarify themes that emerge in the warm-up, again based on movement observation and verbalization from the group. The dance/movement therapist will then allow the group to explore the theme, keeping in mind some of the developmental and psychosocial issues facing teens and any individual or group goals. For example, the theme of identity or "Who am I?" is very common with adolescents. This theme might emerge in teens' verbal comparisons to group members or those outside the group, expressed through remarks such as "She's so smart" or "Everyone likes him." Independence and control is another common theme. The therapist might see this emerge as lack of authentic physical participation and/or statements like "This is silly, I don't want to do this." Other common foci in DMT with adolescents can include getting along with others, expressing feelings in constructive ways, and body image. The exploration section can use varied approaches, from loosely structured free expression or tightly structured specific games to tasks or experiences.

Once the group exploration is brought to a close, the dance/movement therapist begins a cool down or coming back to self through introducing movement and breathing aimed at calming and physically grounding the body and the group's experience. During the closure phase, the therapist encourages discussion of the movement experience with the group, makes connections or observations, and asks questions. Throughout, the dance/movement therapist is observing and responding both verbally and nonverbally to the movement and verbal expressions of the group while continually working on integrating thoughts and feelings. Schmais (1985), one of the original second-generation DMT educators, drew parallels between group DMT and curative factors of verbal group therapy. These included building synchrony, fostering connection through rhythms, allowing for expression, experiencing vitality, integrating mind and body, supporting group cohesion, providing education, and connecting to symbolism.

Synchrony (simultaneous action) can be rhythmic, spatial, and energy-based; it involves moving together, in harmony or often in unison, allowing for trust and connection with others and the therapist. For teens, rhythmic synchrony can offer an opportunity to connect in a safe way that is not too expressive or self-revealing and allows for grounding, connecting, emphasizing, and clarifying. These elements can be directly accomplished by introducing dynamic changes to movement, for example slowing it down or increasing the energy needed to produce the movement. Other changes, such as focus on different body parts and use of space, also assist the ongoing efforts of the dance/movement therapist to modify the movement to help participants clarify feeling states by grounding, connecting, and emphasizing them as they emerge in sessions.

Thus, expression in movement using the body can bring feelings out of the darkness in an appropriate way and allow for discovery. Strong emotions can be less threatening when experienced in a group through symbolic movement that is developed dynamically with input from the group and the therapist. Giving adolescents a chance to practice expressing emotions in a group may make it feel less scary and can be cathartic (Anderson, Kennedy, DeWitt, Anderson, & Wamboldt, 2014).

Dance and movement expression can be vitalizing and make one feel alive, especially teens who are depressed. Experiencing vitality or enjoyment, and connecting through rhythm and synchrony, can bring about energy and positive feelings about oneself (Anderson et al., 2014) underscored by increasing endorphins normally associated with physical activity.

While an ideal for any group, cohesion in DMT can be challenging with adolescents who often want to be autonomous. Joining can be scary because of the developmental need to separate and become more independent, but if teens can become a cohesive unit, it can be quite a powerful experience. They can share in affect, enjoy experiencing together, and understand on a body level that they are not alone.

DMT groups can provide education about self and others through acting or experiencing together, watching, and doing. Teenagers can understand empathy through mirroring, or reflecting another person's movement, or through having someone reflect their own nonverbal expressions to them. Through DMT, symbolism and metaphor can allow for more flexible thinking and creativity (Anderson et al., 2014). DMT can help teens learn to cope with affect and transfer these discoveries to outside groups (Eke & Gent, 2010; Schmais, 1985).

The Challenges of Movement Engagement for Adolescents

Since teenagers' relationship to their developing body is complex, asking them to pay attention to movement—a common technique in DMT—can be both exciting and frightening for them. In a study of DMT graduate students who were reflecting on their own experiences of adolescence, Engelhard (2014) found that two opposing themes emerged: "movement as expression" and "movement as threat" (p. 500). As they discover their new and ever-changing bodies, the influence of hormones and rapid growth can become a source of stress and discomfort. It is no surprise that engagement in a body-based therapy could potentially be difficult for a teen and therefore create a challenge to participation (see Allen & Thomas, this volume). Allowing a teen to lead or make choices within clear structures is often successful at engaging them, as are activities that may be less body-based and more focused outside the self, due to the ambivalent relationship to the body (Engelhard, 2014).

Imus (2016) described an array of DMT interventions with different functions and variations that can be used to adapt to circumstances, settings, needs of clients, and roles of the therapist. This continuum of approaches ranges from pure dance class, performance, and interactive games to teaching coping or social skills and utilizing the creative process to create meaning and bring about transformation and insight. Depending on the needs of the group members, the DMT session may look more like a dance class or just playing games than a traditional therapy session. While working with teenagers, the dance/movement therapist must prepare to be flexible and move from one of these different ways of working to another in order to meet the developmental needs for a group on any given day.

Of course, no discussion of working with adolescents is complete without considering resistance, and engaging teens in movement is no exception. In DMT with adolescents, the importance of the therapeutic relationship is the same as with any other psychotherapy (Eke & Gent, 2010; Engelhard, 2014; Klein, 2015; Sommers-Flanagan et al., 2010). Eke and Gent (2010) and Engelhard (2014) proposed that to be successful with teens, a therapist must acknowledge personal feelings about their own adolescence and continually monitor their own reactions. Therapists use many approaches to understand resistance. For example, Sommers-Flanagan et al. (2010) suggested re-labelling resistance as ambivalence, while Furman and Ahola (1992) noted that resistance can be seen as a "discontent regarding the agenda" (p. 13). They asserted that if a therapist can engage teens by providing clear and flexible leadership, then it is more likely they will reciprocate during treatment.

Likewise, Shechtman (2017) described the balancing of warmth and limit setting that group leaders need to exhibit with adolescents. During the dramatic and rapid changes of adolescence, the therapist and other role models can greatly influence teens. Because of the active nature of DMT, where music, physical action, and expression are valued, therapists are frequently tested around the limits of physical behaviors in sessions. Being clear and direct about those limits is important to the safety of the session, as will be discussed in greater depth in the next section.

Trust is also important to working with resistance. Self-revelation can be a useful tool for building trust or simply providing group members with a positive role model. Offering advice or sharing the therapist's own experience, within limits, can be therapeutic and foster the therapeutic relationship (Klein, 2015). Trust is also impacted by other factors; for example, teenagers have their own culture that is inherently separate from adults. In addition, when the therapist is of a different race than the teens they are working with, it can complicate all aspects of the therapeutic relationship so vital for successful treatment (Choudhuri, Santiago-Rivera, & Garrett, 2012). Ingrained societal issues of racial differences and racism can be evoked when non-minority therapists work with minority clients. For example, minority clients may have trouble trusting a White therapist, and many teens who come to therapy already have issues with trust (Shechtman, 2017). Understanding one's own cultural lens in the context of a system can help the therapist become aware of how clients' cultural perspectives might also be shaped. A therapist who acknowledges culture from a systems perspective can begin to instill trust and show an awareness of difference and a willingness to talk about it and move about it (Choudhuri et al., 2012; Thomas, 2015).

Chang (2016) developed several lists of recommendations for dance/movement therapists to promote awareness and change and to address racial and cultural bias in DMT practice. These recommendations address many levels of practice—personal and individual, institutional, clinical, educational, and scholarly. To highlight just one of her recommendations, DMT practice becomes more viable when "clinicians have avenues to relate to people whose lived experiences are very different from theirs because of skin color, gender identity, country of origin, or socioeconomic background" (p. 273). We propose that because DMT with adolescents involves direct embodied experiences—or close connections as synchrony and mirroring occur between therapist and teen, and between group members—it is even more important for therapists using movement to work specifically on developing the sensitivity and openness Chang described, and for this to be a physical, embodied experience.

Adolescent DMT Experiences

As with any psychotherapy or counseling, emotional safety is important. Since DMT involves the body, physical safety is also important, especially with teens who may become aggressive. One clear way to help establish safety is through structured expression. Since teens can be impulsive, having a structured means of expression can also protect group members from themselves. Allowing teens to be vulnerable but not too vulnerable can allow them the time to express when they are ready. Understanding they have control over how much to express or engage in an activity not only allows for reduced resistance but also for learning some self-assertion and choice-making (Sommers-Flanagan et al., 2010). A structured activity can give a teen something to hold on to or a place to start from to then develop, change, adapt, and go further. Structure can also assist when group members are all expressing different or opposite needs. When there is conflict in a group, structure can help teens focus on and find useful and more adaptive ways to get along.

For example, starting with chairs in a circle and then offering a prop like a ball, scarf, bean bag, or pillow to pass and squeeze, throw, toss, or use in any number of ways is a simple structure that is helpful. The teen can start to think and move as an individual, creatively and expressively but within the limits of the prop, providing both structure and safety (Anderson et al., 2014). One member might hug it, another might punch it, allowing each to express in different ways. In addition, props can allow for connection in a safe way by focusing on the prop as opposed to the self. Teens can be very self-conscious, and a prop can take some of the focus away from the self in a group and move it onto the prop. An item such as a parachute can remind adolescents of their childhood, providing a reflective or regressive element, but also a sense of growth. In the below example, the goal was to encourage trust and safety while encouraging the students to relate in healthier ways.

During a group DMT session for teens with behavioral issues in a high school, a parachute was introduced. Along with laughter and comments about the colors, texture, and smell, one teen stated, "I played this in kindergarten" and others chimed in saying things like "We used to play this in gym class" or "I remember the game cat and mouse," sharing different personal reflections about childhood. The group became more relaxed and playful as a result, allowing them to relate more fluidly to each other. As the group continued exploring the movements of shaking and swaying with varying intensity and timing, they began to switch places under the parachute. They were encouraged to work together to allow two people to switch places. Each teen chose another peer to switch with, providing both structure and choice. Once everyone had a turn, a new way to switch that involved some type of spontaneous greeting underneath the parachute was encouraged.

This began a series of high fives, slapping hands high in the air, but quickly developed into fist bumps, elaborate handshakes, and even spontaneous dances. The permissive structure allowed for nonverbal expressive and creative elements and improvisation to be introduced. The teens communicated without using words as they negotiated these movement transitions. As trust was built in the group, the members began to look like playful kids who were more fully using their bodies. The group allowed the teens to experience a different way of relating with each other as they connected, and a corresponding shift was observed in their affect and behavior that allowed a new challenge to be introduced to the group.

The activity that was introduced involved both risk and trust. One of the goals was to encourage support of each other and demonstrate responsibility and accountability to the group. The parachute was placed on the floor and one teen volunteered to sit in the middle. The surrounding group was instructed by the therapist to roll the parachute close to and all around the teen lying in the center of the parachute. He was then gently lifted off the ground. Everyone was amazed at their power as a group to lift someone. Each person held the responsibility for a peer's safety and the individual being lifted trusted that the group could hold him. Physical, embodied support and responsibility were demonstrated through movement and the body. The lifting naturally led to a swinging motion, much like a hammock, in which the teens were now using more nurturing and calmer movements, and a lullaby was even sung. The prop provided the container for the expression of support, caretaking, nurturance, and responsibility.

In another DMT group, eight teens, 14 and 15 years old, had worked together for several months and entered the room with lots of energy and a lack of focus. The stretch cloth, a large band made of pliable fabric, was introduced to help with grounding and focus. The prop was chosen to help literally contain the energy while still allowing for some connection and interaction. As the group continued to explore with the prop, the idea of a sling shot emerged. One student would lean back into the cloth while the two adjacent students would pull the teen across the circle arriving on the other side to be "caught." This involved significant risk and loss of control, but in a contained way. It allowed both the pullers and catchers to have some responsibility for the safety of the student they were propelling. The person being pulled had to keep their feet moving, could choose when to go and stop, could ask for more or less support, and was encouraged to say what they needed and to be assertive. Although slightly scary at times for participants, overall it was fun and playful movement. Since it involved risk taking and loss of control, it matched the biological and developmental needs of the adolescents.

Risky behavior often arises through peer pressure in unhealthy ways such as taking unsafe physical risks. This DMT activity allowed teens to experience risk by working together in a supportive and nurturing experience. The teens had the responsibility of keeping a classmate safe, which encouraged problem solving and executive functioning. Discussion during and after was about risk taking and the thrill of being out of control, but the need to also have a safety net in case risks went too far. The teens were able to connect the movement experience to areas outside the therapy where they tended to take risks and to note which risks were more likely to end badly.

Competitive games with no winner or loser, often referred to as *cooperative games*, are another way to provide structure and nonverbal connection. The following example involved a group of adolescent boys, ages 14–16 years, attending a special school for children who had severe behavioral problems.

One afternoon they bounded into the DMT room arguing about something that occurred earlier in the day. The dysregulation and frustration expressed by everyone in the group made it difficult for the therapist to contain the energy. In the movement warm-up, activating different body parts, grounding through the feet, and attempting to connect to each other by sharing feelings through a gesture all failed to produce any effect, and the boys were still angry and frustrated.

A very simple cooperative game was introduced with a beach ball. The boys were challenged to keep the ball in the air without it hitting the ground for as long as possible. While standing in a circle, no one could hit the ball more than three times in a row, just like volleyball. A counting element was added to assess progress and offer another layer of challenge. At first, there was a lot of frustration as some of the boys hit the beach ball too hard or jumped all over the room to get it. As the game continued, the group generated ideas about how to be more successful, such as hitting the ball more softly, hitting it three times before passing it, calling for it, staying in one spot, and letting others have a turn. They had to work out aggression before they could calm down enough to problem solve. Eventually, they made 300 consecutive hits and felt very proud of their accomplishment. No one was out, everyone was included, the group felt more connected, and they worked as a team and learned how to problem solve while helping each other along the way.

This game highlighted the need for group leaders to be flexible in their approach. In this example, the DMT became more recreational and educational, allowing time for the boys to calm down, focus on a task, and become more regulated (Imus, 2016). The game provided a container for the members to focus outside of the body while still using it. The dance/movement therapist used her observational skills to focus the group's attention and awareness on noticing the ways in which they used their strengths or changed movement qualities to become more successful in the task. Through the activity they practiced how to work together and communicate. Discussion following the activity focused on cooperation and how to get along with others. The boys mentioned their own contributions and shared observations of others' strengths. They began to recognize that they all needed each other to be successful, and they all appeared much calmer and were no longer focusing on the earlier event that was disruptive to them. The game allowed them to calm down, focus, and co-regulate.

Rhythm can be grounding and can encourage a sense of self through use of the vertical plane and weight effort, which are both associated with presentation of self (Kestenberg, 1995). Rhythm can also be an organizer, connecting self with others in a safe way. Rhythm is culturally based and can be used to emphasize or reinforce one's heritage, which has been shown to be a resiliency factor in teens (Thomas, 2015; Tummala-Narra, Li, Liu, & Wang, 2014). Relational Cultural Theory emphasizes that resiliency can be fostered when a therapist considers culture in the relationship and utilizes it as an aspect of healing (Headley & Sangganjanavanich, 2014). Encouraging clients to explore and express their own cultural dance styles such as drumline, stomping, belly dancing, salsa, hip hop, and others, or using rhythms from those dance traditions, can ground teens and help connect them to personal power, strength, and culture. This linking often occurs during the co-creative process, allowing cultural and personal aspects to emerge within the context of a group.

Line or folk dances can provide safety and structure, and connect to popular and ethnic culture. Dance/movement therapists in Western cultures often work in circles, which offer a holding shape and a way to equalize members and allow for everyone to be seen (Chaiklin & Wengrower, 2016). Since being the center of attention is not necessarily safe or desired for adolescents, line dances can allow group members to dance with others in tandem, side by side, instead of facing one other. There are many line dances to choose from, they are easily learned and performed, and the function is often social and fun. These dances can be a safer way to relate, and they allow for spontaneous expression and discussion. Often teens begin to talk about themselves while dancing together, sharing memories and stories, or choose to participate nonverbally without revealing anything too personal. These moments are valuable in creating trust and fostering safety in a group. Line dances can allow them to have fun together and connect with what is pleasurable about life, which can often be lacking, especially when a teen is in treatment and focusing on what is wrong. Simply dancing together can bring about a change (Acolin, 2016).

Creativity can foster divergent thinking, flexibility and understanding, and tolerating ambiguity—skills teens sometimes lack (Acolin, 2016; Anderson et al., 2014; Metzl & Morrell, 2008). Increased coping can be achieved through creativity and giving a client the chance to practice another way of operating in the world. In groups, teens can 'try out' different roles and practice alternative ways of expressing themselves and showing anger and aggression. Below are some specific dance activities that can foster creativity and expression in teens.

The dance battle is related to an American dance style originating in Los Angeles in the 1990s called *Krumping*. It emphasizes high-intensity, exaggerated movements in an effort to out-dance a partner, and evolved from an effort to reduce gang violence (Craine & Mackrell, 2010). Dance battles allow expression of aggression and competition in structured and safe ways. They can be playful and fun while allowing teens to move with vigor and in forceful ways while remaining physically safe within the symbolic structure of the dance itself.

While working with a group of adolescent boys in residential treatment who mostly struggled with conduct, behavior, and mental health issues, a dance battle structure was introduced to help channel the anger and hurt. The structure allowed each boy a chance to choose an opponent to dance against. Rules included no touching or bumping into each other. The group was encouraged to clap or cheer for either dancer. The boys took turns dancing and trying to "out-dance" each other. Initially, the movements were more aggressive and angry, with scowling faces, and punching and kicking gestures. As each boy had a chance to perform and cheer for others, the therapist made comments and observations about the movement, such as, "That was so powerful," "Whoa, what a high kick," and "Amazing dancing," noticing reactions and what was happening on a movement level while giving encouraging feedback.

As the dancing continued, the movement qualities started to change. The boys started to be more silly and playful, adding shimmies and goofy faces, and trying to make each other laugh. They began to copy one another and take on each other's ideas, slowly beginning to dance in relationship to each other, and to chant and clap for one another. The group members started to dance together and form partnerships, emphasizing reciprocity and give-and-take in the movement. As the session ended, the boys talked about how much fun it was and how they got to know a little about each other. Through the initial "battle," the boys organically became less aggressive and more relational.

Structured dance classes, choreography, and performance with a focus on self-esteem and body-positive messages can improve health and body image, especially among adolescent girls (Anderson et al., 2014; Duberg, Hagberg, Sunvisson, & Möller, 2013; Fourie & Lessing, 2010; Thomas, 2015).

In a school for students with special needs and emotional and behavioral problems, the teenagers in a dance therapy group expressed a wish to showcase their work at the end of the year for their parents and staff to witness. Since it was student-initiated, dances were created based on dance/movement therapy group experiences. One dance involved dancing names, based on a movement activity often used for introductions. Each person chose a movement that represented an aspect of self, a talent, or hobby. The group responded in unison to the nonverbal expression by mirroring the movement and saying the name of the person. In the dance, the name game became more structured and choreographed, with each student presenting their name dance to the audience in a line.

Another dance evolved out of a turn-taking DMT dance structure in which each dancer went into the center of the circle to improvise to recorded music while the members on the outside of the circle clapped encouragement. This organically turned into two people dancing together, with each student choosing when to enter the circle and nonverbally asking to switch with those currently in the middle.

This process emphasized the curative factors of synchrony, rhythm, expression, vitalization, integration, and cohesion (Acolin, 2016; Schmais, 1985). Each dancer had to negotiate space and time to know when to enter the dance, when to leave, and how to engage with another person.

Humor can often ease work with teenagers. Having a sense of humor about oneself and them, admitting mistakes, and playful teasing can sometimes break tension and remind teens in DMT that it is about "playing" with movement and interaction.

During one particularly tense group in a residential treatment facility for girls, a graduate student working under Morningstar's supervision began the group by encouraging each girl to create an "awkward dance" (M. Whyte, personal communication, April 17, 2015). Each participant began by traveling across the circle in a silly way and each girl in turn chose the most strange and silly way to walk she could improvise. It allowed the members to embody their awkward feelings in fun, playful, and safe ways and broke the ice with their discomfort in engaging in movement and dance (Sommers-Flanagan et al., 2010).

The above examples show that DMT can allow for social connection, creative problem solving, expression, and transformation of emotions, catharsis, and self-expression. Group members can learn about what makes them unique and special through connecting the mind and body. By exploring movement together, adolescents can feel less isolated and really embody togetherness. Although DMT groups with teens are often disconnected and can feel a little chaotic to the therapist, this dynamic can reflect the lived experience of the teens over it and can be an opportunity to explore the chaos and gain a sense of mastery. While working with adolescents can be a challenge, the therapist must remember that this is characteristically developmental, not personal. Teens can be incredibly creative, passionate, and engaging given the safety, space, structure, support, and care.

Adapting DMT Approaches and Conclusion

For group therapists who want to incorporate movement approaches into their work, it is vital for them to think first about their own sense of comfort with their body and movement, and to think about safety. Movement can elicit affect and can bring about powerful emotions in a very quick and sometimes surprising manner. Offering a clear and well-thought-out structure to any dance and movement activities will aid in creating a situation conducive to safety. Structure could include rules, adding a physical boundary, or adding a pause or freeze element into whatever action is used. Pausing can allow for control, for example a chance to reflect on what to do next or to slow the action down if it is getting too intense. Allowing teenagers choices and providing ways to reduce participation if they get overwhelmed or feel too vulnerable is advisable.

The therapist's personal comfort level with movement should be considered from several perspectives, including their comfort with having movement taking place in the therapy space. Dance/movement therapists move and dance alongside their clients in a group. Moving with clients can provide important role modeling and make teens feel less self-conscious, especially if the leader makes mistakes or is willing to look silly or awkward. The therapy space needs to be large enough to accommodate moving as a group. One might automatically think of a very large space such as a gymnasium, but a space that is too large can work at cross purposes to the safety of the group. A space where each person has the room to stretch their arms to the sides, front, and back without touching another person when the group stands in a circle, is generally large enough to accommodate some movement while keeping the group safe. If a therapist is used to having teens sit in chairs in session, making the change to moving around the room may be uncomfortable. If that is the case, it is perfectly fine to begin sitting in chairs and introduce movement that can take place while sitting. Such an activity might be passing or tossing a very soft ball and sharing something about themselves or how they are feeling. Alternatively, teens might be asked to introduce a gesture while sitting that sums up their day or week. As the therapist becomes comfortable with introducing movement, the same activities that have been used while sitting can be repeated while standing. Once that seems comfortable, other types of movement and dance activities can be introduced if desired.

Since the body reflects what is happening in the mind and emotions, noticing a client's movement dynamics can aid in understanding and addressing verbalizations. Paying attention to what is going on in the body is important on many levels. If muscle tension or other signs of distress such as very fast changes or increases in movement energy become obvious, the therapist can assist de-escalation with simple breathing exercises (see Biondo, 2017). Also, techniques like mirroring or reflecting movement nonverbally can demonstrate to a teen that the therapist is aligning with them and trying to understand their feelings.

On an inpatient unit or in another type of community setting, the therapist and staff can also introduce a movement or exercise time during the day. It could be a time to introduce a line dance or mini dance party, and the therapist, if comfortable, could join in with the dancing to develop more experience and expertise with introducing dance and movement activities. Staff members can also encourage and lead physical games that are cooperative rather than competitive (Orlick, 2006; Rusch & Imus, 2017). Doing so may help teens see their roles and contributions to the larger group, which in turn can offer opportunities for self-reflection. In community settings, with the support of several staff members, it might also be possible to give adolescents a chance to be creative and put together a show or performance with the emphasis on the process of creating or the making of the show rather than the product or quality of the performance.

Thinking through the goals of adding movement and dance is useful and guides the choice of intervention. Taking a few minutes to observe and assess group members and the stage of group development can aid in choosing how to incorporate a movement activity. For example, if a group is relatively 'new' and more cohesion is the goal, introducing an activity that embodies synchrony such as a line dance or a follow-the-leader, mirroring type of activity will create movement cohesion. If the goal is more appropriate social connection among members, using a prop such as a parachute or a ball provides a bridge for teens to connect from the prop to each other.

The goal of impulse control can be addressed through a move-and-freeze activity in which each participant dances when music is playing and freezes when the music stops. This allows for control of stopping and starting and practicing waiting and listening. The goal of highlighting the advantages of cooperation and working together can be met through using a cooperative game where everyone has the same objective. Creative thinking can be achieved through creating dances, or the developing of new movements can be used to meet a goal of problem solving. In addition, once a goal and initial structure designed to achieve that goal have been initiated, the therapist may find that the group naturally contributes changes to the 'rules' or develops the structure and creative ways that address other group needs and goals.

In conclusion, we would like to bring the reader's attention to the value of DMT and activities derived from DMT, not just for teens but also for the communities that serve them. Regardless of setting, providing opportunities for staff and other adults to observe teens engaged in creative movement and dance can be enriching to the care they are tasked with providing. A phenomenon has been observed by dance/movement therapists in clinical settings since the early years of DMT at St. Elizabeths Hospital in Washington, DC (Chace, 1951/1975) and by us personally. That phenomenon is that both clinical and non-clinical staff members who have the opportunity to observe group DMT in action often notice strengths in clients of which they had been previously unaware, especially when those staff members actually participate in dance and movement groups side-by-side with the clients. This shift happens across all age groups and disability statuses. Truly, the arts, including dance, are humanizing, and interacting with teens in dance and movement can allow the staff who work with them to envision new possibilities for treatment and growth, while simultaneously allowing teens to see the staff as adults who hold the promise of helping with their challenges.

References

Acolin, J. (2016). The mind-body connection in dance/movement therapy: Theory and empirical support. *American Journal of Dance Therapy*, 38(2), 311–333.

Anderson, A., Kennedy, H., DeWitt, P., Anderson, E., & Wamboldt, M. (2014). Dance/movement therapy impacts mood states of adolescents in a psychiatric setting. *The Arts in Psychotherapy*, 41(3), 257–262.

Berrol, C. (2016). Reflections on dance/movement therapy and interpersonal neurobiology: The first 50 years. *American Journal of Dance Therapy, 38*(2), 303–310.

Biondo, J. (2017). De-escalation with dance/movement therapy: A program evaluation. *American Journal of Dance Therapy, 39*(2), 209–225.

Blakemore, S. (2012). Imaging brain development: The adolescent brain, *NeuroImage, 61*(2), 397–406.

Capello, P. P. (2017). Crossing continents: Global pathways of dance/movement therapy. *American Journal of Dance Therapy, 39*(1), 47–60.

Chace, M. (1975). Dance therapy at St. Elizabeths. In H. Chaiklin (Ed.), *Marian Chace: Her papers* (pp. 52–54). Columbia, MD: American Dance Therapy Association. (Original work published 1951)

Chaiklin, S., & Wengrower, H. (2016). *The art and science of dance/movement therapy: Life is dance* (2nd ed.). New York, NY: Routledge.

Chang, M. (2016). Dance/movement therapists of color in the ADTA: The first 50 years. *American Journal of Dance Therapy, 38*(2), 268–278.

Choudhuri, D., Santiago-Rivera, A., & Garrett, M. T. (2012). Multicultural counseling competence. In *Counseling & Diversity* (pp. 301–318). Belmont, CA: Brooks/Cole, Cengage Learning.

Craine, D., & Mackrell, J. (2010). *The Oxford dictionary of dance* (2nd ed.). New York, NY: Oxford University Press.

Cruz, R. F., & Sabers, D. L. (1998). Dance/movement therapy is more effective than previously reported. *The Arts in Psychotherapy, 25*(2), 101–104.

Cruz, R. F. (2002). Perspectives on the profession of dance/movement therapy: Past, present and future. *Bulletin of Psychology and the Arts, 2*(2), 74–78.

Cruz, R. F. (2006). Assessment in dance/movement therapy. In S. Brooke (Ed.), *Creative arts therapies manual: A guide to the history, theoretical approaches, assessment, and work with special populations of art, play, dance, music, drama, and poetry therapies* (pp. 133–143). Springfield, IL: Charles C. Thomas.

Duberg, A., Hagberg, L., Sunvisson, H., & Möller, M. (2013). Influencing self-rated health among adolescent girls with dance intervention. *JAMA Pediatrics, 167*(1), 27–31.

Dulicai, D., & Berger, M. R. (2005). Global dance/movement therapy growth and development. *The Arts in Psychotherapy, 32*(3), 205–216.

Eke, L., & Gent, A. M. (2010). Working with withdrawn adolescents as a moving experience: A community resourced project exploring the usefulness of group dance movement psychotherapy within a school setting. *Body, Movement and Dance in Psychotherapy, 5*(1), 45–57.

Engelhard, E. (2014). Dance/movement therapy during adolescence: Learning about adolescence through the experiential movement of dance/movement therapy students. *The Arts in Psychotherapy, 41*(5), 498–503.

Erikson, E. H. (1963). *Childhood and society.* New York, NY: Norton.

Fourie, J., & Lessing, A. (2010). The influence of dance and movement therapy (DMT) on the body image of female adolescents. *African Journal for Physical Health Education, Recreation and Dance, 16*(2), 297–315.

Furman, B., & Ahola, T. (1992). *Solution talk: Hosting therapeutic conversations.* New York, NY: Norton.

Giedd, J. (2015). The amazing teen brain. *Scientific American, 312*(5), 32–37.

Ginsburg, K. R., & Kinsman, S. B. (2014). *Reaching teens: Strength-based communication strategies to build resilience and support healthy adolescent development.* Elk Grove Village, IL: American Academy of Pediatrics.

Haen, C. (2017). An integrative perspective on group therapy. In C. Haen & S. Aronson (Eds.), *Handbook of child and adolescent group therapy: A practitioner's reference* (pp. 193–202). New York, NY: Routledge.

Headley, J. A., & Sangganjanavanich, V. F. (2014). A recipe for change: Promoting connection through relational-cultural theory. *Journal of Creativity in Mental Health, 9*(2), 245–261.

Herbert, S. E. (2011). Female-to-male transgender adolescents. *Child and Adolescent Psychiatric Clinics of North America, 20*(4), 681–688.

Kestenberg, J. (1995). *Sexuality, body movement and the rhythms of development*, Northvale, NJ: Jason Aronson.

Klein, R. (2015). The nuance of difference in therapeutic relationship. In L. French & R. Klein (Eds.), *Therapeutic practice in schools: Volume two: The contemporary adolescent* (pp. 129–134). London: Routledge.

Koch, S., & Fischman, D. (2011). Embodied enactive dance/movement therapy. *American Journal of Dance Therapy, 33*(1), 57–72.

Koch, S., Kunz, T., Lykou, S., & Cruz, R. F. (2014). Effects of dance movement therapy and dance on health-related psychological outcomes: A meta-analysis. *The Arts in Psychotherapy, 41*(1), 46–64.

Metzl, E. S., & Morrell, M. A. (2008). The role of creativity in models of resilience: Theoretical exploration and practical applications. *Journal of Creativity in Mental Health, 3*(3), 303–318.

Mills, K. L., Goddings, A., Clasen, L. S., Giedd, J. N., & Blakemore, S. (2014). The developmental mismatch in structural brain maturation during adolescence. *Developmental Neuroscience, 36*(3–4), 147–160.

Newman, B. M., & Newman, P. R. (2015). *Development through life: A psychosocial approach* (12th ed.). Belmont CA: Wadsworth Publishing.

Orlick, T. (2006). *Cooperative games and sports: Joyful activities for everyone* (2nd ed.). Champaign, IL: Human Kinetics.

Ritter, M., & Low, K. G. (1996) Effects of dance/movement therapy: A meta-analysis. *The Arts in Psychotherapy, 23*(3), 249–260.

Rogel, A. D., Clark, P. A., & Roemmich, J. N. (2000). Growth and pubertal development in children and adolescents: Effects of diet and physical activity. *The American Journal of Clinical Nutrition, 72*(suppl), 521S–528S.

Rusch, D., & Imus, S. (2017). The same kid in yet another hood—Deep game design as creative arts therapy? In D. C. Rusch, *Making deep games: Designing games with meaning and purpose* (pp. 167–191). Boca Raton, FL: CRC Press.

Samaritter, R. (2009). The use of metaphors in dance movement therapy. *Body, Movement and Dance in Psychotherapy, 4*(1), 33–43.

Schmais, C. (1985). Healing processes in group dance therapy. *American Journal of Dance Therapy, 8*(1), 17–36.

Shechtman, Z. (2017). Bridging the gap between research and practice: How research can guide group leaders. In C. Haen & S. Aronson (Eds.), *Handbook of child and adolescent group therapy: A practitioner's reference* (pp. 52–65). New York, NY: Routledge.

Sommers-Flanagan, J., Richardson, B., & Sommers-Flanagan, R. (2010). A multi-theoretical, evidence-based approach for understanding and managing adolescent resistance to psychotherapy. *Journal of Contemporary Psychotherapy, 41*(2), 69–80.

Swanson, D. P., Cunningham, M., Youngblood, J., & Spencer, M. B. (2009). Racial identity development during childhood. Retrieved from http://respository.upenn.edu/gse_pubs/198.

Thomas, E. (2015). The dance of cultural identity: Exploring race and gender with adolescent girls. *American Journal of Dance Therapy, 37*(2), 176–196.

Tummala-Narra, P., Li, Z., Liu, T., & Wang, Y. (2014). Violence exposure and mental health among adolescents: The role of ethnic identity and help seeking. *Psychological Trauma: Theory, Research, Practice and Policy, 6*(1), 8–24.

7

Adolescent Group Drama Therapy

KRISTIN LONG AND MARK BEAUREGARD

"But is she group-ready?"

The question came as a surprise. I (KL) had never been asked that in the three years I had worked on the adolescent inpatient psychiatric unit. The attending doctor, who was new to the unit, was covering morning hospital rounds. She continued, "Not all kids are ready for group treatment. We need to assess if this patient is developmentally able to tolerate being in a group session."

This idea stayed with me, and for the first time I considered that not all kids should be in group therapy without prior assessment or preparation. On the hospital unit, it was a given that, as part of their treatment plan, all children and adolescents were assigned groups. But is this best practice? As drama therapists, much of our training is group based, and our improvisation skills and clinical training prepare us to do groups in almost any setting, with most populations. Perhaps this expectation to offer groups left us unprepared to ask if individuals were actually 'group-ready.'

This chapter will explore what group therapy is, and why it is a preferred modality for many adolescents in both inpatient and outpatient treatment sites. Also, we will look at what it means to be group-ready, how to assess this, and how to advocate for some clients to not be in group until certain diagnostic criteria are met. Developmental models will be discussed, as well as using drama therapy theory as a proposed template for adolescent group treatment.

What Is Group?

According to the American Group Psychotherapy Association, group therapy is defined as "a special form of therapy in which a small number of people meet together under the guidance of a professionally trained therapist to help themselves and one another" (AGPA, n.d.). While group therapy can be a significant model toward wellness, the therapist must be trained to assess if each individual has the ego strength needed to tolerate group work while maintaining the support needed to prevent individual traumas from eliciting overbearing reactions in others (Long & McKechnie, 2008). Group experiences can bring about major changes in one's superego, both for individuals who have severe pathologies and for those who are not currently experiencing major life or emotional disturbances (Van Dam, 1991). Group therapy can be a time-limited experience, either due to restrictions of the setting (such as acute treatment in a hospital) or a format choice (as in a ten-week fixed group). Other options include an ongoing group, which may or may not accept new members at specific intervals, or open groups, which invite new people to join each session. Group therapy can be a stand-alone treatment or augment individual therapy sessions. Concurrent treatment should be discussed with each clinician to assure best practices in the therapeutic alliance.

Group therapy offers opportunities for practicing many life skills, including increased empathy, a greater sense of universality, improved self-worth, understanding the importance of taking turns, maintaining safe personal/physical boundaries, producing feelings of security and safety, and other interpersonal skills (Goldstein, 2018; Haen, 2005; Scroggs, Bailey, & Fees, 2016). Adults, adolescents, and children can all benefit from sharing experiences with peers in group sessions, and this model of treatment can take many forms, including Cognitive Behavior Therapy (CBT), Dialectical Behavior Therapy (DBT), psychoeducation, psychodynamic treatment, and creative arts therapy, to name a few.

What Does Being Group-Ready Mean for Adolescents?

Some adolescents, especially when admitted to inpatient psychiatric units, may "have difficulty tolerating a group setting as they are adjusting to not only being away from family and home, but also the structure of the unit" (Long & McKechnie, 2008, p. 202). The regressive behaviors these children demonstrate usually indicates that they are not group-ready; rather, they need individual support, if available, to help guide them to a place where they can first tolerate being alone with themselves before being expected to be in the presence of others. For some youth, it is important to consider if group involvement may lead the teenager to abandon individual rationality, as we can see with people who are drawn to cult situations (Van Dam, 1991).

Interpersonal skills are often lacking with adolescents who receive services in hospital and clinic settings. Sometimes this support can be offered within the structure of a group session, but at times the adolescent is so dysregulated that they are not yet able to tolerate a therapy group. This is not the fault of the clinician, as even the most talented group facilitators may not have access to the collateral information needed to assess this in advance. When this is the case, a further assessment by the clinical treatment team may be the best way to determine if group settings are suitable, and if so, which treatment modalities are best for the individual youth.

Even in outpatient settings, complete psychosocial histories are not always obtainable. Clinicians don't always have access to this vital information prior to starting a group session. Groups may be facilitated in non-clinical settings, such as after-school programs or community centers. Because the developmental period of adolescence is known to be a time of much growth and change, and group settings are not always consistent, as therapists we are called upon to use our improvisational skills and assessment strategies to facilitate groups in less-than-ideal situations. Often, we offer treatment to teenagers without knowing much about the systems from which they come. We may or may not meet their parents or know the details of their home life, relationships with siblings or other family members, or school setting. Likewise, we may lack knowledge about the socioeconomic, racial, cultural, and gender differences that intersect between and around each individual patient. As authors, we recognize we will be offering only a segment of possibilities for this work and encourage the readers to explore deeper areas of interest.

A Developmental Model of Group Work

How is adolescent group therapy different from adult or child treatment? Erikson (1956), a developmental psychologist, published concepts about psychosocial stages. During adolescence, the primary developmental challenge was between *Identity* and *Identity Confusion*. He wrote:

> The young adult gains an assured sense of inner continuity and social sameness which will bridge what he was as a child and what he is about to become, and will reconcile his conception of himself and his community's recognition of him.
>
> (Erikson, 1956, pp. 67–68)

Erikson (1977) was also a proponent of play, and he believed that positive experiences with play at an early age with reliable caregivers help young people develop a sense of safety and security. He believed that body exploration was part of improvisational play for children. In drama therapy, we are invested in how to incorporate play at all levels of development. We will explore this later in the chapter.

It's been well-documented that adolescence is a period of life filled with many transitions (Bradley, 2003; Emunah, 1994; Goldstein, 2018; Siegel, 2013; Wise, 2004). Simultaneous rapid change and growth is occurring biologically, socially, and emotionally. In essence, adolescents are "out of sync" (van der Kolk, 2014, p. 338). It's a time in which teens are struggling to resolve conflicts about themselves through a sense of personal identity. Neurologically speaking, adolescence is now considered to be from about 12–25 years of age (Giedd, 2016; Wise, 2004). However, for the purpose of this chapter we will be looking at the age range from 12 to 18 years.

Keeping this in mind, clinicians engaging in group work with adolescents need to be savvy, utilizing a wide range of developmental and social models to inform their practice. The therapeutic needs of 12- and 13-year-olds will look vastly different from those of older adolescents, who are close to being in their college years. Adolescence is also the phase of development when numerous mental illnesses may start to emerge (Giedd, 2016). Knowledge of these are imperative for group practitioners in order to offer referrals outside of group settings, and to provide appropriate treatment based on symptom management.

Every group has its own distinct composition. Each session, the group leaders and members co-create a container for the material that will emerge. The therapist is often a stand-in for the role of primary caregiver, thus offering the members opportunities for reparative relational experiences, if needed. Adolescents are particularly seeking approval from peers, and group sessions with a skilled leader can facilitate this process (Barish, 2004). Drama therapist Cossa (2006) highlighted this possibility:

> As young people move into this period of their lives, they revisit the developmental challenges of childhood, with the peer group assuming a role of support and influence parallel to that held by the family during childhood. With appropriate support from caring adults and connection to a positive peer group, the earlier challenges that have been met can be revisited at a new level of awareness. Additionally, those challenges that have not been successfully negotiated can be revisited and appropriate repairs be made.
>
> (p. 21)

Drama therapy for adolescents can help facilitate a more secure sense of identity. We will now look at the general workings of drama therapy and its effectiveness as a form of treatment for adolescents.

What Is Drama Therapy?

The North American Drama Therapy Association (NADTA) defines drama therapy as "the intentional use of drama and/or theater processes to achieve therapeutic goals" (NADTA, n.d.). This definition can be expanded, adding:

> Drama therapy is active and experiential. This approach can provide the context for participants to tell their stories, set goals and solve problems, express feelings, or achieve catharsis. Through drama, the depth and breadth of inner experience can be actively explored and interpersonal relationship skills can be enhanced. Participants can expand their repertoire of dramatic roles to find that their own life roles have been strengthened.
>
> (NADTA, n.d.)

Drama therapy contains within itself a wide variety of theoretical frameworks and practice approaches (Johnson & Emunah, 2009). A detailed exploration of the breadth of theory and approaches is beyond the scope of this chapter, and we encourage readers to research more closely the specific ways in which drama therapy is utilized and practiced. We will cover a more general understanding of the profession as a whole, briefly describing its history and development. We will also summarize the variety of ways drama therapy is applied in clinical settings, and how the application of group drama therapy methods can be particularly impactful for adolescents.

Drama therapy, and more specifically, the practice of theater as a ritual for social healing and dialogue, can be traced back to ancient Greece. Aristotle had a concept of theatre's function to provide actors and audiences with *catharsis* (Bailey, 2006). Jacob Levy Moreno, creator of Psychodrama, is widely regarded as having had a substantial influence in the development of drama therapy as a field. From Moreno's influence came many individuals who created and paved a way for the separate but closely related profession of drama therapy. Associations were established in both Britain (BADTh.org.uk) and North America (NADTA.org), and drama therapy is now practiced all over the world (Johnson, 2009). For a more in-depth understanding of the historical contexts and development of the profession of drama therapy in the United States and internationally, we refer readers to texts by pioneer leaders in the field, including Johnson and Emunah (2009), Bailey (2006), Landy (1994, 2008), Jones (2007), and Weber and Haen (2005).

Drama therapy is utilized in a large variety of spaces and communities with people across the lifespan. Drama therapists around the world are utilizing their skills to help children, adolescents, their families, and adults of all ages with various needs. These range from emotional and behavioral disorders, life and familial transitions and traumas, social and emotional struggles, academic challenges, and much more. Settings where drama therapy is used directly with adolescents may include inpatient and outpatient mental health programs, educational settings, community centers, shelters, group homes, multi-cultural centers, private practice, home health agencies, hospices, rehabilitative facilities, hospitals, and wellness centers (NADTA, n.d.)

Why Drama Therapy? Can't We Just Talk?

The arts, and in this case drama, give voice to identity and lived experience, sometimes when there is a limited vocabulary or difficulties with articulation. Barish (2004) noted that "observation of the play and fantasy of children, their symbolism and metaphor, offered previously unavailable glimpses of the child's inner world" (p. 386). Working dramatically, which involves story, play, and the use of one's body, can be an alternative to spoken language. Drama becomes another form of self-expression, one that is at times more accessible to the teenager, with which to engage and communicate, connecting body, mind, and affect. As van der Kolk (2014) articulated, the arts and expressive therapies are able to "circumvent the speechlessness" (p. 245) of trauma as a way for initial, challenging experiences to have an outlet.

Drama engages adolescents in particular in a developmentally appropriate way, linking fun, interest, and action, while simultaneously connecting to underlying emotions often in need of release and processing. "Love and hate, aggression and surrender, loyalty and betrayal are all the stuff of theater and the stuff of trauma" (van der Kolk, 2014, p. 337). These traumas include relational and attachment traumas, as well as other more explicit traumatic experiences. Through the more accessible and distanced form of drama, storytelling, and role play, with their emphasis on metaphor, fears of being pathologized or a sense that 'something's wrong' are given space to be explored. Doing so often helps clients work through initial resistances and anxieties around going to therapy.

In addition to addressing resistance, drama provides an active way of externalizing issues, giving teens a medium through which they can give tangible form and shape to internal states, projecting them outside of themselves, in order to better interact and engage with emotional and intrapsychic material. In drama therapy, the group room is the theatrical stage, and the drama therapist facilitating a group session works to encourage everyone to support this process. For adolescents, this may look very different from more traditional play therapy with children, where toys, art materials, and other projective objects are often used. While children may use dolls, puppets, small cars or trucks, and other figurines, adolescents are usually less drawn to these play things. Adolescents have had more time to build up their psychological defenses and are often more inhibited in their play than younger children. Scroggs and colleagues (2016) noted, "It is not the presence of play that changes throughout development but rather it is the type of play" (p. 213). In our experience, adolescent play frequently involves an array of experiences from digital creativity (such as with the use of computer or video games) and projective work (such as oral and/or visual storytelling and masks), to more embodied work (such as improvised or scripted role play).

Drama therapist Pitzruzzella (2017) asserted that there is a strong link between creativity and intersubjectivity. He suggested that group modalities especially foster creativity, even for people who have challenges in trusting others. Cossa (2006) wrote:

> This is the point at which the parallel between Winnicott's (1958) "good-enough" parent and the "good-enough" group leader becomes especially informative. The good-enough parent allows autonomous action while still providing guidance, support, and protection. The good-enough group leader attends with honesty to the emerging "shadows" and allows and supports the conflict and challenges to move into the light, rather than ignoring, resisting, or trying to control them with increased authoritarian fervor based on fears of losing control of the group.
>
> (p. 39)

Improvisation and dramatic play are extremely effective with younger adolescents, who haven't lost their spirited nature nor have developed all the constrictions apparent with older participants (Maden, 2008). Trust games, warm-up activities, and simple 'get to know you' exercises all help adolescents begin to feel comfortable in a group setting, both with the therapist and with other members. Pitre, Mayor, and Johnson (2016) reported, "The core processes of telling one's story and being heard and listened to, resulting in a sense of no longer being alone and holding a shameful or frightening secret, are at work" (p. 172). While they are referring to individual short-term work, the belief translates to group work. Validation, especially from peers, is vital for teens to feel connected and part of a community. Cossa (2006) supported this notion: "Given the primary role that peers play at this time of life, working with adolescents in groups optimizes these interpersonal connections, and provides a kind of support and safety that adults alone, no matter how well intentioned, cannot provide" (p. 21).

Once safety and trust are established, often through the use of games, warm-up activities, and an intentional movement toward increased playfulness and spontaneity, the group can begin to explore and utilize dramatic forms to address and work through concerns and issues. The possibilities for how this takes shape are endless: monologues, body sculptures and tableau images, improvised games, scenes and movement pieces, using existing plays and scripts, co-creating plays and texts, embodied stories and fairy tales, video production, puppetry, mask making, public performance, and so much more. Adolescents become the authors, editors, producers, directors, actors, and storytellers, empowered to create for and with one another in mind. It becomes less important to 'interpret' the meaning of the work, as the therapy process happens throughout the session in metaphor and story (Aron & Atlas, 2018; Kindler, 2017).

Fundamental Concepts Applied to Adolescent Group Drama Therapy

Distancing and Drama Therapy

Distancing is a fundamental concept in understanding how drama process and drama therapy techniques are applied to help clients navigate and work through emotional material. Landy (1994, 2008) has contributed significantly to drama therapy theory in this regard. For Landy, helping individuals achieve a balance between *underdistanced* and *overdistanced* states is imperative to therapeutic growth. An individual who is overdistanced presents as extremely rational and cognitive, devoid of strong affect and detached. An individual who is underdistanced presents as highly emotional, reactive, and impulsive. Landy (1994) described the balance of these two states as *aesthetic distance*, a state that allows an individual to both think and feel simultaneously, and therefore better process and heal safely. It is essential that individuals using drama therapy processes or techniques have in-depth training to understand the power that drama has in order to help regulate clients' ability to tolerate strong emotion, without being affectively flooded. The distance that drama therapy can provide can be enormously impactful in helping adolescents work through difficult emotional material in a safer way. The key is in therapists' ability to be attuned in the process and know how and when to modify drama therapy interventions to best suit individual and group needs.

Different drama therapy techniques or interventions lend themselves to particular levels of emotional distance. As Pitzruzzella (2017) simply put it, "It is necessary to find the right distance" (p. 133). This will look different for each group member, and may even vary day by day, depending on what is happening in the world that may impact group process. In an earlier writing, my co-author and I (KL) discussed how toys of choice changed for children in a New York City hospital setting following the terrorist attacks of September 11 (Long & Weber, 2005). In the current political climate, both authors of this chapter have noted that girls are taking a stronger stance in their play, stating that their voice needs to be heard and that they have a right to say 'no.' During the height of the 2016 American presidential election, we noted increased discussion and exploration of themes of sociopolitical imbalance and concerns about the future causing distress in kids and families. Many of our adolescent clients expressed fear, anger, and a sense of feeling devalued. While adolescents can often address these topics directly in groups, we have found that distance and playing through metaphor have value in their ability to allow safer processing of tenuous information. Distancing techniques must be applied and adjusted to allow clients an ability to tolerate emotion and reason, balancing mind and body. Landy (1994) explained:

Thus, the drama therapist works toward distancing clients from feelings that are too threatening through the use of such projective devices as masks, puppets, and stylized props and dolls. Further, in playing a social type rather than a psychological character, and in telling stories rather than directly dramatizing experiences, the client is able to create distance from potentially overwhelming feelings. Generally speaking, to move from the naturalistic techniques of psychodrama to more stylized projective techniques gives the client more space in which to present his issues safely.

(pp. 87–88)

Therapists utilizing dramatic techniques must possess a keen understanding of the spectrums between fictional and nonfictional play, between fully embodied role play and projective techniques such as masks and puppets, between the therapist being director and facilitator of role play versus being a co-player in the drama, and the impact these elements can have on group members. Such understanding allows group leaders to aim toward achieving aesthetic distance and maximizing therapeutic gains. Figure 7.1 illustrates these four spectrums for therapists to consider when matching appropriate interventions to the group's needs, which we will also reference in a later case example.

Imaginary props such as remote controls that can pause action and use slow motion or fast forward playback can be a wonderful device when working with adolescents to help foster control and balance between impulse and reason. Uses of the body can be structured to minimize or maximize the level of embodiment, thus altering distance and emotion levels, such as when creating *tableau sculptures*

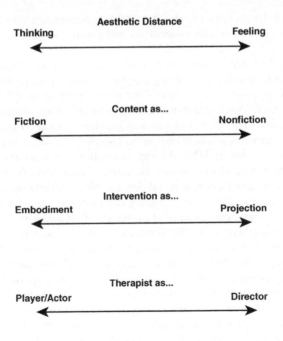

Figure 7.1

(human sculptures in which group members hold a frozen pose for a short period) versus fully acted out or moving scenes. Pitzruzzella (2017) explained: "Embodiment work generally reduces the distance, while projective work enlarges it; role work can be oriented towards identification (reducing the distance) or towards estrangement (enlarging it)" (p. 134). Knowing when and how to use techniques is a complex and multi-layered aspect of the training of a drama therapist, and this takes time and supervised experience to develop; however, many of these creative ideas can be implemented into groups of other modalities.

The Drama Therapy Group as a Playspace for Identity Formation

The adolescent drama therapy group, figuratively held by a supportive and skilled clinician, can serve as an exceptional space for adolescents to experiment with play and to form their sense of self. Emunah (1995) wrote:

> Drama therapy provides a laboratory setting in which adolescents can experiment with numerous roles, without long-term commitment or consequence . . . The fact that one is 'only acting' is liberating; play and pretend offer a protective shield from the real world. In this safe and permissive context, familiar roles can be explored, latent roles can be unearthed, idealized roles can be examined, feared roles can be practiced. Past roles can be reviewed, discarded, or integrated. Future roles can be tried on and previewed.
>
> (p. 159)

The freedom to try on roles and identities without consequence and to experience one's self in various ways with a supportive peer group is an essential therapeutic component at this particular stage of life.

Erikson (1968) highlighted role confusion in his fifth developmental stage *Identity versus Confusion*, emphasizing that for adolescents the primary developmental task is to answer the question "Who am I?" In doing so, it is natural and healthy for them to experience shifts in, and insecurities about, identity. They may feel confused about how they fit into society, and most likely will experiment with different roles, activities, and behaviors before consolidating their various roles into one more coherent identity. While this experimentation is a necessary part of adolescence, it can also be highly charged and scary for many teens (and caregivers!) who fear social judgment, or family and peer rejection. A drama therapy group of supportive members can provide a holding and nurturing place for teenagers to develop a more secure sense of self, and a comfort with multiplicity of identity.

For adolescents, there are real-life demands and social interaction dilemmas that can be challenging on a daily basis. Answering the question "Who am I?" is closely tied to thinking about "With whom do I associate?" or "How should I act?" The drama therapy group can serve as a place for adolescents to grasp both fantasy and reality. Imagination and play are maintained in the improvisational and creative process of collaborative theater making, leading to generating and playing out stories of all kinds. And, as mentioned, that process often provides a therapeutic distance to effectively address 'here and now' dilemmas and dynamics. However, as the members become more cohesive and more comfortable with the ability to play together and share, the group can also move toward a laboratory space for role training and skill building for 'in the moment' dilemmas and challenges—a rehearsal for life. Dramatic content can shift toward exploring themes and scenarios that are less distanced and more directly personal to an individual in the group or the group-as-a-whole, helping to give space to answer and explore the immediate questions of adolescence. This shift in focus addresses a sense of urgency that teens often feel strongly.

Drama therapist Emunah (1994, 1995, 2009), who has written extensively about working with adolescents, developed the Integrative Five Phase Model for drama therapy work, emphasizing a gradual progression from distanced play to the personal realm in developing nonfiction-based scene work and therapeutic performance. We encourage any clinician using drama with adolescents to familiarize themselves with her writings and approach. A similar progression of moving from more distanced play to less distanced personal story will be illustrated in our group case example.

The Role of Group Leader and Co-Leadership

As therapists, we believe that leading and co-leading are different skills, and that an intern or co-leader should never be placed in a group therapy setting without prior training and discussion. Co-leading is often a model for group therapy and can work beautifully while adding additional levels to the experience for all involved. One person may 'hold' the group while another guides the play, either from outside dramatic reality as a director or from the inside as a fellow player. As clinicians who are co-leading, our attunement needs to be channeled differently. Each group leader has a level of awareness that is directed toward the other leader, as well as all the individual members of the group. Co-leading that appears effortless can take practice and time to develop.

Case Example

Let's look at the group process for one outpatient adolescent group. We recognize that this case illustration is but one composite of a group, and while we will speak to the general workings of drama therapy, not all drama therapy interventions are made for all individuals. Group interactions and dynamics will change quickly based on who is in the room and what is happening. Truly, one size does not fit all, and improvisation is the therapist's best friend.

This drama therapy group was a closed group that met for eight weeks for 90 minutes in an urban outpatient child and adolescent mental health clinic. The group comprised six members between 14 and 17 years of age who were of mixed gender and race. Many of the teens worked individually with a primary therapist in the same clinic and had a variety of diagnoses related to depression, anxiety, and severe emotional disturbances. It is not possible to provide a complete history for every member, but many had also experienced significant hardships in their schools, or within their families or communities. In general, there was a common theme of isolation from family and/or peers that was a primary factor in therapists referring their patients, with the premise that a drama therapy group would be helpful in breaking down isolation, building self-esteem, and providing an outlet for emotional expression and skill building.

In this circumstance, because the therapist was receiving referrals from within the clinic, contact was made with each member's individual therapist, which allowed for a better understanding of their history and to determine if they were group-ready. In determining group-readiness, the group therapist and referring individual therapist discussed the adolescent's ability to tolerate being in a peer group, particularly one involving the use of high levels of interpersonal engagement. As such, the potential member's interpersonal skills were an important piece to consider, wanting to be sure that each person had enough ability to engage with and tolerate group interaction, while also identifying the specific areas of need the group could serve. The group therapist was also able to work with a member's individual therapist when important issues would arise over the course of the group.

Often, though not always, drama therapy groups follow a triphasic structure that involves *warm-up*, *action*, and *closure*. The warm-up quite literally warms the members up to one another, loosens them up, and help them get more into their bodies and the space, and often serves as a jumping-off-point for further dramatic exploration in the action phase of the group. The action phase is often considered the 'working through' portion of the session when dramatic action is the focus of the group. Closure refers to the processing of the group experience, making connections to the work that was done, and preparing the group to transition to the rest of their day. These three phases may happen both in the group over time, or in each session.

While reading through the forthcoming clinical material, we ask you to keep in mind the importance of improvisation as a group therapist. This spontaneity facilitates a sense of play within the group, but even more important, it demonstrates to the members that the therapist is present. By being fully engaged in the 'here and now,' the group leader basically states, "*I see what is happening and will guide us, as needed.*" This level of attunement allows members to feel truly seen and increases the changes for personal sharing while creating an atmosphere of respect for all involved.

Readers may find written resources for using improvisation and drama with groups very helpful in structuring sessions and developing rapport. Books by Boal (2003), Cossa (2006), Emunah (1994), Fox (2010), Nelson and Finneran (2006), Spolin (1999), and Wiener (1994) provide wonderful guides to developing creative group interventions. Many of the exercises and games referenced in this case example can be found in these books.

Session 1

In the beginning sessions, we recommend using warm-up games with the aim of starting to co-create a sense of trust and security. This feeling takes time to develop, and clinicians must keep in mind that just announcing that a space is safe does not make it so. Rather, a sense of safety generally unfolds as group cohesion builds.

After engaging in some basic name games and warm-up exercises, we set guidelines for the group as well, regardless of whether the group is ongoing or meeting with all the same members just once (as often happens in inpatient hospital settings). Announcing guidelines and establishing group expectations gives the group session a sense of form, which is one method for safety to start to develop.

Together as a group we answered the questions, "*Do we have rules in this group?*," "*What do we need from one another?*," and "*What do we want from this group?*" It was established that no one had to do anything they weren't comfortable with, and that being "in the audience" or "behind the scenes" is just as important as being "on stage." Enforcing confidentiality is tricky in group settings, when the burden of confidentiality is really on the therapist, not the members. The request can be made, however, and discussed in group as a way to inform members to take responsibility for maintaining a sense of respect and kindness for the disclosures of others. Breaches of confidentiality should be brought back to the group for discussion.

The rest of this group was spent engaging in drama games and warm-ups to help bring the members closer and begin to experience what it is like to play with others. Common warm-up games included *Zip-Zap-Zop* (where group members pass a hand-clap around the circle while following the sequence of saying "zip-zap-zop," focusing on connection, speed, and rhythm), *The Wind Blows*, and other improvisational games. (In The Wind Blows, group members sit in a circle of chairs with one member standing in the middle. This person states: "The wind blows for anyone who . . .," finishing with a true statement about themselves. Other group members are instructed to find a new seat if the statement is true for them as well. This is played in rotation, is fast-paced and fun, and develops connection.) Verbal processing as a group at the end focused on asking members what their experience of playing with others was like and what, if anything, might have surprised them in the process. The group ended with a ritual closing where they brought down an imaginary 'magic box' from the ceiling, and each member was invited to pretend to take something from it that they wanted for themselves—a gift for the week ahead of them.

Session 2

The next session began with the therapist introducing a ritual exercise for the start of each group meeting. Members were invited to 'throw' into the middle of the circle anything they would like to put away for the moment to better allow themselves to be present to the group. These 'tosses' into the middle ranged in responses: "*stupid boyfriend*," "*mom stress*," "*stomach ache*," "*worries*," and so on. Once each member took a turn naming something and physicalizing throwing it in, the group collectively decided what to do with the responses—how to transform the pile (e.g., throw it out the window, or squash it into the floor, or send it up to the clouds, or set it on fire and toast marshmallows). This was a way to bring the group together with immediacy, by sharing personal struggles and harnessing creative problem solving collectively.

The rest of the session continued with more warm-up activities and drama games, focusing on connecting members, bringing in playful interactions, and increasing emotional expression. Common improvisation games were used, including The

Wind Blows, mirroring exercises in pairs, *Hot Seat* (a singing free-association game in which one person enters the middle of the group circle and starts singing, and other members are encouraged to take the place of the person in the middle in turn by singing whatever comes to mind), and *Complete the Image*. (During the last game, one person creates a frozen tableau with their body, and group members are encouraged to then come up and create a complimentary pose in connection to it, telling some kind of story or showing a relationship. Group members are invited to rotate in and out of images, and those in the audience can also be invited to elaborate stories based on what they see.)

These games were used as a means to warm-up to more embodied scene work through the use of the game *Freeze*, in which two group members begin an improvised scene. At any point in the scene when an audience group member has an impulse, they call out "freeze" and tap one of the players out. They take that member's place and begin a whole new scene. Freeze allowed for members to start to play with more distanced, embodied scene work, creating fictional characters and scenarios that transformed quickly through free association.

In closing, the group members processed the experience of improvising and making choices, reflecting on being in the scenes with one another as well as how they felt they related or did not relate to characters and situations that were portrayed. Excessive verbal processing or interpretation, as in connecting the drama work too personally to their lives beyond what they noticed, was intentionally avoided at this phase by the therapist. It was more important in this initial stage to let the sense of play increase and allow the focus to remain on the activity of theatre-making and ensemble-building. Creative collaboration was not completely natural for most of the members, who were at times reluctant, anxious, or guarded. The session then closed with the familiar magic box ritual.

Session 3

The third session began with the ritual beginning and then again moved into improvisation games focusing on connection and being present to each other, going back to paired and then group mirroring exercises. Wanting to increase the group's range of emotional expression with one another, the leader engaged them in *Emotional Greetings* (group members are asked to create a list of emotions and invited to walk around the space. When each emotion is called out, members are invited to embody that emotion as they go around and greet one another, emphasizing both physical and verbal ways of expressing each emotion. Actual words can be used, as a script, or simply gibberish). They also played *Group Mood* (one member volunteers to leave the room while the rest of the group decides on a collective emotion/mood they will play out. The member comes back in and must observe and interact with individuals in the room to try to guess the mood).

The improv game *Expert* was then used, a format where two people are enroled as experts on a talk show and must speak about a topic, each saying one word (or sentence) at a time, while being interviewed by a host. The other members in the audience provided topics: "*Love expert*," "*How to get out of school*," "*Dealing with annoying people and parents*," "*Peer pressure*." This was a significant moment in which humor (there was a lot of laughter) and real-life scenarios were intersecting and surfacing for the group. Group members were able to use one another as advisors, albeit through comedic interaction. It marked a shift in the group, in which the members' own knowledge and feedback for one another was emphasized and considered an essential part of the group process. The material from this game then became inspiration for the group to break into smaller groups, creating scenes around these themes. In closing, they processed feelings and connections, and again brought down the magic box and took something they needed for the coming week.

Session 4

After the ritual opening and warm-ups to free the body and mind through group sound and movement exercises, the members decided they wanted to embark on creating a piece as a whole group. The group therapist honored this impulse, acting as a guide in helping them organize themselves by way of selecting a subject matter, creating a storyline, and casting roles. In this way, the therapist played an important role in modeling leadership, organization, and fostering collaborative communication, encouraging group members to express their individual interests while also contributing toward a group goal.

Members showed interest in creating a video that could be shown to other kids to address issues related to gang affiliation and peer pressure. While all the members were drawn to the idea of using video, not everyone wanted to be on camera. The idea to use puppets was established as a means of not being on film, and emphasis was placed on the various tasks that were required beyond acting. These included making scenery and title pages, constructing puppets, and of course the countless roles needed for video production, such as director, set dresser, cinematographer, sound engineers, actors, and editors. In essence, every role is an essential and significant part of the completion of the piece. The task of creating a film was highly energizing for the group, bringing them together in a focused way. The rest of the group time was dedicated to creating a loose script and plot line based on a modern-day Romeo and Juliet twist, with the plan of filming during the following session.

Session 5

The following week, the group began production. This was the first time the camera came into the room. The camera in many ways becomes another group member, and there must be sensitivity to how it is handled and used. Therapists must be aware of the power dynamics and vulnerabilities that cameras can illicit. The role of cinematographer must be carefully chosen, and until it was clear who the right person for that job would be, the group therapist played the role, holding the camera initially and reiterating the importance of trust and responsibility that comes with the role. The group as a whole was warmed up to the camera by passing it around the circle and letting each member hold and play with it *without* recording. This was followed by having the group create a group video piece in which each person had one moving shot, adding on from the person before them, involving no people but only objects in the room. The therapist acted as a creative assistant of sorts as each member worked on their individual piece, helping technically if/as needed, while the rest of the group were in the roles of witnesses and curious observers of the choices and creativity of their peers.

Once warmed up to the technical element of the equipment and creative impulses were beginning to emerge, the group began production, assigning the on- and off-camera roles, with the ability to shift roles throughout the process as needed to allow everyone to be part of the assembly in different ways. The group proceeded to create the video, at times needing to take different shots or re-takes.

Collaborative video-making process helps to increase skills of negotiation, focus, and shared accountability in attending to the needs and visions of oneself and the group, while at the same time working toward a common purpose. In this instance, the footage was played back at the end of the group in its raw format with no editing, and the group processed the experience of creating and watching the piece. They explored if the short movie came out the way they wanted, and how they related to it and the messages it contained.

Sessions 6 and 7

Over the next two sessions, there was a shift in the group in regard to personal sharing. Members expressed enjoying the video-making format and wanted to continue, deciding to work on documentary-style vignettes. After quick group warm-ups, the members were invited to find an object that they had on them that day and to write a mini-monologue from the point of view of that object. The objects were then filmed, with monologues read in voice-over style. As is always the case, members were given the artistic freedom around the choices they made, whether they wanted it to be their voice or that of a peer, and what kind of shots would be taken. The objects of members in the group (keys, phones, backpacks, jewelry) held stories that provided a slightly distanced and yet extremely intimate understanding of each adolescent.

It was decided that the group would work on "A Day in the Life" vignettes centering on something they wanted to share with the group—a moment or happening in their life. Most vignettes centered either on events that brought them into therapy or topics they were addressing in therapy. Group members who wished to be the director of their piece were encouraged to play that role, with other members being cast as needed. They were given the option to incorporate any music into their pieces at the end while the credits rolled. Scenes were shot, with the group assisting each person to create the story they wished to tell.

Group members chose various stories to share. For example, one created a short video about their family members not accepting their goth dress and emo identity, saying they wanted them to stop saying, "It's just a phase." The final scene of the piece was a conversation the teen wanted to have with their mother about this. Similarly, another member focused on representing the immense pressure that she felt from her family to be perfect, and to do better than her parents had done. Yet another created a piece about an anger management group they were mandated to attend, and how they would lead the group differently if they were the therapist.

A few members chose to create videos showing their experiences of intense anxiety, the adults who connected them to therapy (family and school counselors), and how coming to treatment has been helpful to them. Another shared about his experience of a recent school assault and resulting feelings of depression and anxiety around the incident. This video included his subsequent change of schools, and dealing with being the 'new kid.' Each vignette was given a title by its author/director. It was not required that each member create a piece, though everyone had the opportunity.

It was clear that through collaborating, and in the telling of each other's stories, there was a tremendous bond fostered and healing occurred. Between these two sessions and the final one, the therapist edited together the video footage into one video with distinct segments and corresponding music/sound elements, as well as creating a bloopers segment of interactions and funny moments shared by the group members throughout the whole process.

Session 8

The group began the final session as usual and then moved into watching the various video pieces and reflecting on them. They discussed the experience they had in playing the roles, sharing and being witness to the stories, and how they related to the process and themes. In closing, members were asked to think of three words to describe themselves: one for the day they came to group, one for that day, and one for their future. Members were then invited to create three group tableaus representing these collective words. The session closed with the magic box, this time offering imaginary gifts to others in the room and taking a gift for themselves moving forward.

Summary

It is our belief that successful adolescent group therapy requires a clinician who is playful, well-attuned, and able to establish an atmosphere of creativity and respect. Group is a form of therapy that requires specific training to be successful, in this case an understanding of adolescent development and group process, as well as an appreciation that certain participants may need individual treatment and/or a medication consultation before they are able to tolerate and engage in group modalities. Group treatment may be one of the most passion-filled and stimulating ways to work with teens. Their innate curiosity, liveliness, and often thought-provoking character traits mean the group leader must be ready for almost anything. Peer and clinical supervision help group clinicians keep their countertransference responses in mind while facilitating sessions. Drama therapy groups provide a powerful way for adolescents to engage in a therapeutic process that is developmentally appropriate and simultaneously fun and productive for helping them master the identity formation and life tasks ahead of them.

References

American Group Psychotherapy Association. (n.d.). *What is group psychotherapy?* Retrieved from www.agpa.org/home/practice-resources/what-is-group-psychotherapy-

Aron, L., & Atlas, G. (2018). *Dramatic dialogue: Contemporary clinical practice.* New York, NY: Routledge.

Bailey, S. (2006). Ancient and modern roots of drama therapy. In S. Brooke (Ed.), *Creative arts therapies manual: A guide to the history, theoretical approaches, assessment, and work with special populations of art, play, dance, music, drama, and poetry therapies* (pp. 214–222). Springfield, IL: Charles C. Thomas.

Barish, K. (2004). What is therapeutic in child therapy?: I. Therapeutic engagement. *Psychoanalytic Psychology, 21,* 385–401.

Boal, A. (2003). *Games for actors and non-actors* (2nd ed.). New York, NY: Routledge.

Bradley, M. (2003). *Yes, your teen is crazy! Loving your kid without losing your mind.* Gig Harbor, WA: Harbor Press.

Cossa, M. (2006). *Rebels with a cause: Working with adolescents using action techniques.* London: Jessica Kingsley.

Emunah, R. (1994). *Acting for real: Drama therapy process, technique, and performance.* Levittown, PA: Brunner/Mazel.

Emunah, R. (1995). From adolescent trauma to adolescent drama: Group drama therapy with emotionally disturbed youth. In S. Jennings (Ed.), *Dramatherapy with children and adolescents* (pp. 150–168). London: Routledge.

Emunah, R. (2009). The integrative five phase model of drama therapy. In D. R. Johnson & R. Emunah (Eds.), *Current approaches in drama therapy* (2nd ed., pp. 37–65). Springfield, IL: Charles C. Thomas.

Erikson, E. H. (1956). The problem of ego identity. *Journal of the American Psychoanalytic Association, 4,* 56–12.

Erikson, E. H. (1968). *Identity: Youth and crisis.* New York, NY: Norton.

Erikson, E. H. (1977). *Toys and reasons: Stages in the ritualization of experience.* New York, NY: Norton.

Fox, H. (2010). *Zoomy zoomy: Improv games and exercises for groups.* New Paltz, NY: Tusitala Publishing.

Giedd, J. (2016, May). The amazing teen brain. *Scientific American Mind, 25*(2), 32–27.

Goldstein, B. (2018). Cultivating curiosity, creativity, confidence, and self-awareness through mindful group therapy for children and adolescents. In T. Marks-Tarlow, M. Solomon & D. Siegel (Eds.), *Play and creativity in psychotherapy* (pp. 338–358). New York, NY: Norton.

Haen, C. (2005). Group therapy in a children's inpatient psychiatric setting. In C. Haen & A. M. Weber (Eds.), *Clinical applications of drama therapy in child and adolescent treatment* (pp. 189–203). New York, NY: Routledge.

Johnson, D. R. (2009). The history and development of the field of drama therapy in North America. In D. R. Johnson & R. Emunah (Eds.), *Current approaches in drama therapy* (2nd ed., pp. 5–16). Springfield, IL: Charles C. Thomas.

Johnson, D. R., & Emunah, R. (Eds.). (2009). *Current approaches in drama therapy.* (2nd ed.). Springfield, IL: Charles C. Thomas.

Jones, P. (2007). *Drama as therapy: Theory, practice and research* (2nd ed.). London: Routledge.

Kindler, R. C. (2017). Shame and its undoing: A performer's desire to be found. In G. Hagman (Ed.), *Art, creativity, and psychoanalysis: Perspectives from analyst-artists* (pp. 47–56). New York, NY: Routledge

Landy, R. (1994). *Drama therapy: Concepts, theories and practices* (2nd ed.). Springfield, IL: Charles C. Thomas.

Landy, R. (2008). *The couch and the stage: Integrating words and action in psychotherapy.* Lanham, MD: Jason Aronson.

Long, K., & McKechnie, B. (2008). No time to say hello, good-bye: Drama therapy with children on an inpatient psychiatric unit. In S. Brooke (Ed.), *The use of the creative therapies with survivors of domestic violence* (pp. 199–222). Springfield, IL: Charles C. Thomas.

Long, K., & Weber, A. M. (2005). Through the eyes of the therapists and children: Drama therapy during and after September 11th. In C. Haen & A. M. Weber (Eds.), *Clinical applications of drama therapy in child and adolescent treatment* (pp. 261–279). New York, NY: Routledge.

Maden, A. (2008). Ma mere et moi: Creative arts in a group treatment. In S. Brooke (Ed.), *The use of the creative therapies with survivors of domestic violence* (pp. 270–296). Springfield, IL: Charles C. Thomas.

Nelson, L., & Finneran, L. (2006). *Drama and the adolescent journey: Warm-ups and activities to address teen issues.* Portsmouth NH: Heinemann.

North American Drama Therapy Association. (n.d.). *Drama therapy with children and adolescents.* Retrieved from www.nadta.org/assets/documents/children-adolescent-fact-sheet.pdf

North American Drama Therapy Association. (n.d.). *What is drama therapy?* Retrieved from www.nadta.org/what-is-drama-therapy.html

Pitre, R., Mayor, C., & Johnson, D. R. (2016). Developmental transformations short-form as a stress reduction method for children. *Drama Therapy Review, 2*(2), 167–181.

Pitzruzzella, S. (2017). *Drama, creativity and intersubjectivity: The roots of change in dramatherapy.* New York, NY: Routledge.

Scroggs, B., Bailey, S., & Fees, B. (2016). The impact of participation in creative drama on empathy levels in emerging adulthood: A pilot study. *Drama Therapy Review, 2*(2), 211–221.

Siegel, D. J. (2013). *Brainstorm: The power and purpose of the teenage brain.* New York, NY: Penguin.

Spolin, V. (1999). *Improvisation for the theater* (3rd ed.). Evanston, IL: Northwestern University Press.

Van Dam, H. (1991). Vulnerability of adolescents and young adults to "cult" phenomena. In S. Greenspan and G. Pollock (Eds.), *The course of life: Volume IV: Adolescence* (pp. 301–311). Madison, CT: International Universities Press.

van Der Kolk, B. A. (2014). *The body keeps the score: Brain, mind, and body in the healing of trauma.* New York, NY: Penguin.

Weber, A. M., & Haen, C. (Eds.). (2005). *Clinical applications of drama therapy in child and adolescent treatment.* New York, NY: Routledge.

Wiener, D. (1994). *Rehearsals for growth: Theater improvisation for psychotherapists.* New York, NY: Norton.

Wise, I. (2004). *Adolescence.* London: Karnac.

8
Music Therapy in Adolescent Groups

KATRINA SKEWES MCFERRAN

Introduction

This chapter will provide an overview of the ways that music therapists have been working with groups of adolescents across a range of contexts. This necessarily involves diverse theoretical approaches, as well as the use of a range of specific music therapy methods and techniques. Despite this diversity, I posit that a humanistic orientation is central to most approaches, which involves the therapist focusing on the inherent potential that is not always outwardly apparent in adolescent groups. Emotional connectedness is another priority, whereby music affords ongoing access to emotional material that is then integrated into the therapeutic process.

The chapter will begin with my perspective on the historical development of music therapy practice with adolescents and the influences that appear to have been more prominent in different decades and different continents. It will then describe the research that has been conducted in the context of music therapy with adolescents, beginning with case studies and then moving to interview and arts-based studies, followed by a movement toward collaborative and participatory approaches, and finally toward objective measurement. The second part of the chapter presents three illustrative vignettes, each describing the use of the three dominant methods in music therapy group work with adolescents, namely song sharing, improvisation, and songwriting. Each vignette is grounded in a particular theoretical orientation—but is followed by a discussion of how that method could also be used in a different way with the same group if the therapist chose to adopt a different orientation. I conclude by noting the relevance of integrating performances into music therapy with adolescents, as well as the changing practice trend toward brief rather than long-term therapy.

Historical Overview of Music Therapy With Adolescents

The professional practice of music therapy began across a range of continents following World War II, although the use of music for therapeutic and healing purposes has existed in many cultures for far longer and continues in parallel. The initial forms of professional practice were closely linked to the dominant approaches in each context where it emerged, so that work in mental and physical health aligned with a medical model, and work in schools aligned with the popular educational approaches of the time. Although adolescents were seen in a range of contexts, they were typically not distinguished from either children or adults in the literature. Despite this, music therapists were working with adolescents, and often reported that adolescents in their practices required different approaches, both therapeutically and musically. I was one of those music therapists, beginning in the early 1990s.

While conducting my doctoral dissertation on group work with bereaved adolescents between 1998 and 2001, I searched the literature feverishly, seeking guidance that I might have missed in my earlier readings. I discovered a number of case studies that described practices with young people who had experienced trauma (Cassity, 1981; Clendenon-Wallen, 1991; Flower, 1993; Lehrer-Carle, 1973; Lindberg, 1995; Robarts, 2000) and some descriptions of behavioral approaches with young people who had severe and profound multiple disabilities (Boswell & Vidret, 1993; Holloway, 1980; Spencer, 1988), as well as a small number of descriptive chapters about group work in particular contexts, such as working predominantly with Black Americans in the north-east corner of the United States in the 1970s and 1980s (Brooks, 1989; Ragland & Apprey, 1974; Well & Stevens, 1984). All of this work provided useful insights into individual music therapists' practices with adolescents, but did not seem to capture the unique aspects that I had noted in my practice and knew to be similar to other music therapists working with teenagers in the early 2000s. This signaled to me that a change was occurring in therapeutic practice, where adolescents were beginning to be seen as a unique cohort of therapy clients who warranted explanations that were contextualized in terms of their developmental stage.

Over the next two decades, this gap in the literature was addressed through research and practice articles that more closely reflected ways of being with young people that seemed familiar to me. Authors seemed to adopt a broadly humanistic orientation demonstrated by a keen interest in the preferred music of the young people themselves, as well as very flexible ways of engaging adolescents in group processes in relation to both the structure and content of sessions. There was an interesting confluence of international perspectives here.

Jukka Tervo (2001), from Finland, contributed an important descriptive article to professionals in clinical child psychology and psychiatry, and my own contributions about processing grief and loss work in groups in Australia emphasized a number of the same issues (McFerran & Grocke, 2000). British music therapist Tuulia Nicholls (2002) provided a surprisingly similar description of working with adolescents who had severe learning disabilities, emphasizing choice and freedom and not seeming to be restricted to a particular theoretical approach to music therapy practice. This was further consolidated through Phillipa Derrington's (2005) descriptions of songs written in therapy with adolescents identified as having emotional and behavioral difficulties (a term which has since been changed to 'adolescents having difficulties with social interaction,' and/or 'emotional regulation,' and/or 'experiencing mental health needs' [SEMH]). Although all four of us positioned our practices as psychodynamic, many aspects of our descriptions contradicted a typical analytic approach and focused more on working with social relationships and aspirations for the future, rather than on the resolution of past traumas or interpretation of dynamics. There was clearly need for more research in the field to unravel the common elements of different music therapists' approaches to group work, as well as the benefits of this work.

Empirical research began in earnest at this time, building on the case studies and descriptions of practice that had previously been dominant. Many of these studies were qualitative, which seemed congruent with the predominantly humanistic orientation. Investigators focused on listening to young people's voices and documenting what adolescents believed, not only about addressing the issues that brought them to therapy but also about the particular role that music therapy could play in their lives. Young people described how the combination afforded by shared *musicking* for both choice and control were important to them (McFerran, 2001). They also described how it was important that the sessions were fun and interactive, while simultaneously providing ways to express complex emotional experiences that were holding them back (McFerran, 2010b). The paradoxes that have often been noted about the adolescent stage of development were also clearly present in their explanations of music therapy, and again, this contradicted past approaches that had emphasized high levels of structure and restrictive uses of preferred music.

Clinical researchers working in adolescent mental health used interviews with young people to develop initial theories about how music therapy might promote young people's identities and facilitate recovery. This approach consolidated the humanistic orientation that had become more prominent and highlighted how music therapists focused on the construction of a health-based identity, as well as supporting social participation (Hense, McFerran, & McGorry, 2014). This in turn extended to theorizing about the value of the powerful emotional connections that music offered to youth with mental health problems (Cheong-Clinch & McFerran, 2016).

Such research, as well as further investigations that included young people with depression (McFerran & Saarikallio, 2013), also highlighted how adolescents' uses of music were not always helpful in relation to their mental health. We began to recognize how mental illness might produce uses of music that reinforced unhealthy patterns of thinking such as rumination, isolation, and intensifying emotions. This shift in perspective provided an important counter-balance to the strengths and resource orientation that had become more dominant in the literature, and highlighted the importance of incorporating psychodynamic tenets into engaging and strengths-oriented practice.

In addition to using interviews to listen to young people's voices, researchers around this time also turned their attention to other sources of knowledge such as the musical material generated in therapy. Tom Dalton and Robert Krout (2006) undertook a comprehensive analysis of songs written by bereaved teenagers and used their findings to develop a grief processing scale that had a strong emphasis on emotional work. I conducted a retrospective analysis of songs written with young women hospitalized for eating disorders (McFerran, Baker, Patton, & Sawyer, 2006), from which we found issues related to identity formation were most prominent, incorporating a particularly large set of lyrics with a future orientation that involved exploring new behaviors and positive self-talk. An investigation of pre-adolescents (Roberts, 2009) suggested that this orientation toward identity was specific to adolescents, as younger people wrote more concrete or alternately highly imaginative tales.

Ideas about identity in songwriting were further consolidated by the emphasis on metaphor that emerged in Mike Viega's (2008) analysis of songs that teenagers bring to therapy, and became clear when we attempted to analyze lyrics published in the literature without any inside knowledge of the obtuse meanings that were present in many songs written in therapy (McFerran, Baker, & Krout, 2011).

In addition to lyric analysis, Susan Gardstrom (Gardstrom, 2004) and I (McFerran & Wigram, 2005) both explored the musical material generated by improvising adolescents in music therapy using Bruscia's (1987) Improvisation Assessment Profiles. In both cases, the young people's reflections on the meaning of their improvisations were quite different from the features identified by the therapist's analysis and clarified that it was difficult to understand the meaning of the musical material to young people without their own interpretations being incorporated. It was clear, however, that emotional expression was considered important, and that young people felt they could connect with and release the emotions they were struggling with through the music (McFerran-Skewes, 2000).

Supplementing these qualitative and musically focused studies were a series of action research projects conducted by researchers in the southern hemisphere. These authors drew back the lens of their investigations to consider the influence of context on music therapy practices with young people, as well as attempting to engage adolescents as players in shaping the kinds of practices they wished to participate in. From the outset, it became clear that young people were not particularly interested in taking a role as co-researcher (Hunt, 2005) and would often only engage in providing this level of feedback if it occurred through musical means, such as songwriting (McFerran, Roberts, & O'Grady, 2010). However, it was very helpful to listen to adolescents' desires from the outset of processes, rather than gathering their perspectives only at the end, and this supported relationship building during therapy (Wang, 2008).

Adolescents seemed to desire opportunities to perform their music, and projects often (but not always) included performances to closed audiences or for the purposes of recording (Bolger, 2015; McFerran & Hunt, 2008). This dimension was subsequently investigated by Fairchild, Thompson, and McFerran (2016), who discovered that children experienced intense, but mixed, emotions related to performances, and that the audience played an active and important role in the experience of performance. In addition to the performative dimension that was highlighted in these action research studies, researchers also recognized that it was essential to listen to the perspectives of other adult stakeholders in schools, hospitals, and community settings. These people were gate keepers who shaped the ways young people could engage in music therapy research and practice in the first place, and reinforced the kinds of hierarchical relationships that music therapy often sought to usurp.

This strong emphasis on empowering approaches to practice and research has gradually been supplemented by quantitative studies, perhaps in response to the demands of research funders as well as a desire to prove that the benefits young people reported from engaging with music clinically could also be measured by adults. The first meta-analysis of quantitative investigations of music therapy with children and adolescents with psychopathology (Gold, Voracek, & Wigram, 2004) confirmed the idea that music therapy did have a significantly positive effect on relevant clinical outcomes. It also suggested that benefits were easier to measure for behavioral and developmental disorders than socioemotional issues, and that eclectic, psychodynamic, and humanistic approaches were most effective. Indeed, researchers have faced a number of challenges in quantifying the outcomes described as helpful by distressed adolescents with social and emotional issues, but data from validated measures did not confirm this perception (Derrington, 2012; McFerran et al., 2010).

Improvements in depression have been detected reasonably consistently, however, with an RCT in the United Kingdom capturing improvements (Porter et al., 2012), as well as a study of group improvisation in Venezuela (Albornoz, 2011), and a pre-post study with young people in Australia presenting with depression for the first time (McFerran, Hense, Koike, & Rickwood, 2017). Improvements have also been captured in pre-post testing of levels of motor impulsivity in young people with ADHD (Rickson, 2006), and emotional and physical well-being in adolescents who have been traumatically injured (Robb, 2003). In addition, results have been found in studies of adolescents participating in a violence prevention program in Germany that compared music therapy to a treatment condition focused on aggression and conflict regulation (Wölfl, 2014).

The research and practice literature provides many insights into music therapy with adolescents, although not all of it is focused on group work. In fact, a systematic analysis of the literature (McFerran, 2010a) showed that less than 40% of music therapy publications through 2008 described group work, despite its obvious relevance to adolescence. Further analysis suggested a reasonably similar number of methods were being used in group and individual sessions, with group work more often including receptive methods in addition to the use of live songs and improvisation. Descriptions of songwriting only began to achieve prominence around this time, although it has been increasingly common. The following section will focus on describing songwriting and the other most common methods, as well as the particular issues and features of the various approaches in different contexts.

Music Therapy Methods in Adolescent Group Work

The three dominant methods used in adolescent group work are *songwriting*, *song sharing*, and *improvisation*. The ways in which these methods are offered by the therapist vary depending on their context and the theoretical orientation of the music therapist, which is often predominantly humanistic, but also incorporates psychodynamic, developmental, cognitive–behavioral, and ecological influences. In order to illustrate how these methods are introduced and facilitated by the therapist, I will provide a series of vignettes that are then discussed to illustrate what differences might be observed if a different orientation was adopted. Obviously, these are only indicative, and would vary in many ways depending on the individual therapist and their own culturally informed beliefs about practice.

Group Song Sharing

Steve sits with a group of five young people who are lounging around on bean bags, couches, and cushions. They are participating in a series of ten workshops that are intended to support their recovery from substance abuse by attending to lingering grief and loss issues. Most of the young people have agreed to attend voluntarily, although a lot of support is required for the sessions to happen—including workers picking up all the individuals from their supported, community-based housing. Eight young people are listed as participants, but there are rarely as many as five there on any given week.

Steve asks whether anyone has a song that is meaningful to them that they would be willing to share with the group and offers to plug anyone's phone into the portable amp he has provided. The young people look around at one another furtively, and no one looks ready to volunteer. Steve reminds the group that he anticipated this activity last week and was hoping that they might have spent some time thinking about and choosing a song. After some further silence, one of the most extroverted young people stands up and tosses his phone toward Steve, nodding that he should plug it into the amp. He begins to describe his favorite electronic artist and how much he likes the fat bass lines and the dub drops. Steve accepts this music-oriented explanation and doesn't probe further, but simply hits play on the phone that had been thrown to him.

The group sits around listening to the song, which lasts for nearly six minutes. At times, the group members talk to one another, although Steve is modeling attentive listening. At other times, the contributor begins wandering around, talking loudly about how great this track is and looking a little uncomfortable about some of the lyrics that can be heard describing violent fantasies and some misogynistic themes. After the song has finished, Steve carefully unplugs the phone before the next track begins and then turns back to the group and hands the phone to the young man. "So, what does that song mean to you?" he asks.

In the ensuing conversation, the young man continues to emphasize the music more than the meaning, so Steve probes a little more. "I noticed some pretty dark themes in there. What was it like to share that with these guys?" The young man is defensive about the possibility of being judged and explains in an animated way how it is just imaginary, and people don't take that stuff too seriously. A number of the group agrees. Steve repeats one of the lyric lines that had made him uncomfortable and asks whether or not it sounds like an endorsement of rape culture. The group declines to answer, so Steve softens his approach and offers a potential solution. "Not everyone takes the lyrics of songs very seriously," he says. "Had you even noticed that line before?"

"Well, I have now!" the young man replies, "But that doesn't make me a rapist!" The group continues to process the song and to discuss both the appealing and less comfortable aspects alternately, with Steve carefully watching to see how much the group, and the young man, can tolerate. After a few moments, he decides it is enough and asks if anyone else has a song to share. This time a young woman offers to have a turn. "Well, it's not about rape, but it is about a very ugly breakup," she says, and the group settles in once again to listen and see what comes next.

Although song sharing sounds like a relatively innocuous method, both because it involves receptive rather than active participation and because the material has been created elsewhere rather than in the session, it can be very confronting. Young people usually have strong attachments and loyalty to their favorite tracks, although this may vary widely from month to month as new songs come into favor. But at any one moment, their preferred song can be both a badge of identity and a connection to their inner world. This means that sharing songs is simultaneously a bold statement and a moment of intense vulnerability. Young people anticipate correctly that others may not like their songs and that they may be misunderstood based on what song they present. The role of the therapist is to understand the intense flood of emotions that might be felt as the young person suddenly realizes how much they have revealed to the group simply by playing their chosen song. How the therapist responds to this varies quite significantly between settings and orientations.

In the vignette provided, Steve is working with a psychodynamic lens, and the song is understood to be a vehicle for projection. He does not assume to know what the young man is projecting through his own listening, but instead relies on a dialogue to draw out the meaning. Some of the song's meaning will already be known to the group member, and new realizations also tend to occur through the therapeutic process of sharing with the group. Depending on the individual, they might find it more or less easy to articulate the feelings and associations that are triggered by the song, and so the therapist might provide some language for consideration—trying to put words to what the contributor might be experiencing so they are able to accept or reject the proffered interpretation. The music therapist is particularly sensitive to the stereotypes that might be associated with specific genres, such as Rap and Metal, which often inspire fear and concern in the hearts of adults.

While research has repeatedly shown that music does not cause people to act in the ways portrayed in songs (North & Hargreaves, 2005), there is a connection between emotional needs and the emotional nature of songs, which needs to be explored. The psychodynamic therapist might draw on their own countertransference reactions to do this, but not leap to stereotypical assumptions that offensive lyrics mean the contributor is an offender, as highlighted in the vignette. Rather, they will explore what the lyrics mean to the individual and the group, often taking the young person's social world into account, where bravado and toughness may be a critical survival strategy, or it might be that their own experiences have normalized abusive behaviors. In any case, the songs being shared often provide a lot of material for consideration.

At other times, or in other contexts, the therapist might not offer so many, or such challenging, interpretations. They may choose to stay with the adolescent's focus, which is often to describe the musical material itself and why they like that genre of music. This is a more strongly humanistic approach, with a focus on validating the identity representations of the young person by offering unconditional positive regard. The act of sharing might be seen as challenging enough, and the group members would be encouraged to also show respect for diverse contributions. Here the group process would be focused on empathy and kindness, rather than on meaning making and interpretation.

If the group was working in a more behaviorally focused way, group song sharing affords a number of opportunities for developing social skills. The expectation that members might sit and listen through an entire song without interrupting would certainly provide a challenge for many young people. The facilitator might focus the commentary on the reactions of group members to another's song, and their ability to listen or not. They could even stop the song if group members started talking and ask them to consider how that might feel for the contributing group member. The song sharing could be followed by a series of activities, such as generating a list of words that describe the emotions that each group member felt or heard in the song. This could be used as a way of identifying and labeling emotions and developing an increased vocabulary for expressing emotional material.

In order to achieve more sustainable outcomes from the experience, the therapist might focus on developing the young people's capacity to use music as an ongoing coping strategy by integrating educative elements into the groups. Raising young people's awareness of the ways music can trigger strong emotional responses is an important part of promoting the use of music as a resource, and this often involves explaining how music can work. Adolescents are frequently unaware that particular songs can become associated with traumatic experiences, complex memories, or coping behaviors that are unhelpful (such as self-harm), and therefore continue to listen to music even when they feel worse after listening. Discussing responses to particular songs in the group can be sufficient for making this more conscious, while creating playlists together as a group, or individually within the group, can be a productive way to reinforce this understanding. Group playlists tend to build memories of the group and connectedness between members, whereas individual playlists provide the opportunity to compare and discuss habits of music use, and one person's insights can trigger increasing understanding for another (Bibb & McFerran, 2018).

Although these different ways of describing the use of group song sharing make the approaches sound distinct, a therapist might also interweave different levels into their approach on different days, or depending on different group members' capacities. Not all young people are ready for challenging insights, and not all are satisfied by straight-forward validation. Even more common is that a behavioral intention might be softened during the actual session, and that the therapist may decide to tolerate less compliant behavior in service of the development of group bonding or emotional expression, which are often dominant where music is concerned.

Group Improvisation

Maria is working with a group of young people in an alternative school setting. They meet on a weekly basis to use music as way of addressing the personal and social capabilities listed in the curriculum guidelines. These include self-awareness and management through recognition and expression of emotions and the development of resilience. Social awareness and management are also included, with relationships and diversity being highlighted. In developing classroom goals for the year, Maria had proposed the extended use of group improvisation to the teaching team, who meet regularly to discuss this small class and to ensure their individual educational goals are being achieved. The team liked the idea that it would move away from more verbally demanding activities, such as generating lyrics for songs, to focus on an embodied experience of managing self and relationships. Maria warned them that it might be a powerful process, and they might need to work together to process some of the responses that the young people have to the extended group process, and the team agreed to provide the necessary supports when times get tough.

After six weeks of playing the instruments, the group has, indeed, reached a point of group development where tension is high. As Maria instigates the second improvisation of the 45-min session, she tries to focus the young people on the purpose of the week. "This time, try to choose an instrument that you can play to express anger," she says, "and consider experimenting with something you haven't played before." The group looks resistant, but gradually moves forward and picks instruments from the various hand percussion options available. A number of people choose djembes and doumbeks, and one young woman chooses the large gong. Another member selects some finger cymbals, while others take tambourines, a metallophone, and a cabasa. Maria is relieved to see the spread of instruments across melodic, headed drums and other forms of percussion, since she knows that diversity will allow for a more nuanced emotional portrayal than if everyone had chosen the drums.

"Just begin when you're ready," Maria calls, and then sits back to wait and see who will begin. She doesn't have to wait long. One of the group members begins to thump their drum, repeatedly and loudly. Others quickly join in, and a wall of sound is created through which it becomes difficult to hear anything more than the thick texture and the intensity of the timbre. After about a minute, some people begin to quiet, and it becomes possible to hear the different lines. One person is playing the cabasa strongly and quickly, with no gaps in the sound they are creating. Another is playing similarly on a hand drum, while yet another plays up and down the notes of the metallophone without ceasing. The gong is sounded randomly, but momentarily dominates the sound, while the finger cymbal player taps gently but persistently in the background. The remaining players contribute sporadically, playing then stopping, until they eventually come to a close. At one point, one of the group members had stood up and gone to a nearby shelf to procure a bike helmet, which they put on their head in a way that covers their eyes, before continuing to play the doumbek. This player and the sounds of the metallophone continue long after everyone else had ceased, only coming to a stop when Maria stands up and gestures to finish.

The group remains still for some time after the sound has finished. Maria passes out some pieces of blank paper and asks them to draw about the sound of the 'angry' improvisation. The group members remain silent during this activity, but draw actively for around five minutes. When they come to a stop, Maria asks them to turn their page over and to write a story about what they have drawn. When this is finished, she suggests they give the story a title. They then take turns around the circle, with each group member describing what they had heard, drawn, and written to one another, with the group remaining quiet while each person speaks.

At the end of the exercise, Maria asks each member to comment on what they had noticed about another person. No one mentions the bike helmet, which is still being worn by the doumbek player, but some people do comment on the intensity of some of the playing and how clearly they felt it represented one type of anger. Others comment on the way that anger seemed to come and go for some people, and how it remained consistent for others. Each of these comments is noted by Maria, who moves to close out the end of the session by suggesting a relaxation exercise while she improvises on the guitar. This is the usual way the group closes, so members agree readily and position themselves comfortably in their chairs as the music begins.

In this vignette, the music therapist has adopted a humanistic lens within the school context. Although the group is using music as a way of working with emotional material, it has a learning orientation. Expressing and embodying emotions is part of the learning, but the emphasis is on using a creative and nonverbal medium to elicit self and social awareness, while remaining focused on intellectual understandings and verbal processing. By using a phenomenological technique for experiencing at multiple levels, further material is generated for reflection than through using a single medium. It also provides the space for the young people to process individually before they combine their learnings together to generate more language and constructs for understanding themselves and one another.

This exercise can readily be moved into a more psychodynamic orientation, however. It would not require a lot of variation for the therapist to pursue more meaning making and to probe for insights about the origins of such intense emotional expression. The amount of time devoted to the expression of anger by some of the group members is worthy of note, as are the different ways it is expressed, and possibly experienced. Sustained and unrelenting expression, as opposed to sporadic and occasional playing, might say something about the degree of anger being held by the young person. It may also be useful to explore how comfortable group members are with even recognizing anger, and whether they believe it is helpful to hear it, or play it, or whether they consider it something that is better avoided and controlled. This topic might be processed with words and further improvisations, and members might be encouraged to explore other instruments and to experience the different ways that anger can be played.

A more cognitive–behavioral orientation might integrate role plays into the processing of this initial exploration of anger. The subsequent discussion might be used to identify situations in which anger can be triggered, and then the group could explore using the instruments as a way of rehearsing alternative reactions or testing how others might react if anger were expressed in particular ways. The therapist might be active in making suggestions in this context about what behaviors to explore, and to help the group consider alternatives. This could involve setting homework, particularly within the school context, where the group members are asked to observe their anger during the week and come back with examples of their experience to be processed musically in the following session. Each of these strategies would be oriented toward helping the young people develop a repertoire of behaviors in response to being able to recognize their own emotional reactions, particularly with peers.

An alternative to this kind of free and expressive improvisation is a more structured approach to improvising together. This would involve focusing less on the latent emotional content and more on the interactive experience between members of the group. Drum circles are often used when the development of self-control is prioritized, since this allows for simultaneous playing and listening to others, requiring heightened self and other awareness and compliance. A successful drumming experience such as this can be rewarding, since bonding is promoted in a way that is aesthetically satisfying and bodily experienced. It can provide a relief from the constant experience of emotions, as the group members lose themselves in the flow of playing together and have the opportunity to be connected in a peaceful and concentrated way. In addition, the production of a great shared sound can be a powerful reward for the benefits of team work, and it is quite common for participants to enjoy the experience so much that they are happy to do it repeatedly. In this case, the complexity of the playing can be gradually sequenced to introduce more and more musical challenges, thereby maintaining a steady sense of competence development, bringing further rewards.

Once again, it is common for therapists to move between these different approaches with different groups in the same context, or different weeks with the same group, or even different parts of the session, since a structured improvisation can be as relaxing as a receptive music listening experience. However, the intention is quite different, and the belief about how music can be most powerfully used varies substantially between free and structured improvisations. Music therapists are therefore influenced by both their own beliefs and experiences with music and the expectations and needs of the young people they are working with in particular contexts.

Group Songwriting

Juyoung stands in front of the whiteboard with a marker in her hand, facilitating a brain-storming session with the group about ideas for their song. The group members are all hospitalized due to weight loss issues, and most have been diagnosed with eating disorders. The acute context, combined with the extreme weight loss, means that the medical team focuses on weight stabilization and coping during the group members' hospital stay. There is an assumption that each patient will access more long-term therapy after discharge from the pediatric hospital and will be supported in their recovery through a mental health service. This trajectory influences the music therapy program, and the music therapist's role is to contribute to the goal of minimizing the adolescents' length of stay in the hospital and to motivate them to go home. To this end, Juyoung has suggested writing a song about their experience of being in the hospital. Her intention is to encourage connectedness between the young people by highlighting their shared experiences, as well as focusing on the prospect of release and discharge.

The group members have been readily contributing words that describe how they feel about the hospital admission: "It sucks!" "Like a rat in a cage." "I want to get out of here!" "I miss my parents . . ." "They force you to eat the disgusting hospital food." "I hate being controlled like this." "I want to escape." "It's not fair!" "The nurses are pretty nice." "I want to go home . . ." The young people call out words and Juyoung writes them on the board, accepting everything that is suggested during the initial brainstorming. Once the volley of sounds has finished, she turns back to the group and suggests a focus by circling the words relevant to the idea of going home. "Look at this," she says. "What is it you are most looking forward to when you go home?"

The group members begin calling out more words, and this time Juyoung uses a different color to write up the next set of ideas. The young patients describe their dogs, their own comfortable beds, their family members, their freedoms, and their favorite things. The board is now covered in ideas and the general mood of the group is quite high.

Juyoung decides it is the right moment to introduce the musical side of songwriting, and that they will return to lyric generation later. She asks the group members to suggest a style of music, and most seem to have a preference for pop music, particularly songs that integrate some rapping. Juyoung poses a number of options to the group about how they might create the music—using beats on the iPad, using guitars and drum kits, singing acapella with someone beatboxing, or using the keyboard with a drum sound to accompany it. After Juyoung has described what would be involved with each, the group members choose the combination of keyboard and drumbeats and then spend some time listening to different voices/sounds on the keyboard and a range of pop drumbeats to make a specific selection. Most of the young people start to lose interest after about ten minutes and Juyoung then draws their attention back to the whiteboard.

"Now that we've decided on the sound and the style, let's create a story out of these words" she says. "First, let's decide what ideas we put in the chorus. This will be central to the song, because they keep coming back after each verse. How about we make it something general about how good it is to get out of hospital?" The group agrees and make suggestions about which words they could use. After some discussion and some active facilitation by Juyoung, a chorus is created:

I can't wait to go home, it's a great place to be
I can have all my things, they're surrounding me
When I need some support, people I love are near
And when I feel like crap, they will help quell my fear

The group members are surprised by their success in writing the lyrics and motivated to continue. Juyoung again uses the extra energy to refocus on the music and starts playing the chosen drumbeat on the keyboard while experimenting with some simple chord progressions using the sounds chosen earlier. "How about this? Do you think this would sound good behind it?" The group laughs and nods, so Juyoung makes up a melody and sings the chorus to the group. "That sounds great!" they say.

"Hmmm, maybe," replies Juyoung, "or it could sound more like this?" This time she sings with a much higher pitch and with a different style to her voice.

"I like that better," call a couple of girls, and the others agree.

"Okay then. Sing along with me." Juyoung sings the second version of the chorus through a number of times, and the group members sing quietly in the background, shy at first, but then gradually growing louder.

Once they become bored of singing the chorus, Juyoung again takes the group back to work on the lyrics—this time focusing on the verses. She encourages them to tell different stories about their own experiences in each verse, and before long the song has six verses to represent each of them. The group practices singing through the chorus and then each group member rapping their own verse. Again, there is some shyness, but the general confidence of the group gradually increases. As the hour-long session comes toward the end, Juyoung suggests they record the song and consider who might be an audience for hearing it.

Creating an original song in a single group session is an impressive effort in music therapy, both for the facilitator and the members. In this case, the music therapist uses a directive approach to facilitate the speed of the process, which is congruent with an expert medical model in which the adult is assumed to know what is best for the young people, who are the recipients of care. The goal has been predetermined and is aligned with the intentions of the medical team, and the topic of the song and focus of the decision making within the songwriting process is deductive. Despite the therapist deciding on the focus, there are still myriad opportunities for choice and control, which illuminates how a humanistic dimension is often integrated into music therapy group work with adolescents.

A less expert-driven approach would take longer, and the therapist would allow the focus to emerge from the material of the young people. Rather than having a pre-set idea about what the song would address, the music therapist could offer inductively derived suggestions, based on what ideas have been produced during brainstorming, both in the words themselves and in the therapist's perception of the meaning behind the words. The more these ideas come from the young people, the better. However, this would involve more space and silence, and the facilitator would be required to hold a sense of discomfort and uncertainty in the group as they contemplate what they might like to focus on and how to do that—in relation to lyrics, style/genre of music, and the details of instrumentation, performance, and every other detail.

As in all group processes, reaching consensus about this might reveal an array of group dynamics between members. Rather than a smooth process where young people end up feeling impressed with what they have managed to achieve, a psychodynamic orientation would foster a range of more complex and authentic responses that reflect the actual dynamics between individuals in the room. These would need to be processed and would require as much attention as the material generated through the songwriting process.

The balance of focus between music and words is always interesting and can vary significantly between therapists and contexts, and depending on the purpose of using songwriting. A more cognitive-behavioral focus demands an emphasis on the intellectual processing of the material, and hence the words would be prioritized. A psychodynamic lens would emphasize what happens between the words and music, particularly in relation to the here-and-now interaction between group members, and facilitate processing of that material. A more humanistic approach would suggest a greater focus on the creative process of composition and performance of the song, where more time was spent in playing the music and jamming on different ideas. It would also lead more readily into the performance of the song to an audience or via recording, which introduces a more ecological orientation that is less centered on the therapy room and more interested in how young people impact their circumstances directly. Taking a recording of the song to the medical team is one way of doing that, and this aspect could have been more emphasized from the beginning of the process, allowing space for the young people to actively protest about their restrictive context and to have their voices heard.

Concluding Comments

This chapter began by providing a historical context for practice and research with adolescents in music therapy groups. The three case illustrations then provide examples of the most common methods used in music therapy groups, although there are many more variations on these approaches than those highlighted. The focus has been on dismantling an assumption that a particular method is most appropriate for a specific goal, instead emphasizing how a combination of theoretical orientation and context shape the ways in which song sharing, improvisation, and songwriting can be used.

The final illustration of songwriting highlights an issue that has been interrogated in music therapy practice around the globe and is related to performance. From a psychodynamic perspective, performance of therapy materials beyond the room generates a range of boundary issues, not least of which has to do with the basic tenet of confidentiality. However, an ecological perspective, which has been highlighted through a discourse on community music therapy, suggests that moving beyond the bounds of the therapy room has several potentials. In particular, musical performance gives voice to adolescents and provides a vehicle for their protests and experiences to be witnessed. It also affords opportunities for development of social and musical capacities that can become a resource beyond the internal experiences of therapy and into the future of the young person. This development can occur both through group members' realization that they can express themselves publicly through musical means, and through a desire to continue to do so, independent of the therapist, through open-mic nights, karaoke experiences, choir participation, or deciding to study an instrument. Thus, while the idea of performance is dangerous and counter-intuitive from a psychodynamic perspective, it holds enormous potential from a humanistic and ecological position.

Another issue highlighted across the three vignettes is related to the length of engagement in therapy. Brief interventions have become common in many of the systems where music therapists meet adolescents. Patients can be discharged from acute pediatric hospitals with minimal notice, meaning that each session needs to be treated as though it could be the last (Yalom, 1983). Inpatient mental health settings are relatively rare for adolescents, since the focus is often on maintaining a connection to family. Workshops are often hosted by community-based organizations who do not perceive a need for ongoing music therapy, but who want to provide creative opportunities for their clientele. Young people themselves may not wish to continue in group therapy for a long time and, when given the choice, are often quite sporadic in their attendance, for a range of reasons. The idea of a group process that extends more than ten weeks is relatively rare in music therapy practice with adolescents, and mostly occurs in school contexts, where the young people are timetabled to attend therapy, often for an entire year. This shortened duration has an impact on what kind of process is facilitated, and a higher degree of structure and directedness by the therapist is often required to manage brief processes.

Finally, it is worth noting that a distinction between different theoretical approaches is useful for reflecting on practice but is necessarily an abstract construct. When practicing, the therapist is usually present and focused on the emerging needs of the adolescent, and therefore moving fluidly and organically between different interactions without pausing to consider whether that statement or action is aligned with a psychodynamic, humanistic, or ecological approach. In our best moments, we transcend any particular theoretical orientation and integrate everything that the therapist knows, both consciously and unconsciously, into the encounter. Reflections on practice and research inform these moments, but they are separate.

The experience of group music therapy has been described by many adolescents as engaging and satisfying. Perhaps more than the therapists themselves, young people have faith in the affordances of music, particularly for emotional expression and the establishment of a sense of identity. They describe feeling better, having fun, and being connected, sometimes despite a therapeutic orientation that might have been more focused on cognitive processing or increasing awareness of unconscious materials. The emphasis on positive regard for young people's capacities to flourish, given conducive circumstances, tends to dominate many music therapy groups and seems to be in response to what young people seek from shared musicking. They want to recover. They need opportunities to feel good about themselves. They love their music.

Although the actual experience of facilitating a music therapy group with adolescents can be draining and confusing for the professional, research shows that the group members typically find it much more helpful than they reveal in the moment. Thus, the music therapy experience reflects the ambiguity of adolescent life quite authentically, and the group therapist who chooses to journey there is often one with great courage and tenacity as well as a shared love of the musical preferences of young people themselves. It can be great fun, and it can be exhausting. Welcome to adolescence.

References

Albornoz, Y. (2011). The effects of group improvisational music therapy on depression in adolescents and adults with substance abuse: A randomized controlled trial. *Nordic Journal of Music Therapy, 20*(3), 208–224.

Bibb, J., & McFerran, K. S. (2018). Musical recovery: The role of group singing in regaining healthy relationships with music to promote mental health recovery. *Nordic Journal of Music Therapy.* Advance online publication. doi: 10.1080/08098131.2018.1432676

Bolger, L. (2015). Understanding collaboration in participatory music projects with communities supporting marginalised young people. *Qualitative Inquiries in Music Therapy, 10*(3), 77–126.

Boswell, B., & Vidret, M. (1993). Rhythmic movement and music for adolescents with severe and profound disabilities. *Music Therapy Perspectives, 11*, 37–41.

Brooks, D. (1989). Music therapy enhances treatment with adolescents. *Music Therapy Perspectives, 6*, 37–39.

Bruscia, K. (1987). *Improvisational models of music therapy.* Springfield, IL: Charles C. Thomas.

Cassity, M. D. (1981). The influence of a socially valued skill on peer acceptance in a music therapy group. *Journal of Music Therapy, 18*(3), 148–154.

Cheong-Clinch, C., & McFerran, K. S. (2016). Musical diaries: Examining the daily preferred music listening of Australian young people with mental illness. *Journal of Applied Youth Studies, 1*(2), 77–94.

Clendenon-Wallen, J. (1991). The use of music therapy to influence the self-confidence and self-esteem of adolescents who are sexually abused. *Music Therapy Perspectives, 9*, 73–81.

Dalton, T. A., & Krout, R. E. (2006). The grief song-writing process with bereaved adolescents: An integrated grief model and music therapy protocol. *Music Therapy Perspectives, 24*, 94–107.

Derrington, P. (2005). Teenagers and songwriting: Supporting students in a mainstream secondary school. In F. Baker & T. Wigram (Eds.), *Songwriting: Methods, techniques and clinical applications for music therapy clinicians, educators and students* (pp. 66–81). London: Jessica Kingsley.

Derrington, P. (2012). *Music therapy for youth at risk: An exploration of clinical practice through research.* (Unpublished doctoral dissertation). Anglia Ruskin University, Cambridge.

Fairchild, R., Thompson, G., & McFerran, K. S. (2016). Exploring the meaning of a performance in music therapy for children and their families experiencing homelessness and family violence. *Music Therapy Perspectives, 35*(1), 36–49.

Flower, C. (1993). Control and creativity: Music therapy with adolescents in secure care. In M. Heal & T. Wigram (Eds.), *Music therapy in health and education* (pp. 40–45). London: Jessica Kingsley.

Gardstrom, S. (2004). An investigation of meaning in clinical music improvisation with troubled adolescents. In B. Abrams (Ed.), *Qualitative inquiries in music therapy: A monograph series* (Vol. 1, pp. 77–105). Gilsum, NH: Barcelona Publishers.

Gold, C., Voracek, M., & Wigram, T. (2004). Effects of music therapy for children and adolescents with psychopathology: A meta-analysis. *Journal of Child Psychology and Psychiatry, 45*(6), 1054–1059.

Hense, C., McFerran, K. S., & McGorry, P. (2014). Constructing a grounded theory of young people's recovery of musical identity in mental illness. *The Arts in Psychotherapy, 41*, 594–603.

Holloway, M. S. (1980). A comparison of passive and active music reinforcement to increase preacademic and motor skills in severely retarded children and adolescents. *Journal of Music Therapy, 17*(2), 58–69.

Hunt, M. (2005). Action research and music therapy: Group music therapy with young refugees in a school community. *Voices: A World Forum for Music Therapy, 5*(2). Retrieved from www.voices.no/mainissues/mi40005000184.html

Lehrer-Carle, I. (1973). Group dynamics as applied to the use of music with schizophrenic adolescents. *British Journal of Music Therapy, 4*(2), 2–10.

Lindberg, K. A. (1995). Songs of healing: Songwriting with an abused adolescent. *Music Therapy, 13*(1), 93–108.

McFerran, K. S. (2001). *The experience of group music therapy for six younger bereaved adolescents.* (Unpublished doctoral dissertation). University of Melbourne, Melbourne, Australia.

McFerran, K. S. (2010a). *Adolescents, music and music therapy: Methods and techniques for clinicians, educators and students.* London: Jessica Kingsley.

McFerran, K. S. (2010b). Tipping the scales: A substantive theory on the value of group music therapy for supporting grieving teenagers. *Qualitative Inquiries in Music Therapy (A Monograph Series), 5*, 2–49.

McFerran, K. S., Baker, F., & Krout, R. (2011). What's in the lyrics? A discussion paper describing the complexities of systematically analysing lyrics in music therapy. *Canadian Journal of Music Therapy, 17*(1), 35–54.

McFerran, K., Baker, F., Patton, G. C., & Sawyer, S. M. (2006). A retrospective lyrical analysis of songs written by adolescents with anorexia nervosa. *European Eating Disorders Review, 14*, 297–403.

McFerran, K. S., & Grocke, D. (2000). What does group music therapy offer to bereaved young people? A rounded approach to the grieving adolescent. *Grief Matters: The Australian Journal of Grief and Bereavement, 3*(3), 54–61.

McFerran, K. S., Hense, C., Koike, A., & Rickwood, D. (2017). Intentional music use to reduce psychological distress in adolescents accessing primary mental health care. Manuscript submitted for publication.

McFerran, K. S., & Hunt, M. (2008). Learning from experiences in action: Music in schools for coping with grief and loss. *Educational Action Research, 16*(1), 43–53.

McFerran, K. S., Roberts, M., & O'Grady, L. (2010). Music therapy with bereaved teenagers: A mixed methods perspective. *Death Studies, 34*(6), 541–565.

McFerran, K. S., & Saarikallio, S. (2013). Depending on music to make me feel better: Who is responsible for the ways young people appropriate music for health benefits. *The Arts in Psychotherapy, 41*(1), 89–97.

McFerran, K. S., & Wigram, T. (2005). Articulating the dynamics of music therapy group improvisations. *Nordic Journal of Music Therapy, 14*(1), 33–46.

McFerran-Skewes, K. (2000). From the mouths of babes: The response of six younger bereaved teenagers to the experience of psychodynamic group music therapy. *Australian Journal of Music Therapy, 11*, 3–22.

Nicholls, T. (2002). 'Could I play a different role?' Group music therapy with severely learning disabled adolescents. In A. Davies & E. Richards (Eds.), *Music Therapy and Group Work—Sound Company* (pp. 231–246). London: Jessica Kingsley.

North, A. C., & Hargreaves, D. J. (2005). Brief report: Labelling effects on the perceived deleterious consequences of pop music listening. *Journal of Adolescence, 28*, 433–440.

Porter, S., Holmes, V., McLaughlin, K., Lynn, F., Cardwell, C., Braiden, H. J., . . . Rogan, S. (2012). Music in mind, a randomized controlled trial of music therapy for young people with behavioural and emotional problems: Study protocol. *Journal of Advanced Nursing, 68*(10), 2349–2358.

Ragland, Z., & Apprey, M. (1974). Community music therapy with adolescents. *Journal of Music Therapy, 11*(3), 147–155.

Rickson, D. J. (2006). Instructional and improvisational models of music therapy with adolescents who have attention deficit hyperactivity disorder (ADHD): A comparison of the effects on motor impulsivity. *Journal of Music Therapy, 43*(1), 39–62.

Robarts, J. Z. (2000). Music therapy and adolescents with anorexia nervosa. *Nordic Journal of Music Therapy, 9*(1), 3–12.

Robb, S. L. (2003). Designing music therapy interventions for hospitalized children and adolescents using a contextual support model of music therapy. *Music Therapy Perspectives, 21*, 27–40.

Roberts, M. (2009). *A mixed-methods content analysis of song lyrics composed by bereaved pre-adolescent children during individual music therapy.* (Unpublished master's thesis). The University of Melbourne, Melbourne, Australia.

Spencer, S. L. (1988). The efficiency of instrumental and movement activities in developing mentally retarded adolescents' ability to follow directions. *Journal of Music Therapy, 25*(1), 44–50.

Tervo, J. (2001). Music therapy for adolescents. *Clinical Child Psychology and Psychiatry, 6*(1), 79–91.

Viega, M. (2008). *Conceptualizing the lived experience of three adolescents through the interpretation of the core metaphors in their preferred music.* (Unpublished master's thesis). Temple University, Philadelphia, PA.

Wang, T. (2008). *Action research: Improving my music therapy practice with hospitalised adolescents through building relationships and meeting their developmental needs.* (Unpublished master's thesis). New Zealand School of Music, Wellington, New Zealand.

Well, N. F., & Stevens, T. (1984). Music as a stimulus for creative fantasy in group psychotherapy with young adolescents. *The Arts in Psychotherapy, 11*, 71–76.

Wölfl, A. (2014). *Gewaltprävention mit Musik: Empirische Wirkungsanalyse eines musiktherapeutischen Projektmodells.* Wiesbaden, Germany: Reichert-Verlag.

Yalom, I. D. (1983). *Inpatient group psychotherapy.* New York, NY: Basic Books.

9

Group Poetry and Writing Therapy With Adolescents

NANCY S. SCHERLONG AND LAURA SANTNER

Introduction

Poetry therapy techniques and elements of therapeutic journal writing can help adolescents in groups to clarify and express issues of identity and belonging, find and use their individual and collective voices, and connect and work with one another to increase engagement and resilience. Literature can offer a "witnessing ear" to some of life's most shameful or isolating problems. Poetry allows for indirect and symbolic expression through the vehicle of metaphor. Through writing, young people can externalize and transform painful introjects, concretize the abstract, and 're-write' their self-perceptions or life stories. Poetry therapy can be utilized with diverse populations and in a variety of settings, including but not limited to: schools, detention centers, hospitals, treatment and recovery programs, community centers, and clinical private practice. Language matters. Throughout this chapter, though the pronouns utilized will be *he* and *she*, it is important that we not restrict others with labels, but instead inquire about each person's pronouns.

Attention will be given to the developmental aspects of group process when using writing, as well as to clinical models of practice. We will offer a brief history of the interactive process of biblio-poetry therapy and its theoretical underpinnings, examine considerations for planning and literature selection, including how to differentially formulate writing activities for teens in groups, and explore an overview of the current literature. Through the presentation of clinical case material and sample session plans, therapists of all disciplines will likely find something of use for their practices.

It is important to note that the fields of therapeutic journal writing and poetry therapy have extensive training programs. We offer an introduction to this work with the foreknowledge that each practitioner will act within the ethics and professional boundaries of his or her education and training. The following clinical exercises are specifically geared toward teens; however, adjustments can be made to tailor activities to suit other age groups as well. Suggestions for clinical consideration and potential pitfalls are explored. Collaboration with a trained poetry or journal therapist (resources can be found at the end of this chapter), as well as creative arts practitioners from other disciplines, may be useful to deepen one's understanding of the method or to troubleshoot difficulties should they arise.

What Is Poetry Therapy?

For centuries, people from a variety of cultures have found healing in both the written and spoken word. Poetry therapy is defined by Mazza (2012), the field's most prolific scholar, as "the use of language, symbol and story in therapeutic, educational, and community-building capacities" (p. 1434). Poetry therapy need not always even include traditional poetic forms and may incorporate examination of song lyrics, contemporary and unstructured verse, and prose or spoken word poems. The field of poetry therapy is currently considered inclusive of biblio-therapy (its root origin) and journal and narrative therapies, although each now has its own distinct training and practice methods (Mazza, 2017).

An Interactive Process

A prominent librarian and one of the original pioneers in the field, Arleen McCarty Hynes, and her daughter Mary Hynes-Berry (1994), added early on that biblio-poetry therapies are "interactive," with a focus on "the triad of participant–literature–facilitator" (p. 11). This configuration differs from the traditional literature-based classroom (Figure 9.1a) where the teacher is the facilitator of the interaction, not the literature itself (Figure 9.1b) (Sawyer, 2013, p. 76–77).

This distinction signifies an important paradigm shift given that many people, but particularly school-aged children, may have experienced shame or criticism about what a work of literature "means" rather than the more personal, dynamic, and therapeutic 'knowing' of what the literature inspires in him or her. In poetry

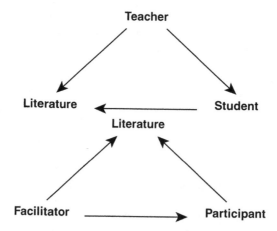

Figure 9.1 Configurations of (a) traditional literature-based classroom and (b) one in which the teacher is the facilitator

© 2013. Joy Roulier Sawyer, from "Liberating Beauty: The Hynes and Hynes-Berry Bibliotherapy Model" in Expressive Writing: Foundations of Practice, K. Adams, Ed. Lanham MD: Rowman & Littlefield Publishing Group.

therapy, the participant's reaction and subjective communication with the literature, as well as with self and other about this felt experience, is paramount and the
cornerstone of its healing power. Hynes and Hynes-Berry (2012) posited that most
therapeutic writing or poetry therapy follows a four-stage sequence of:

- *Recognition* (identification with the theme/literature/self in the group).
- *Examination* (deepening connection: using questions who, what, when, why, how much).
- *Juxtaposition* (comparison, holding of opposites, shifting awareness, expansion).
- *Application to self* (evaluation, integration, and carrying forth into action).

This sequence is a helpful structure to be mindful of when facilitating responses to
literature and serves as a map to guide group interaction.

Theoretical Foundations: A Practice Model of Poetry Therapy (RES)

Poetry therapy's roots in psychological and literary theory are many and deep and
have continued to grow since its formal inception in the early nineteenth century.
Theories from the psychoanalytic, Jungian, Adlerian, cognitive–behavioral, existen-
tial, gestalt, narrative, and constructivist traditions are all present in the progressive
development of the field, which is both interdisciplinary and international (Mazza,
2017). An individual, group, family, or community session may involve any or all of
the following components from Mazza's (1999) RES poetry therapy practice model:

- *Receptive/prescriptive*: Pre-existing poetry/literature sparks the interactive process.
- *Expressive/creative*: Generative writing occurs through a variety of prompts or questions.
- *Symbolic/ceremonial*: Metaphors, ritual, and storytelling enliven and enrich connections.

All of the creative arts therapies share these same thematic elements (Mazza & Hayton, 2013) and can be viewed through this tri-partite lens. More detailed instruction
for applying these components to poetry and journal work with adolescents will
be offered later through clinical vignettes. Most often, discussion and examination
precede writing about a poem or work of art in order to facilitate identification and
a deeper understanding. The writing process may expand or solidify meaning making and personal relevance, frequently extending beyond one's conscious awareness.
The RES model is not necessarily sequential in nature, as both group warm-up and
closure activities may contain elements of ritual or symbolism, as may the reading
or writing portions of sessions.

Overview of Literature

Though 30 years have passed since Pennebaker's landmark study with college students demonstrated a positive correlation between emotional disclosure through

expressive writing and improvement in health and functioning (Pennebaker & Beall, 1986), the research base since then has gained great breadth and depth. Subsequent studies also found health benefits from writing about intensely positive experiences (Burton & King, 2003). There are many additional explorations of the physical, social, and emotional benefits associated with poetry therapy and writing interventions (Adams, 2013a; Mazza, 2017). Particularly significant bodies of work have been written on the interface of expressive writing and trauma (Pennebaker, 2004), resilience (Pennebaker & Evans, 2014), and health improvements and reduction of emotional pain (Pennebaker & Smyth, 2016).

One must be cautious, of course, in generalizing results from studies conducted with adults to teens who have different cognitive, neurological, and developmental aptitudes and concerns. As we cannot provide an overview of all relevant literature, particular attention will be given to studies involving narrative and symbolic methods, interventions with at-risk youth, and specific health effects for adolescents engaged in writing interventions. Narratives, be they verbally, manually, or digitally transferred, are frequently incorporated into counseling interactions with school-aged children to encourage positive identity development and behavior change (Kloser, 2013; Sawyer & Willis, 2011).

According to Jirek (2017), assisting trauma survivors to "create a more coherent narrative, through trauma-related writing, conversation and self-reflection, may encourage the development of post-traumatic growth" (p. 166). One university social work program used a play written by a local child care worker to tap into area foster care teens' writing, speaking, and acting abilities, creating a program called *The Foster Care Chronicles* (Nsonwu, Dennison, & Long, 2015). Another study found a combined art and poetry program to significantly alleviate many symptoms of depression (poetry) and post-traumatic stress disorder (art) in abused adolescents (Brillantes-Evangelista, 2013). With rapidly changing technology and so many ways for one to tell one's story, adolescents may need to be made aware of the potential pitfalls of publication, blogging, and generally going public with a vulnerable story before they are ready for such visibility.

Adolescents appear to glean some positive emotional and physical health effects similar to those gained by adults who participated in prior expressive writing trials. In a study with adolescents diagnosed with asthma, emotional and behavioral symptoms were lessened through written disclosure (Warner et al., 2005, p. 557), conceivably because of a more positive affect and fewer instances of internalizing, factors that may contribute to the exacerbation of a condition like asthma. In another study involving adolescents diagnosed with HIV, participants were reported to have increased self-expression, decreased isolation, and behavioral improvements after participating in the creative writing program *Teens Out Loud* (Fair, Connor, Albright, Wise, & Jones, 2012), although there were concerns about disclosure of such sensitive topics.

In general, it appears that expressive and narrative writing exercises frequently yield positive results "at the level of universal prevention, targeted prevention and intervention levels" (Taylor, Jouriles, Brown, & Goforth, 2016, p. 57). Most participants experienced small but significant reductions in somatic complaints, as well as improved school adjustment, participation, and performance (Travagin, Margola, & Revenson, 2015, p. 53). Few published experimental studies are conducted by trained creative arts practitioners. It is an exciting time to pursue research in poetry therapy and therapeutic writing with an eye toward the specific intervention needs of adolescents.

Why Group?

Creative approaches in group work can concretely facilitate a group's achievement of developmental tasks, from formation and bonding to termination (Gladding, 2016). Innovative interventions that directly involve a young person through activity may increase opportunities for mutual aid and decrease potential difficulties with engagement (Mogro-Wilson, Letendre, Toi, & Bryan, 2013). Group work is the modality of choice for many when working with adolescents. Developmentally, teens have a strong drive toward peer affiliation. Simultaneously, adolescence is an explorative and sometimes divisive period regarding issues of identity and sexuality, values clarification, preparation for the future, and familial individuation/separation (Malekoff, 2014).

Adolescents are most frequently referred to group treatment settings by adults, be they parents or helping professionals. Already feeling disempowered by their lack of independent access to resources, some young people may enter therapy with a fair amount of treatment-resistant behavior. It is helpful if facilitators join with group members in validating their feelings as well as sensitively adapting activities in response to changing needs. There are positive correlations between in-session engagement and productive therapy outcomes both in and out of sessions (Orkibi, Azoulay, Regev, & Snir, 2017). Interactive and creative therapies, with their projective techniques and distancing yet playful devices for identification, can be powerful in lowering such aggression or defensiveness (Shechtman, 2017).

Teens, by nature spontaneous and innovative but sometimes reticent or impacted by traumatic experience, can often be further engaged in group process with the addition of expressive arts activities (Haen, 2015). There are rich opportunities in a group setting to encourage collaborative works, for members to become an observing ego for the other, to provide positive peer support, to enhance empathic listening, and to increase one's repertoire of potential coping skills; the development of a reading or writing practice is just one of them. Groups are social microcosms with rich opportunities to learn social skills, including the incorporation of improved self-concept into transactional peer relations. The multi-layered models of poetry therapy and therapeutic writing provide a doorway through which there are many ways to enter.

Setting the Stage for Writing Interventions

Poetic License: Role of the Facilitator and the Group Members

Whether conducting adjustment-focused, life-stage work or a clinical psychotherapy group, a biblio-therapeutic facilitator should uphold the basic tenets of good counseling: *respect, confidentiality, empathy*, and *genuineness*. Because the interactive process of poetry therapy involves the additional risk of reading (sometimes orally) and writing (sometimes sharing aloud), perhaps most important is the creation of a non-judgmental atmosphere. Members always retain the right to pass up opportunities to read or to share their work. One can always choose to share about the process rather than the content of writing. Providing this option can significantly increase the safety of participation. Poetry therapy is neither a writing workshop nor a setting appropriate for writing critique of any kind, though participants may be deeply moved and comment on one another's images or words. Well facilitated, poetry therapy can help improve the capacity to respond, increase self-understanding, and clarify personal relationships (Hynes & Hynes-Berry, 1986/1994).

Adolescents, with their acute sense of self-consciousness, may be especially hesitant to write, and even more so in a group setting. For this reason, establishing group norms is particularly crucial. At a developmental stage in which the focus of common core instruction is on product more than process and form overrides content, inspiring creative abandonment among young people may be challenging. One tool to assist this is the following "Poetic License," developed by Reiter (2000), an item with which many facilitators begin a first meeting (see Figure 9.2).

This certificate acts as a transitional object to strengthen the therapeutic alliance among members as well as with the facilitator. Therapeutic writing sessions thereby become a forum where young people can experience freedom from many constraints through creativity while still experiencing the safety of structure through

Poetic License

I have the write to use black and white to create or destroy, dream and scheme, transform heroes into villains, and victims into victors, disguise the good, the bad, the happy, the sad. I have the write to turn up into down, and out into in, to turn truth into lie, and good into sin. I surprise, disguise and even use lies whenever I choose, I have the write to conceal or reveal. This poetic license gives me the right to express, to digress, to confess or finesse – and even to jest. Yes, I have the write.

Signature: _____ Date: _____

Figure 9.2 Poetic license

the container of writing. It is not always useful to use the term "poetry therapy" with adolescents as the connotation is restrictive and can be off-putting. Using descriptions such as *writing circle* or *expressive writing group* may result in more effective recruitment of teens. We have found that allowing teens to create a name for the group such as "Write to be Me" may also make membership more inviting to peers. When group attendance is open or voluntary, young people are often the best recruiters of additional group members and can create and distribute flyers about the group's structure, purpose, and next meeting.

One way to foster cooperation, cohesion, and a sense of belonging is to make setting group guidelines a playful task by writing a collaborative poem (Chavis, 2011; Mazza, 2017).

On the first day of a social skills group with adolescent boys ages 11 to 12 years in a local mental health clinic, each boy completed a sentence stem with "this group is _____," adding a quality or hope that he had for how meetings would be conducted and how communication and behavior would be structured. The facilitator acted as scribe, noting their responses on a flip chart at the front of the room. Not only did the poem allow for discussion of some basic ground rules (confidentiality, safety, self-expression), it then became a living document that changed as the group changed, with additions as new guidelines were addressed and incorporated.

Suggestions for Literature Selection

One of the most challenging and complex aspects of poetry therapy practice centers on the issue of planning literature selection and usage (Mazza, 2017). Attunement to themes and needs in the group, both latent and manifest, as well as to the literature's content and form, are ingredients essential to a facilitator's skill set. One will want to have a degree of cultural competence when making selections and an awareness of literacy levels, though many a powerful group has been facilitated with those who cannot read or write by having an assigned scribe or reader.

Some general qualities that make a particular work a good selection include: universality of relatable emotion, clear and understandable language, striking or memorable imagery, compelling rhythm, and adequate complexity (Hynes & Hynes-Berry, 2012). In poetry therapy, the poem serves as an object of projection, a canvas blank enough to invite participants' own experiences, yet rich enough to inspire a feeling response. Poetry therapy pioneer Leedy (1973) emphasized the *iso principle*, borrowed from music therapy, which entails matching or mirroring the client's emotional state while leaving room for an affective shift (Leedy, 1973). Poetry therapists may at times edit out a particularly activating or non-therapeutic element of a work (such as glorification of violence, encouraging suicide, or an ending without hope) and note with an ellipsis that a portion had been omitted and an excerpt has been offered. Practitioners are careful to attribute works to their appropriate authors and sources and mark the bottom of each copy *for educational and/or therapeutic use only* to demonstrate ethical intent.

While specific recommendations are given within clinical exercises later in this chapter, some youth-friendly modern writers to consider include but are not limited to: Julia Alvarez, Billy Collins, Carolyn Forche, Terrance Hayes, Jane Hirsh-field, Cathy Park Hong, Anna Journey, Christopher Soto (Loma), Claudia Rankine, Solmaz Sharif, Naomi Shihab Nye, Shel Silverstein, Natasha Tretheway, and Ocean Vuong. Rap and spoken word poetry have much to offer in therapeutic interventions with youth, particularly rap that positively explores coping skills and solutions (Tyson, 2002). Most powerful is when young people include themselves in the selection process, bringing in works by songwriters and poets that are meaningful to them (Reynaga-Abiko, 2008).

Sample Questions to Prompt Initial Discussion

- *Before even reading it, how does the poem look to you on the page?*
- *Let's read the title. What does it bring to mind?*
- *If you wrote your own poem, with the same title, how would it be different? The same?*
- *Let's read the poem. Let's try reading it again. What does this poem mean for/ to you?*
- *What do you like or not like about it?*
- *Can you relate and do you agree or disagree with the message?*
- *Where do you feel its impact in your body/soul?*
- *Is there an image/section/line that holds particular meaning for you? Which one/why?*
- *What would you say to the author about this poem?*
- *If you were to change how this poem ends, what would your new ending be?*

When and How Do We Write? Structure, Pacing and Containment: The Journal Ladder

Not every poetry therapy session will necessarily involve the inspiration of a poem or work of literature. Sometimes writing itself is the primary intervention. Although journal and poetry therapy have somewhat different approaches and separate training programs, the field of therapeutic journal writing contributes immeasurable clinical wisdom in crafting well-thought-out writing exercises. Adams (1998), journal therapy pioneer, poetry therapist, and founder and director of The Center for Journal Therapy, offers the organizational structure of a ladder, with exercises moving from the most concrete lower rungs (sentence stems) to the most abstract upper ones (free writing). Each technique is described briefly (see Table 9.1) and cast within the larger context of the whole, a journey from information to insight to intuition (see Figure 9.3).

The most commonly used writing technique by therapists without training tends to be free writing, which is the least structured, potentially most overwhelming, and least appropriate first choice for clients struggling with trauma or emotional difficulty. These clients often need containment or titrated activities so as not to become flooded or overwhelmed. Additionally, perhaps one of the most important contributors to meaningful therapeutic outcomes using writing involves the addition of the reflection write (a technique used in Pennebaker's original studies) and the way in which writing to one's self about one's writing inspires the synthesis of awareness, perceptual shifts, and insight (Adams, 2013a).

Sample Session Plans and Clinical Vignettes

The following session plans are examples of what has worked for us in group settings. Please adjust them accordingly to suit your particular setting's requirements, with cultural curiosity and attunement to your clients' readiness for creative work. The exercises also follow a developmental trajectory in terms of the beginning, middle, and end phases of group and address warm-up, activity, and sharing/closure aspects of the session itself.

"I Am" Poetry: Identity Sentence Stems

Goals: Introduction/Inclusion, Concept of a Personal Identity/Voice, Discovering Group Themes

Much has been written about sentence-completion exercises as generative and direct methods to facilitate idea expression (Adams, 1990; Gold, 2014; Koch, 1973; Mazza, 1999). Their pithy, non-threatening format make writing feel and look less intimidating, with an inherent unifying structure that can be ideal for groups. Because each member is able to individually craft his or her own response in silence, this method allows for autonomy and individuation, ultimately improving self-assurance. During the processing/sharing stage, there is rich opportunity for integration and connection. Additional resources are noted at the end of the exercise should you wish to use poems as an introduction to the concept of identity and voice.

Expressive/creative: Provide each group member with paper and pen or pencil. Also have a larger piece of paper available near the front of the group's circle to capture collective responses during sharing for the creation of a collaborative poem. You may use the inventory of statements below (adapted by Santner) or create your own. Allow for 5–7 minutes for individuals to complete the sentence stems. Consider completing your own first as an example

Sharing/closure: Once complete, have participants review their own responses silently and consider what they would like to share with the group (all, part, or none) and mark these sections for ease of reading. With group guidelines of respect, confidentiality, and safety in mind, allow members one at a time to stand and share their declarative "I am" statements.

Encourage participants to listen only, without comment or applause and with the response of "thank you." If the group contains more than six to eight members, you may want to consider having them share first with a partner and then a few selections with the full group. Processing questions might include: *How was that experience? Did you learn anything about yourself or a group member that you didn't know? What was it like to find and hear your own voice?* Processing and sharing can

Table 9.1 The Journal Toolbox: 14 Writing Techniques on the Journal Ladder

Technique on Ladder, Bottom to Top	Description
Sentence Stems	A sentence-completion process. Fill in the blank with a word or phrase. May be very universal (*Right now I feel—*) or highly customized to an individual's immediate question, problem, or interest.
Five-Minute Sprint	A timed writing process designed to bring focus and intensity in short bursts. Excellent for those who are resistant or aversive to journal writing, or who are uncertain about how to start, or who state they do not have time to write journals.
Inventory	A problem-solving/goal-setting approach to quickly identify an area of difficulty, the goal or vision for resolution, and a brainstormed list of action steps to take.
Structured Write	A series of Sentence Stems grouped and sequenced to reveal consistently deepening layers of information and awareness.
Clustering	Visual free-association from a central word or phrase. Lines and circles connect key thoughts and associations to the central core. Work quickly to maximize results. Cluster until a felt-sense shift (usually 3–7 minutes), then switch to a 5-minute sprint to synthesize findings.
List of 100	A list of 100 items, many of which will probably be repetitions, on a predetermined theme or topic. Repetition is an important part of the process. Topics can be about any current issue (for example: 100 Things I'm Sad About; 100 Things I Need or Want to Do; 100 Places I Would Like to See). At the end of the list, group the responses into themes or topics and count up entries for each.
Alpha Poem	Write the alphabet, A–Z, or any collection of letters, vertically down the side of a

Technique on Ladder, Bottom to Top	Description
	page. Then write a poem in which each successive line begins with the next letter. Alternatively, use a word or phrase as the poem's spine. Excellent for groups as it promotes a high level of participation and sharing. Adolescents and reluctant writers respond well.
Captured Moments	Vignettes capturing the sensations of a particularly meaningful or emotional experience. Written from the senses with strong descriptors. Captured Moments of beauty, joy, blessing, calm can add balance, hope, and perspective to a challenging time.
Unsent Letter	A metaphoric communication to another that is written with the specific intention that it will not be shared.
Character Sketch	A written portrait of another person, an aspect of the self, or an intangible such as an emotion or an obstacle. Describe outward appearance as well as actual or imagined personality characteristics, motivations, fears, needs, desires, etc.
Dialogue	A metaphoric conversation written in two voices. Anyone or anything is an appropriate dialogue partner. There is no constriction by time, space, physical reality, or literal voice (Prog off 1992).
Perspectives	An alteration in point of view that provides a different perspective on an event or situation.
Springboards	A free-write with a prompt (question, thought, focus). Otherwise, no structure, pacing, or containment.
Free Writing	Unboundaried, unstructured, unpaced narrative writing. Useful for creative flow or spontaneous writing sessions. Can be structured by adding a time limit or page limit.

© 2013. Kathleen Adams LPC, from "The Journal Ladder" in *Expressive Writing: Foundations of Practice*, K. Adams, Ed. Lanham MD: Rowman & Littlefield Publishing Group. Adapted from Adams, K., Writing as Therapy, *Counseling and Human Development*. Denver: Love Publishing, Jan 1999

(Adapted from Adams 1999)

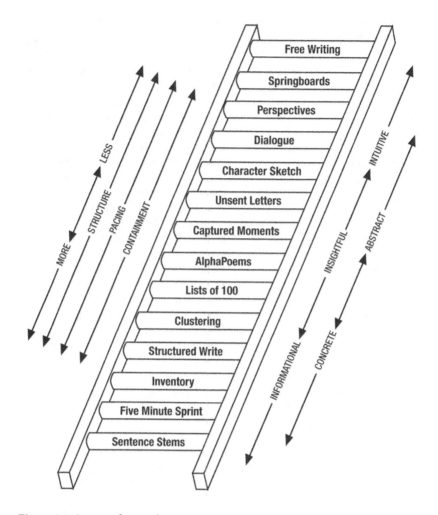

Figure 9.3 Journey from information to insight to intuition

be done verbally or in writing, or both. As the facilitator, capture and share group themes, careful to pay equal attention to each member.

I am (your name) _____ I am from (place) _____
I am (relationship to another person) _____
I am like (compare to an object) _____ because _____
I am (two characteristics) _____ and _____
I believe life is _____ I value _____
I hope to _____ I try to _____
I often dream about _____
I am (adjective) _____ and my name is _____

This is also an exercise that can be repeated over time as self-perception is a dynamic construct. There is a unifying and equalizing quality to having each group member following the same structure, even if some may not choose to share their responses in full.

Clinical Vignette: *In a suburban school of 120 12- and 13-year-olds, a variation of this exercise was used in coordinating an assembly project about identity and development called "Being 13." As a push-in to the English curriculum on poetry and language arts, all students were supplied a worksheet including statements like "You see that I _____ but you don't know me. You would know me if _____ you knew how hard it was _____ or you knew how I sometimes feel _____" (Gold, 2014, p. 58). The program was inclusion-based and offered workshop space to every student in crafting their pieces and in practicing their performances. On the third day, a school assembly was held for the entire grade and related staff. Every student performed in some way, whether by reading a title only, choosing a stand-in reader, or by writing and performing collaboratively, some in rap form. This experience was a good example of creative flexibility. The event would have been valued differently had students who chose a reader or written a title only been viewed as resistant or noncompliant. In this case, students felt supported and encouraged toward individualized and differential participation, allowing their unique voices to be heard.*

Additional resources on this theme: There are many poems available on the theme of identity and claiming one's name. A few to explore include: "My Name" by Sandra Cisneros (1984), Emily Dickinson's (1976) "I'm Nobody! Who Are You?," "Ego Tripping" by Nikki Giovanni (1973), George Ella Lyon's (1999) "Where I'm From," "If I Had Been Called Sabrina or Ann, She Said" by Marge Piercy (1985), and Philip Schultz's (2007) "What I Like and Don't Like."

What's Your Credo?: Symbolic Life Metaphors

Goals: Building Connections, Values Clarification, Introduction to the Concept of Resilience

Adolescence is a particularly crucial time for young people to examine and clarify values. They are often attempting to individuate and separate from parental and societal influences in order to affiliate more with peer groups. The following exercise is inspired by a writing project in which high school seniors identify the laws or values by which they live (Banyard, Hamby, & Grych, 2016; Stepney, Elias, & Epstein, 2015; Templeton, 1994) as well as the tenets of positive psychology in wellness coaching (Arloski, 2014). All the creative arts build on the concept of metaphoric identification and communication (Dean & Landis, 2017; Mazza & Hayton, 2013), and the uses and power of metaphor in psychotherapy has been lauded for decades.

Symbolic/ceremonial: This activity can follow the aforementioned *I Am* exercise or can stand alone. Brainstorm with the group on a chalkboard or flip chart (or use prior results from their sentence completions) responses to the statement: life is _____. Common metaphors or themes that may arise will likely include: life is a race, a battle, a journey, a stage, a test, or an adventure. Many may sound cliché, and that is fine as the exercise will serve to allow for personalization.

Receptive/prescriptive: If your group is open to movement and is large enough (eight or more participants), choose three or four of the metaphors and place each on a sign taped to various locations around the room. Instruct members to take a moment to reflect and then select a sign to stand under that represents their most commonly held life view. Subgroups will form, so you will need to allow for a brief discussion period (no more than three or four minutes) with members responding to questions such as: *Why did you choose this position? From whom/what did you obtain this life view? Does this life view fit your life now?* As a facilitator, you may need to encourage member distribution with a rule such as no more than three people under each sign so that the entire group is not gathered in one location. Allow group members to make a second choice based on a life view that they hold less frequently and to discuss with subgroup members, noting how it feels to have chosen a different position.

Expressive/creative: After returning to their seats, allow for a five-minute writing sprint where there is reflection about their two choices. You might encourage them to choose two of the following possible prompts for writing: *What was it like to complete this exercise? What was it like to share your views with others? Hear theirs? Do the two choices you made inform each other or change your life-law for today? How would you change your choices now? Is there a larger story connected to the life-law you chose or are holding right now in this moment? Maybe a difficult time you had or overcame? If so, note what the title of that story would be.*

Sharing/closure: To deepen this exercise, ask participants to re-read their own writing and to write a two- to three-minute self-reflection about either the content, the process, something that surprised them, or how this activity will impact their interactions with others as they move through their day. Verbal sharing and closure may include spoken reflections about the exercise, reading aloud one's responses, sharing the reflection writing, or sharing a one-word summary or reaction. It is important to give everyone an opportunity to share at whatever level he or she chooses. This is an exercise that can be repeated over time and expanded to demonstrate the nature of changing values based on members' life experiences.

Clinical Vignette: *In an urban outpatient clinic, a group of 18 severely and persistently mentally ill adolescents explored the metaphor of "what is life?" They began with discussion of the question "When you think about what life is, what do you think?" Then participants performed an internet search to find quotations about the meaning of life. They were asked to use the sentence stem "Life is____" for their own writing, with encouragement to incorporate a word or line(s) from items they found. Those requiring more structure were advised to write an acrostic, a poetic device that spells out a word vertically and then uses each beginning letter to create a new line (Collom & Noethe, 2005). Participants wrote and shared, providing each other with support and encouragement. They exhibited active listening skills and remained positive. The group chose to end the session with the following collaboratively constructed group poem:*

> *Life is beautiful like a rose, it is about learning new things*
> *It is a struggle and a sense of humor*
> *It is joy, fate, good, fantastic, hard*
> *It has its ups and downs but it is what it is*
> *Have forgiveness, life is using your mind, it is forever.*

Facilitator focus was not on traditional grammar and punctuation, as the emphasis is on the creative and therapeutic process. The exercise was well received by the group, with members citing an increased level of relaxation and motivation.

Additional resources/ideas on this theme: Lessons on life metaphors may create an opening for accompanying art activities. Participants may create thematic collages or journal covers with selected scrapbook materials or magazine words/pictures and preserve them with clear adhesive book covers as laminate.

Defenses and Coats of Armor: Lists and Directions

Goals: Creating Awareness, Exploring Relationship With Self/Others, Working Through Anger

Adolescence is a time of rapid growth, change, and development and can leave many teens feeling ill equipped to handle the resultant myriad physiological, psychological, and social stressors (Hutchison, 2011). This lack of readiness for coping may weaken their already compromised defense systems. In times challenged with unspeakable violence, bullying, and a thinner veil than ever between adulthood and adolescent responsibility, creating space and giving voice to unexpressed fears and anger is even more crucial. Writing and poetry can serve as the containers to hold these sometimes overwhelming experiences and as an introduction to additional, deeper conversations.

Warm-up/ceremonial: Build an emotional vocabulary by brainstorming a list of feeling words on a board that the group can see. Invite conversation, without evaluation or judgment, about stereotypes regarding which feelings are easiest or most difficult for people to manage and why. Allow for a five-minute sprint write so that each person has private expression time and a two-minute reflection write to glean any particular relevance or meaning. The results can be shared in community or not, depending upon time.

Receptive/prescriptive: Using the poem "*Directions to the Armorer*" by Elder Olson (1959), have two different readers read the poem aloud for variety. Though it cannot be reprinted in full here, this is a poem in which a man has a conversation with an armorer, requesting a sword and shield and set of armor for protection, later realizing some of the needed protection is internal (Adams & Rojcewicz, 2003). Engage the group in discussion using some of the following questions, or craft your own: *What do you think of the directions to the armorer? Are they clear? What does the speaker really want? Do you have a favorite line or image? Why? Where do you relate most to the poem? What more could you say about that?* If you are going to have the group do some writing, here is a good time to shift their focus toward personalizing and deepening their responses.

Expressive/creative: This poem presents many possible options for writing. Because the topic is emotionally big and potentially charged, writing structures from the bottom or middle rungs of the Journal Ladder may be most appropriate. Good choices for structure would be list making, stepping stones, or *clustering* (a graphic form of brainstorming or mind-mapping). There is also a poetic device centering around recipe writing (Collom & Noethe, 2005) wherein participants could write a set of directions to his or her own imagined armorer.

Some potential questions for timed writes (of about 10–12 minutes) that could result in lists or clusters might include: *What kind of armor do you have or need? What does it look like? How does your armor help you? What feelings or situations or people do you need protection from? How do you currently protect or shield yourself from what bothers you? What changes would you like to make in how you do things? Are there ways in which you are your own enemy? Who or what can help you with your enemies?* Caution: there is a chance that this exercise, though therapeutic and powerfully useful, can call forth painful introjects. It is for this reason in a group setting that shortened writing and warm-up times are recommended for emotional regulation.

Symbolic/ceremonial: This activity opens itself nicely to artwork in the creation and decoration of shields as a form of extended and concrete metaphor.

Sharing/closure: Invite participants to re-read their own writing, providing them with an additional two- to three-minute time to write a self-reflection. This reflection could center on what most surprised them, a reaction to the overall exercise, a new realization about their defenses, self-advice, or a kinesthetic reaction to any part of the exercise. Reminding the group of behavioral ground rules for sharing, save at least 15 minutes for sharing one's writing or reflections and to process activity closure.

Clinical Vignette: *In an inpatient psychiatric unit, a small group of ten clinically depressed male and female adolescents, ages 14–18, explored the theme of masks. The session began with brainstorming the topic of hiding the self. The group read and discussed the poem "Hiding in the Mask" by Ellen Bauer (1999), a poem formatted on the page in two vertical columns and designed to be read in two voices. First, two males read the poem aloud, and then two females. The group expressed a desire to hear it read from multiple perspectives in exploration of the inner and outer self. Participants felt comfortable writing and sharing, taking off their own "masks," and were receptive to feedback and peer support. They discussed the need for and purpose of defense mechanisms and what allows us to take the risk to be vulnerable.*

Additional resources/ideas on this theme: Two classic poems on the theme of defenses/masks are Stephen Crane's (reprinted, 1970) "If I Should Cast Off This Tattered Coat" and Paul Laurence Dunbar's (reprinted, 2010) "We Wear the Mask."

The lyrics from "Fight Song" by Rachel Platten (2015) have also provided additional inspiration to teens throughout exploration of this theme. The conversational tone of writing recipe directions also lends itself to performance or spoken word poetry, a form sometimes more appealing for teens. Facilitator openness to integrating items from youth culture increases engagement and teens' ability to create work that is relevant and therapeutically meaningful to them.

Conversations with Grief: Dialogue, Letters and Character Sketches

Goals: Externalization, Extended Metaphor, Psychoeducation on the Grieving Process

The process of development itself is marked by continuous loss and gain. Many young people face tremendous grief as a consequence of divorce, relocation, illness, physical death of a loved one or pet, or consequences of substance use or peer suicide, to name just a few. Adolescents experience grief as profoundly personal and may continue to be affected by its impact throughout several subsequent developmental stages. Because of grief's heightened impact on teens, the continuity and connection offered by creative arts approaches in a group setting are especially powerful (Slyter, 2012).

Warm-up/ceremonial: Brainstorm different types of grief (you may choose to capture them for the group as a list poem). Allow each member to name one thing/person lost and a response/feeling word. If you have time to pre-plan this activity, it can be helpful to encourage each member to bring a totem like a photo, coin, or jewel that signifies the connection as a touchstone for talking, for symbolic interaction and as a way to decrease object loss.

Receptive/prescriptive: Using the poem "Talking to Grief" by Denise Levertov (1982), have participants read it aloud. You may want to change readers by stanzas or proceed until he or she hits end punctuation, or even try having the group read it in unison. For optimal response, read the work twice to allow the imagery to settle in. The poem describes a woman who is treating her grief like a homeless dog, though she is aware that it belongs to her, needs a home, and is living under her porch.

Although this is an abstract poem that makes use of extended metaphor, many teens of various ages can relate to the notion of personifying a feeling or an animal representing their difficulty, or joy. Allow for some time to discuss the poem and react to its imagery. Some possible questions might include: *What kind of animal is your grief? Where is it now? What is it trying to say to you? What do you have to say to it? What do you think it needs or wants from you? What helps you to get distance or relief from your pain?* (This will likely bring up both healthy and unhealthy coping skills.)

Expressive/creative: Writing in response to this poem can take many forms. Some teens may wish to write a dialogue with their grief, using the poem as an example, taking turns between the voice of the self and the voice of the grief. Others may prefer to craft an unsent letter to the person/place/thing that they are missing, expressing all that has been left unspoken. And still others may wish to create a character to represent their grief, personifying features and personality characteristics. An excellent resource guide for examples of 78 different feeling states portrayed as characters is Gendler's (1988) *Book of Qualities*.

As this is more of a process piece, you will want to allow a timeframe long enough for expression (15–20 minutes) but not so long that emotional flooding occurs. It may be wise to have a brief conversation about positive coping skills (some of which may have been generated in the discussion portion) in preparation for writing. Prompt participants as they near the end of the writing time (with five minutes left) to bring their work to closure and to say the last things that need saying so they are feeling more complete at time's end.

Sharing/closure: Encourage the participants to re-read what they have written. Allow three minutes for reflection writing and identification of a section of writing they may like to share. With reminders about group guidelines, invite and note the range of responses. Many groups create a group poem representative of the theme at a final session. Creating a composite *Grief Is* poem and distributing copies to members honors the diverse range of responses while creating a transitional object and keepsake for members to carry forward once the group has adjourned.

Clinical Vignette: *In a transitional foster care facility, this exercise was used during a multi-gender sibling grief group with nine teens ages 13 to 17 years possessing myriad concrete and ambiguous losses. In addition to writing, the teens decided they wished to perform their pieces. Those who wrote letters chose to read them aloud to an empty chair or picked a group member to hold the role of the lost person/place/situation. Those who wrote dialogue either played both roles using different nonverbal positions and body postures or chose a partner actor. Those creating character sketches chose to embody their character in a brief monologue. One member was not comfortable with performance, so held the role of audience and participated fully in the processing. Enactment provided an additional opportunity for release and nervous system completion for those who felt comfortable. Members were also invited to speak briefly from the role of other, making certain to end their piece in their own role with last remarks.*

Additional resources/ideas on this theme: As providing multiple perspectives is often facilitative for healing traumatic grief and loss, an additional activity includes either writing or performing from a past or future position such as one year ago or five years into the future. A few additional poems on the theme of loss include: Denise Levertov's (1967) "The Fountain," "The Peace of Wild Things" by Wendell Berry (1984), "Autumn" by Rainer Marie Rilke (1995), and "The Rainy Day" by Henry Wadsworth Longfellow (1842).

Concluding Comments

Group poetry and therapeutic writing are expressive art forms that can serve as either a therapeutic adjunct or a primary modality, when facilitated within one's scope of practice and training (Haen, 2015). The powerful and forgiving nature of poetry's metaphors and the complexity of its juxtapositions allow teens a place to explore ambivalence, enhance self-esteem, and increase positive coping and distress tolerance. The group writing experience can therefore be both containing and expansive, allowing for individual and collaborative expression. Though research indicates that expressive writing with adolescents often tends to produce improvements in well-being, more specific study is warranted, with increasingly diverse populations and in a variety of settings.

Online Resources and Support

Poetry and Journal Therapy Organizations/Training

International Federation for Biblio/Poetry Therapy: ifbpt.org

National Association for Poetry Therapy: www.poetrytherapy.org

The Center for Journal Therapy: www.journaltherapy.com

Therapeutic Writing Institute: twinstitute.net

Poetry and Literature

Academy of American Poets:
www.poets.org/academy-american-poets/home

Button Performance Poetry:
buttonpoetry.com

Lyric finder:
www.lyricfinder.org

Poetry Foundation:
www.poetryfoundation.org

Poetry Spoken Here:
www.poetryspokenhere.com

Poets.org:
www.poets.org

Power Poetry:
www.powerpoetry.org

Teen Ink:
www.teenink.com/poetry

Yellow Rage Spoken Word Poetry:
www.yellowrage.com

Writing Resource Programs/Projects

Healing Story Alliance:
www.healingstory.org

Pongo Teen Writing Project:
www.pongoteenwriting.org

Public Domain Poetry:
www.public-domain-poetry.com

Writer's Corps:
Bronx www.bronxarts.org;
Washington DC www.dcwriterscorps.org;
San Francisco www.writerscorps-sf.org

Teachers and Writers Collaborative:
www.twc.org

Transformative Language Arts Network:
TLANetwork.org

Academic Journals

Journal of Creativity in Mental Health (Routledge):
www.tandfonline.com/loi/wcmh20

Journal of Poetry Therapy (Routledge):
www.tandfonline.com/toc/tjpt20/current

Psychology of Aesthetics, Creativity and the Arts (APA):
www.apa.org/pubs/journals/aca

The Arts in Psychotherapy (Elsevier):
www.journals.elsevier.com/the-arts-in-psychotherapy

References

Adams, K. (1990). *Journal to the self: 22 paths to personal growth.* New York, NY: Warner.

Adams, K. (1998). *The way of the journal: A journal therapy workbook for healing.* Lutherville, MD: Sidran.

Adams, K. (2013a). *Expressive writing: Foundations of practice.* Lanham, MD: Rowman & Littlefield.

Adams, K. (2013b). The journal ladder. In K. Adams (Ed.), *Expressive writing: Foundations of practice* (pp. 43–51). Lanham, MD: Rowman & Littlefield.

Adams, K., & Rojcewicz, S. (2003). Mindfulness on the journey ahead. In G. G. Chavis & L. L. Weisberger (Eds.), *The healing fountain: Poetry therapy for life's journey* (pp. 7–35). St. Cloud, MN: North Star Press.

Arloski, M. (2014). *Wellness coaching for lasting lifestyle change* (2nd ed.). Duluth, MN: Whole Person Associates.

Banyard, V., Hamby, S., & Grych, J. (2016). Using values narratives to promote youth well-being in schools: An exploratory quantitative evaluation of the Laws of Life Essay. *School Social Work Journal, 40*(2), 1–16.

Bauer, E. (1999). Hiding in the mask. *University Alaska Anchorage/Alaska Dispatch News creative writing contest.* Retrieved from www.litsite.org/data/index.cfm?fa=article&ContentId=1297.

Berry, W. (1984). The peace of wild things. In *Collected poems of Wendell Berry, 1957–1982* (p. 69). New York, NY: Harper Collins.

Brillantes-Evangelista, G. (2013). An evaluation of visual arts and poetry as therapeutic interventions with abused adolescents. *The Arts in Psychotherapy, 40*(1), 71–84.

Burton, C. M., & King, L. A. (2003). The health benefits of writing about intensely positive experiences. *Journal of Research in Personality, 38*(2), 150–163.

Chavis, G. (2011). *Poetry and story therapy: The healing power of creative expression.* London: Jessica Kingsley.

Cisneros, S. (1984). My name. In *The house on mango street* (pp. 10–11). Houston, TX: Arte Pubilico Press.

Collom, J., & Noethe, S. (2005). *Poetry everywhere: Teaching poetry writing in school and in the community* (2nd ed.). New York, NY: Teachers & Writer's Collaborative.

Crane, S. (1970). If I should cast off this tattered coat. In A. Dore (Ed.), *The premier book of major poets* (p. 288). Greenwich, CT: Fawcett. (Original work published 1895)

Dean, M. E., & Landis, H. (2017). Creative arts based approaches with adolescent groups. In C. Haen & S. Aronson (Eds.), *Handbook of child and adolescent group therapy: A practitioner's reference* (pp. 124–136). New York, NY: Routledge.

Dickinson, E. (1976). I'm nobody! Who are you? In T. H. Johnson (Ed.), *The Complete Poems of Emily Dickinson* (p. 288). New York, NY: Doubleday. (Original work published 1890)

Dunbar, P. L. (2010). We wear the mask. In W. J. Harrell Jr. (Ed.), *Dunbar and the politics of representative reality.* Kent, OH: Kent State University Press (poem in public domain).

Fair, C. D., Connor, L., Albright, J., Wise, E., & Jones, K. (2012). I'm positive, I have something to say: Assessing the impact of a creative writing group for adolescents living with HIV. *The Arts in Psychotherapy, 39*(5), 383–389.

Gendler, J. R. (1988). *The book of qualities.* New York, NY: Harper Collins.

Giovanni, N. (1973). Ego-tripping. In *Ego-tripping and other poems for young people* (pp. 3–5). New York, NY: Lawrence Hill.

Gladding, S. T. (2016). *Groups: A counseling specialty* (7th ed.). Boston, MA: Pearson.

Gold, R. (2014). *Writing with at-risk youth: The pongo teen writing method.* Lanham, MD: Rowman & Littlefield.

Haen, C. (2015). Fostering change when safety is fleeting: Expressive therapy groups for adolescents with complex trauma. In N. B. Webb (Ed.), *Play therapy with children and adolescents in crisis* (4th ed., pp. 239–256). New York, NY: Guilford.

Hutchison, E. D. (2011). *Dimensions of human behavior: Person and environment* (4th ed.). Thousand Oaks, CA: Sage.

Hynes, A., & Hynes-Berry, M. (1994). *Bibliotherapy—The interactive process: A handbook* (2nd ed.). St. Cloud, MN: North Star Press.

Hynes, A. M., & Hynes-Berry, M. (2012). *Biblio-poetry therapy: The interactive process: A handbook* (3rd ed.). St. Cloud, MN: North Star Press.

Jirek, S. L. (2017). Narrative reconstruction and post-traumatic growth among trauma survivors: The importance of narrative in social work research and practice. *Qualitative Social Work, 16*(2), 166–188.

Kloser, K. (2013). Positive youth development through the use of poetry therapy: The contributing effects of language arts in mental health counseling with school-age children. *Journal of Poetry Therapy, 26*(4), 237–253.

Koch, K. (1973). *Rose, where did you get that red?* New York, NY: Random House.

Leedy, J. J. (1973). *Poetry the healer.* Philadelphia, PA: Lippincott.

Levertov, D. (1967). The fountain. In *Denise Levertov poems 1960–1967* (p. 57). New York, NY: New Directions.

Levertov, D. (1982). Talking to grief. In *Denise Levertov poems 1972–1982* (p. 111). New York, NY: New Directions.

Longfellow, H. W. (1842). The rainy day. In *Ballads and other poems* (p. 19). Cambridge: J. Owen.

Lyon, G. E. (1999). Where I'm from. In *Where I'm from: Where poems come from* (p. 3). Spring, TX: Absey.

Malekoff, A. (2014). *Group work with adolescents: Principles and practice* (3rd ed.). New York, NY: Guilford.

Mazza, N. (1999). *Poetry therapy: Interface of the arts and psychology.* Boca Raton, FL: CRC Press.

Mazza, N. (2012). Therapy and poetry. In R. Greene & S. Cushman (Eds.), *The Princeton encyclopedia of poetry and poetics* (pp. 1434–1435). Princeton, NJ: Princeton University Press.

Mazza, N. (2017). *Poetry therapy: Theory and practice* (2nd ed.). New York, NY: Routledge.

Mazza, N., & Hayton, C. (2013). Poetry therapy: An investigation of a multidimensional clinical model. *The Arts in Psychotherapy, 40*(1), 53–60.

Mogro-Wilson, C., Letendre, J., Toi, H., & Bryan, J. (2013). Utilizing mutual aid in reducing adolescent substance use and developing group engagement. *Research on Social Work Practice, 25*(1), 129–138.

Nsonwu, M. B., Dennison, S., & Long, J. (2015). Foster care chronicles: Use of the arts for teens aging out of the foster care system. *Journal of Creativity in Mental Health, 10*(1), 18–33.

Olson, E. (1959, November 14). Directions to the armorer. *The New Yorker* (p. 191). Retrieved from www.newyorker.com/magazine/1959/11/14/directions-to-the-armorer

Orkibi, H., Azoulay, B., Regev, D., & Snir, S. (2017). Adolescents' dramatic engagement predicts their in-session productive behaviors: A psychodrama change process study. *The Arts in Psychotherapy, 55*, 46–53.

Pennebaker, J. W. (2004). *Writing to heal: A guided journal for recovering from trauma and emotional upheaval.* Oakland, CA: New Harbinger.

Pennebaker, J. W., & Beall, S. K. (1986). Confronting a traumatic event: Toward an understanding of inhibition and disease. *Journal of Abnormal Psychology, 95*(3), 274–281.

Pennebaker, J. W., & Evans, J. F. (2014). *Expressive writing: Words that heal.* Enumclaw, WA: Idyll Arbor.

Pennebaker, J. W., & Smyth, J. M. (2016). *Opening up by writing it down* (3rd ed.). New York, NY: Guilford.

Piercy, M. (1985). If I had been called Sabrina or Ann, she said. In *My mother's body* (p. 122). New York, NY: Knopf.

Platten, R. (2015). Fight song. On *Wildfire* [record]. New York, NY: Columbia Music Label.

Reiter, S. (2000). *The creative "righting": A curriculum guidebook for the helping professional.* Cincinnati, OH: Union Institute Graduate College.

Reynaga-Abiko, G. (2008). Culturally competent group therapy with Latina adolescents and young adults with eating disturbance: The use of poetry and music. In S. Brooke (Ed.), *The creative therapies and eating disorders* (pp. 159–172). Springfield, IL: Charles C. Thomas.

Rilke, R. M. (1995). Autumn day. In *Ahead of all parting: The selected poetry and prose of Rainer Maria Rilke* (p. 15). New York, NY: Harper & Row.

Sawyer, C. B., & Willis, J. M. (2011). Introducing digital storytelling to influence the behavior of children and adolescents. *Journal of Creativity in Mental Health, 6*(4), 274–283.

Sawyer, J. R. (2013). Liberating beauty: The Hynes and Hynes-Berry bibliotherapy model. In K. Adams (Ed.), *Expressive writing: Foundations of practice* (pp. 69–87). Lanham, MD: Rowman & Littlefield Education.

Schultz, P. (2007). What I like and don't like. In *Failure* (p. 31). San Diego, CA: Harcourt.

Shechtman, Z. (2017). Group intervention with aggressive children and youth through bibliotherapy. *International Journal of Group Psychotherapy, 67*(1), 47–67.

Slyter, M. (2012). Creative counseling interventions for grieving adolescents. *Journal of Creativity in Mental Health, 7*(1), 17–34.

Stepney, C. T., Elias, M. J., & Epstein, Y. M. (2015). What's important to me: Identifying at-risk and resilient students through narrative writing about personal values. *Journal of Character Education, 11*, 129–147. Retrieved from www.character.org

Taylor, E., Jouriles, E. N., Brown, R., & Goforth, K. (2016). Narrative writing exercises for promoting health among adolescents: Promises and pitfalls. *Psychology of Violence, 6*(1), 57–63.

Templeton, J. M. (1994). *Discovering the laws of life.* West Conshohocken, PA: Templeton Foundation Press.

Travagin, G., Margola, D., & Revenson, T. A. (2015). How effective are expressive writing interventions for adolescents? A meta-analytic review. *Clinical Psychology Review, 36*, 42–55.

Tyson, E. H. (2002). Hip hop therapy: An explanatory study of a rap music intervention with at-risk delinquent youth. *Journal of Poetry Therapy, 15*(3), 131–144.

Warner, L. J., Lumley, M. A., Casey, R. J., Pierantoni, W., Salazar, R., Zoratti, E., . . . Simon, M. R. (2005). Health effects of written emotional disclosure in adolescents with asthma: A randomized, controlled trial. *Journal of Pediatric Psychology, 31*(6), 557–568.

Section 3
Clinical Applications

10

Creative Arts-Based Approaches to Working With Adolescent Resistance

HEIDI LANDIS AND BRITTON WILLIAMS

Introduction

It's the first day of my (HL) new job and I'm beginning four new drama therapy groups with high school students. The staff is excited to have a drama therapist on staff and ready for the students to be "fixed" with the groups. In fact, they are so excited that they have been fighting over which classrooms get to have group first. The desks have been moved out of the way, the chairs are set in a circle, the teacher in the room smiles as the first bell rings.

Alex walks into the room, slams his backpack on one of the pushed-away desks, takes the chair out of the circle and places it back behind the desk, sits in it and puts his head down. Jose and Steven enter playfully talking, but stop when they see the chairs in a circle and roll their eyes. Jose grabs a bathroom pass and exits loudly. Marco pushes open the door and then walks back out again exclaiming, "Aw, hell no." As the rest of the group enters, some reluctantly take seats in the circle, some sit at the perimeter of the room, some pretend they don't see me, and some ask the teacher if they can get a computer to work on. I smile on the outside and panic on the inside.

When we think about adolescence, we can often think about resistance as a normal developmental rite of passage. However, in group work many clinicians often feel stuck when resistance enters the room. This chapter provides an overview of how to work with adolescent resistance in group treatment. Current research, viewpoints, and practice methods on utilizing the creative arts therapies to work with resistance are explored. Clinicians will learn creative arts-based approaches and interventions for working through and with resistance in adolescent groups.

What Is Resistance Anyway?

As noted by Stauss (2009), Freud (1912/2010) gave birth to the discussion of resistance in treatment; he theorized that as unconscious memories began to move to the surface, patient resistance was an attempt to avoid painful feelings (Freud, 1923/2010). Freud (1900/2010) furthered that "whatever interrupts the progress of analytic work is a resistance" (p. 517). Freud's original theories of resistance have been elaborated on by a multitude of theorists and practitioners across and throughout the mental health field. While the historical viewpoint of resistance has been a "judgmental" stance (Altman, Briggs, Frankel, Gensler, & Pantone, 2010) that suggests the client is somehow avoiding or blocking treatment, others (Bischoff & Tracey, 1995; Kemper, 1994; Newman, 1994) have broadened this perspective and characterized resistance as an indication of progress or valuable information in treatment. Rogers (1951) offered a client-centered viewpoint that asserted resistance was not an inherent aspect of therapy but possibly the result of the therapist's mis-attunements, lack of skills in working with the client, and desire to rush certain aspects of treatment that the client is not yet prepared to explore.

Pushing against the idea that resistance "interrupts" the treatment allows the clinician to consider every action or inaction as important information regarding who the client is and what they need. Discussing and exploring the most sensitive and challenging experiences of one's life can feel and indeed be threatening to adolescents, who are also deep in the process of trying to discover who they are and how they fit into the world around them. For teens with mental health challenges and/or a history of trauma, the distress of disclosure might be compounded. Resistance can manifest in myriad ways from passive engagement in the group and refusal to participate, to verbal and physical aggression toward the facilitator(s) and/or members. The behaviors associated with resistance quite often signal the need for additional warm-up (Emunah, 1994) and deeper establishment of trust (Malekoff, 2016). Clinicians have found that adolescent clients have a desire to share and engage in therapy; however, for this to happen, therapists must be adept at establishing a safe enough space for clients to engage (Barker & Crenshaw, 2011). It is important that adolescent group leaders work in collaboration with the members to establish the culture of the group so that the adolescents have and feel ownership of and investment in the group.

Adolescence and Resistance

Adolescence is a time of self-discovery and exploration; a big part of this exploratory phase is rebelling against parental and authority figures in an attempt to find one's own voice. According to Emunah (2005), adolescence is an intense time of emotional, psychological, and physiological changes. Furthermore, she noted, due to the chaotic nature of this maturation phase, "adolescent resistance to treatment often can be confused with age-appropriate and healthy rebelliousness" (p. 109). Siegel (2015) posited that during adolescence teens experience a developmental surge that is unlike any other phase in life. He explained that cascading changes in the brain set the stage for four qualities of the adolescent mind: *novelty seeking, social engagement, increased emotional intensity,* and *creative exploration.*

The benefits of novelty seeking include a desire to explore new things and engage actively and creatively with life. The challenges can include risky behaviors in search of thrill and excitement that ignore the dangers and consequences of these choices. The importance of social engagement heightens in adolescence, when teens often begin to privilege relationships with their peers, which can help to create a feeling of connectedness and belonging while supporting the separation and individuation process (Schwarz et al., 2012). Increased emotional intensity brings with it an energy and engagement with one's feelings, though it can also lead to "impulsivity, moodiness, and extreme, sometimes unhelpful, reactivity" (Siegel, 2015, p. 8). Creative exploration, according to Siegel, is the adolescent's ability to think in a broadened and abstract manner. This way of thinking can lend itself to a 'crisis of identity,' feelings of insecurity and lack of focus or direction, and succumbing to pressures from peers. It also creates the potential for imagining new possibilities and exploring novel experiences and the wider world.

While adolescence is wrought with various and conflicting psychological, physiological, and emotional experiences, it is also a time of great possibility. Siegel (2015) asserted that adolescence is the phase in life that has the most potential for "courage" and "creativity" (p. 6). The creative arts therapies allow for this courage and creativity to be fostered and channeled in action while encouraging unique modes of expression and offering new opportunities for exploration.

Working With Resistance in Adolescent Treatment Groups

My co-leader and I (BW) once walked into an adolescent group and were immediately met with a cacophonous greeting of dismay that included "Oh no, not you," "Go away," and "Uhhh, not this group again." We could have certainly responded to this (un)welcome by imploring the members to settle down and prepare for group. Yet, our response was to say, "I know . . . can you believe it? We are back . . . isn't it just the worst!" with a playful tone and manner. The group carried on about how unfortunate our arrival was, but started to mirror our playfulness while getting grander in their protests about our presence. So, we asked the participants what the worst part of being in group with us was, to which one member said, "We start this group the same way each time. It's the same old thing. We should change it up."

It was, in fact, true that each week the group started with a check-in in which the members shared their name, how they were doing, and a third thing about themselves. So, we said, "Okay, let's change it up. How should we begin?" There was a long and quiet pause as it washed over the group that there was a genuine invitation for them to decide how the group should warm-up. Group members decided, "We should do a check out!" My partner and I responded with: "Great, how should our check out work?" Interestingly, the "check out" was surprisingly similar to the check-in, and the group members led this familiar, though self-initiated, way of moving into the group.

If resistance is the pushing away of something, pushing back will certainly cause a block, a stand-still, or an impasse. Working creatively allows space for a full range of expression in group, with the chosen arts modality offering a frame and container. Being met with resistance can bring about feelings of uncertainty and insecurity in the facilitator, especially if they have a lack of experience in this domain (Kemper, 1994). As Emunah (2005) pointed out, facilitators will often attempt to assert their authority and yield their way when met with resistance; this tactic rarely works as it typically results in a power struggle. Emunah's (2005) solution to this dilemma is to welcome the resistance through creative play.

This *moving with* that Emunah (2005) suggested is similar to a concept in martial arts, which encourages moving *with* force as opposed to pushing against it to avoid a harmful impact and to continue the flow of motion. Doyle (2005) incorporated aikido theory and techniques into his drama therapy practice. He shared that when under attack, centeredness and nonresistance beget a situation where there is no struggle. Vickers (2013) furthered:

> Aikido embodies the art of conflict. Instead of resisting an attacker or fleeing the scene, one fully engages the situation, moving toward the oncoming energy and accepting that energy as a gift. Then, stepping off the line of attack, one redirects the energy instead of opposing it head-on. This approach is referred to as blending—the Aikidoist blends with the attack energy and channels it in a new direction, often by executing a turn that leaves both people facing the same way. One is now looking at the situation from the attacker's point of view, without giving up one's own.
>
> (p. 2)

Consider again the example offered above where the leaders were rebuked by the adolescent group. We wholly engaged the encounter with the youth, then moved "off the line" of rebuke through our playfulness. In turning with the group to look at their complaint, the members were able to move in a new direction: one in which there was channeled energy and renewed engagement. There was an acceptance on our part that this was where the group was; we fully met them in that place and together (facilitators and clients) navigated our way through the group. According to Doyle (2005), it is important for therapists to communicate their acceptance to the client(s), and he noted that the act of acceptance is at the heart of *blending*.

Vickers (2013) compared the idea of blending with the "Yes, and . . ." stance of improvisation, in which all offers are accepted and built upon, and explored ways in which the tenets of these practices can align with and lend themselves to the therapeutic process. He further reminded that the therapist too may have a role in any resistances that arise in the work. The cause of a perceived impasse cannot be assumed to be the result of the group's resistance. In fact, many group members who are deemed difficult arrive at this role through the contributions of the leaders and their peers in the group, and they may be serving an important purpose for the group in that moment (Gans & Alonso, 1998). It is therefore imperative that therapists explore their own beliefs about, experiences with, and feelings toward the group (Williams, 2017), as well as the potential value of resistant members.

Using Arts-Based Approaches for Addressing Resistance

Effective interventions for working with and mitigating resistance in group therapy with adolescents are rare. Verbal psychotherapy conducted in a traditional setting often falls short of reaching the teen who is already struggling with the desire to avoid treatment. Adolescents are often brought into therapy because someone else—usually a parent, teacher, or officer of the law—has mandated they attend. This can be a setup for a resistance as the adolescent searches for control in what feels like an out-of-control situation. This behavior is then connected with the objection of the adolescent to engage in therapy, and is believed to be a potential threat to the conclusion of successful treatment. Moreover, the structure of traditional psycho-therapy often expects adolescents to think and respond like adults, often placing them in a position of failure from the beginning. As Twemlow, Sacco, and Fonagy (2008) noted, "Language routes into the conflicted areas are often very circuitous, demand trust, and a capacity for abstraction and psychological mindedness, two qualities that are often not present when beginning work with adolescents" (p. 11). The limits and boundaries of traditional approaches often do not meet the adoles-cents where they are; therefore, engaging teens in psychotherapy often requires a more active and intentional role on the part of the therapist.

In contrast to the traditional paradigm, the creative arts therapies make space for both the containment and expression of more difficult and possibly darker experi-ences alongside the positive ones (Haen, 2015). Through embodiment and move-ment, art making, storytelling, and symbolic play, the arts allow for new inroads to exploring troublesome experiences. Crenshaw (2008) suggested that "psychother-apy at its best is part science and part art" (p. 166). Research and science inform and guide clinical practice, but once an adolescent enters the treatment space, the unique human encounter is as much art as it is science. It stands to reason that the creative arts therapies offer an enticing form of engagement that allows for safe expression of difficult feelings and experiences. In addition, the arts often have the ability to cut through resistances, create connections, increase mind–body aware-ness, and provide a more thorough and effective means of accessing information and insight.

Advantages of Working With Resistance in Group Rather than Individual Therapy

Adolescents who are labeled resistant can greatly benefit from the collective nature of the group process. Group work is a naturally creative endeavor. Leaders who employ arts-based techniques can mine the individual and collective creativity that lives in the group. The non-deliberative essence of the creative arts therapies lets adolescents express themselves using artful, action-based forms and symbols that bring to light "competences of the person other than those prominent in delibera-tive problem-solving" (Lang, 2016, p. 107). In this way, group members often model for each other different role possibilities. Subsequently, if the container of the group is safe enough, the resistant adolescent may be able to step out of their current role and try on something new without feeling the pressure of negative consequences.

When a group is functioning well, it can also allow for the experience of all voices being heard without judgment. Collective art making, whether based in the-ater, art, dance, poetry, or music, fosters a sense of community building. Group members must work together in the process of creation. This act of creation not only fosters personal connections but also allows for the group itself to become the container of the individual and collective experiences (Dean & Landis, 2017). The metaphor created by the group serves as the connective device for the individual experience, allowing for shared projection. In addition, there is often a communal sense of responsibility in the process of art making. Adolescents show up for each other in ways that they may not be willing or able to do with a therapist alone.

Although members need to feel safe, they also need to experience some measure of anxiety in order to motivate them to make changes in their lives. According to Moon (2016), "when clients feel safe they experience the art-based therapy group as a protective shelter in which their anxieties provide the energy needed to promote their desired life changes" (p. 49). In this case it is the job of the therapist to help facilitate creative connections among the members, thus creating an environment of safety, success, pride, and ownership in the group participants. This means that in order to create space for all voices, the therapist might reduce the number of structured exercises in favor of fostering spontaneity and mutual aid (Malekoff, 2016).

It is important to note that that there are a few key strategies to working successfully with resistance in group treatment, outlined here and explained in more detail following. First and foremost, the group leader must understand who they are working with and why the resistances are present. Second, leaders should learn to creatively and spontaneously join the resistance they encounter as opposed to fighting against it. Lastly, they should be adept at helping the group members create connections, allowing them to become their own therapeutic agents.

Three Arts-Based Principles for Working With Resistance in Groups

Understand Who You Are Working With

When we think of a resistant adolescent, we often imagine a teenager who refuses to do what they are asked to do simply out a desire to be obstinate: sitting with crossed arms and a scowl on their face. It is easy when we are faced with the closed-off adolescent (or a group of them!) to take a punitive and often shaming stance. However, when we truly understand who is sitting across from us, we can shift how we engage in the treatment process.

Many of the adolescents whom we come in contact with have experienced complex trauma. Although not every adolescent has experienced trauma, many teens who find themselves in treatment have been exposed to traumatic events. We will use work with traumatized teens to exemplify how group therapists' understanding of their members can help to reframe resistance.

Complex trauma, as defined by the National Child Traumatic Stress Network (NCTSN, 2007), describes both children's exposure to multiple traumatic events— often of an invasive, interpersonal nature—and the wide-ranging, long-term effects of this exposure. These events are severe and pervasive, such as abuse or profound neglect. They usually occur early in life and can disrupt many aspects of the child's development and the formation of a sense of self. Since these events often occur with a caregiver, they interfere with the child's ability to form a secure attachment. Many aspects of a child's healthy physical and mental development rely on this primary source of safety and stability (NCTSN, 2007).

Complex trauma can affect adolescents in a number of ways, including influencing behavioral control, affect regulation, attachment, and self-concept. When we understand that behaviors in the group room may be connected to trauma, and that resistance is a defense that often emanates from fear of vulnerability, then we can approach the treatment with compassion and empathy instead of feeling blocked at every turn. The adolescent member can take comfort in the often 'no-rules' feeling of arts approaches (Dean & Landis, 2017), while the leader can thoughtfully choose the type of arts interventions that will most allow for exploration with each particular group of adolescents. In addition, leaning on the distance and metaphor that the arts offer allows for a safer way to process experiences when direct interpretation and analysis may be too overwhelming. Finally, we are learning that the creative arts therapies, in particular, are helpful in "creating healing pathways to earlier damaged attachment experiences and giving form and grace to the whole self" (Twemlow et al., 2008, p. 11).

CASE EXAMPLE

Teens struggling with substance abuse problems and school truancy were required to come to a weekly therapy group. Before one session, a teacher approached the group leaders to let them know that this particular class had all received detention for a verbal fight that happened in a previous class. When the leaders entered the room, there was a heavy feeling and most participants were sitting with their arms crossed and their heads down. The group members had no desire to participate, let alone engage with each other. The group leaders spoke aloud the perceived feelings in the room: anger, frustration, exhaustion. Group members grunted in agreement with anger and frustration.

With the understanding that most of them had experienced complex trauma and struggled with behavioral control, the therapists knew that the punitive response to their behavior had affected the members on a deeper level. The group did not feel safe enough for participation at this point, and the task of the group leaders was to create a space in which those feelings could be explored without fear of judgment or punishment. Since full verbal expression was not an option at this point, group leaders asked members to share a song that either expressed how they were feeling in the moment or that they liked to listen to when feeling this way. As song titles were expressed, the group leaders played them from the internet, allowing the music listening to awaken a different sense in the room. Therapists made note of each song and the themes arising. As the music played, the teens began to come alive and there was excitement to share their song. By the end of the group, a playlist had been created that served as a jumping-off-point for future creative projects.

Join the Resistance

More often than not, a "resistant" teen can induce panic in the most stable and experienced of therapists. A first instinct may be to try to disarm the teen or create a therapeutic alliance. Although ultimately both of those strategies are important, as mentioned previously, when we understand resistance as coming from a place of protection we can appreciate the *why* of it, and work *with* the resistance as opposed to against it. When we 'join the resistance,' we are accepting the adolescent for who they are and the reasons they have come to therapy. We are able to see the see the world and the present moment as the adolescent sees it (Rogers, 1951) and validate their experiences. Group leaders can use the creative arts therapies in a playful way to work with what is in the room.

J. L. Moreno (1940/1987), the founder of psychodrama, often pointed to the fact that resistance itself is a tension between somatic and mental processes. When more of the whole person is brought into play, then pathological tensions and barriers are often swept away. He expounded on the fact that continually coming back to the warm-up phase of a group may help the subject be ready for spontaneous action (Fox, 1987). Using this idea, we can ascertain that the responsibility to move into action in the therapeutic space does not belong solely to the client or clients with whom we are working. Responsibility for the warm-up is shared with the therapist in a process of co-creation. With the pressure off, so to speak, the client can begin in a place that doesn't feel forced or pressured.

Warming up, using any of the creative arts therapies modalities, can help elicit group themes, facilitate mind–body connection, and begin to create group member associations, making the space a safer place to work. Therapists must access their own spontaneous and playful self to be able to enter a place of joining.

CASE EXAMPLE

As the therapists entered the room, the group exclaimed, "Oh no, not this group! We hate this group. This is the worst group we have." Without missing a beat, the therapists, accessing their own creativity and spontaneity, exclaimed, "Really? This is the worst group of all the groups you've had? You have group every day, and this is the worst? Wow, we win! We are the worst group of all the groups!"

The group members, sensing the playfulness of the leaders, began to laugh and play along: "Yes, Miss, you win the award for not only the worst group, but the worst group leaders we have ever had." Responding playfully, one group leader retorted, "Well, do we get an award for being the worst group ever?" "Yes!" another group member shouted, "I will present it to you." Another group member volunteered to be the camera operator at the awards ceremony, and another the host of the show. Before they knew it, the group had co-created an awards ceremony with each member finding their part in the process. After the leaders received their awards, they were able to ask the members to create awards and ceremonies for each other. The leaders asked each group member what they would like to receive an award for. One member chose to get an award for excelling in a sport, another for being a good friend, and yet another for getting through a difficult situation. As each adolescent chose their award, other members jumped up to play out the different pieces of each ceremony.

Create Connections

Adolescents are often referred to a therapeutic group because they have expressed feeling isolated. Group therapy can be beneficial because of the collective nature of the experience. Adolescents in particular have an opportunity to see that others may have experienced similar situations, and to learn empathy. Moreover, the cooperative nature of group work produces a framework in which interpersonal disconnections can be explored and understood, and ultimately countered by experiences of connections being formed, deepened, and appreciated (Sassen, Spencer, & Curtin, 2005).

Most of the creative arts therapies are innately relational. Improvisational work in therapy requires listening and responding to those with whom one is co-creating, while collective art making encourages connecting individual pieces to make a whole. The role of the group therapist when working with resistance can be one of co-creator and facilitator, rather than all-knowing authority figure, allowing for shared power within and ownership over the treatment process. Over time, the group itself can become its own therapeutic agent; in other words, the more the group members are engaged in the process of art making, the easier that play can happen (Nash & Haen, 2005). The therapist can foster this dynamic by providing ideas and feedback in order to help the members connect during the art making process, and by offering encouraging statements such as "*You are the artists (playwright, poets, dancer), and as a group you have the power to make the decisions about what happens next.*" In addition, using the arts in group work can help to generate metaphors that lead to conversations and connections among members that may not have been present before (Drass, 2016). The skilled therapist can then work to bridge connections (Ormont, 1990) in the process, allowing for the group to develop their inner resources as they negotiate and undertake problem solving, conflict resolution, and mutual support.

CASE EXAMPLE

In a group held in a high school where the adolescent members were identified by staff to participate, the rest of the class had a free period in which they could do an activity of their choosing. This was already a set-up for the group, as the selected kids felt singled out and did not want to be associated with the other kids in the group. Creating connections among members was therefore difficult, but giving them autonomy became the key.

In one early session, the group was working with drama and creating a metaphorical story about things that were important to teens. This particular story was about needing freedom from authority figures. There were two members who became energized by creating a story about two teens running away from home but the other members, although contributing ideas during the story's creation, did not want to act. The group leaders asked the group how they might incorporate the other members. One of them remarked, "Selena likes to write. Maybe she could write the script down as we improvise it." Selena, feeling seen, instantly agreed to be the group scribe. Another member said they would draw pictures of the important scenes so they could remember them, and a third agreed, with the encouragement of the group leader, to be an assistant director. By letting the group negotiate their own roles within the art making, everyone found connections not only to the story but also to each other.

A Range of Arts-Based Techniques for Use With Resistant Adolescents

Superhero/Supervillain

Rationale: Characters that have super powers often garner energy among adolescents and allow for the exploration of several themes, including: power, control, overcoming, and connection–disconnection (Haen, 2011).

Ask the group to consider: "*If you could have any super power what would it be?*" This question usually generates a lot of energy within the group. Once all have shared their power, invite members to create a superhero (or supervillain) who has this power. Have the participants determine their super character's name, power, and weakness/Achilles heel/kryptonite. Once everyone has their character in mind, invite participants to introduce their characters to the group, share their origin story, and (if appropriate) take questions from other characters while in role.

> **Story Variation:** Participants can introduce their character's name, power, weakness, and origin story. Group members can then collaborate to create a group story where these characters are called upon to work together.
>
> **Art Variation:** Participants can draw or paint their superhero or supervillain. They can also draw a comic book version of their character's story or create superhero/villain masks.
>
> **Poetry Variation:** Using the super powers that group members express, the leader can facilitate a collaborative poem by offering stem sentences for the group to respond to. (For example: *I have the power to/of* _____, *I can* _____; *With my power I have* _____; *With my power I will* _____; *My power makes me feel* _____.) The facilitator becomes the scribe for the group and reads the final piece back, making sure to write the words of the group exactly as they are offered. This exercise can also be facilitated as individual poems that are later shared.
>
> **Writing Variation:** Participants can write the story of their superhero or supervillain and, if they choose, share with the group all or part of what they have written. After individual stories have been shared, ask the group to create a new story where their heroes or villains interact.

The Gripe

> *Rationale: Allows for safe and contained expression of all difficult feelings without judgment.*

If the group is blatantly communicating their resistance, invite each member to take one to two minutes to tell a story called "The Gripe" that explores their discontent about being in the group (excluding anything regarding other members), or whatever "complaint" they might be having. The gripe can be told as a story in the past, present, or future and should be set in a place that represents the person's experience. Explain to participants that their goal is to use the full allotted time to gripe. If, for some reason, they run out of gripes in the story and have more time on the clock, tell participants this time should be filled with either things the character likes about the group (or can at least tolerate) and/or what they wish the group could be and/or do. After the two minutes, the facilitator might ask participants to share a post-script (for example, what happens in the future for the character or the group).

> **Music Variation:** The Gripe can be presented in the form of a song or rap.
> **Writing Variation:** The story can be written or it can be scribed as a complaint speech, letter, or monologue. Group members would write for a certain

amount of time and then read all or part of their writing to the group if they choose. If the prompt is to write the complaint as a speech, participants should determine where the speech is being shared and who is in the audience.

Art Variation: Provide art materials to the group. Ask them to draw, paint, or sculpt their gripe or complaint. *If the complaint had a body or personality, what would it look like?*

Fortunately, Unfortunately

> *Rationale: Group members have the opportunity to express both positive and difficult statements while working with group cohesion and creativity.*

With group members sitting in a circle, proceed to tell a story, with each person saying one sentence at a time. Each sentence must start with either "fortunately" or "unfortunately," always alternating.

Drama Variation: Have half of the group tell the story and the other half spontaneously act it out as it is being told. Make sure to switch groups.

Movement Variation: Do not use words but only movements or body sculpts to tell the story.

Music Variation: Provide the group with a variety of rhythm instruments. Invite one or two group members to underscore the story as it is being told.

Case Example

It was in a mandated, school-based treatment group about one year into my (BW) professional career where I encountered one of the most "resistant" adolescent groups I had yet experienced. From the first day, it was clear that the group members were more than disinterested in being part of this therapy group, which situated itself at the start of their school day. Their dismay was not reflected by crossed arms, scowls, or verbal aggression. It was also not expressed in silent refusals to engage. On the contrary, this group was highly engaged and talkative. Each week my co-leader and I would arrange a circle of chairs for the group upon arrival. The members consistently sat outside of the circle we would config-ure, huddled together about the room, immersed in deep discussion. Whenever we made any attempts to join these discussions, conversation would immediately cease.

For several weeks, my partner and I tried to connect with the members only to be shunned with silence, and even at times outbursts imploring, "Leave us alone!" We eventually came to the conclusion that the members were not yet in a space where they were ready and/or able to be a group. Our resistance to imagining new and different entry points for connection blocked our ability to meet the particular needs of this group. It was also likely our own defense against feeling like we were somehow inept as clinicians, and an unwillingness to grapple with the insecurities that arise when being met with a strong rebuke. Yet, in our sweeping assessment, we failed to consider who our group was and what they needed. We were so defended against their resistance that we were not yet willing to join with it.

Around this time, a colleague shared her use of break-in scenes with me during a supervision group. In this technique, the therapists enter the group room as characters who are already engaged in an interaction. This method is one that brings dramatic play directly to the client. I discussed the technique with my co-therapist and we decided to give it a try. We arrived at our next session and walked into the classroom already in role and deeply embroiled in a fictional argument between friends; we chose issues for the scene that we knew would interest the group members. They initially remained disengaged but as they realized what was happening, the teens gradually shifted focus and began watching the conflict unfold.

Through our character roles we began to reach out to the members, asking their advice and seeking guidance regarding what we should do. Participants naturally gravitated to the friend that they either sided with or to whom they felt they could offer some wisdom. They counseled us, "stop yelling at each other," "you have to listen," and "calm down." Through the group members' guidance, the friends were eventually able to restore their friendship before the scene came to an end.

As we moved to close the session, my partner and I invited the group to sit in the circle so we could process the drama and reflect on the themes that emerged. From our viewpoint, this was an important step before closing, and necessary for it to be considered a successful session. The participants immediately and quickly fled the circle at our attempt, no longer engaging with our prompts. It was clear that my partner and I needed to reevaluate our approach and really take in what the group was communicating to us about their needs. In any group it is necessary to establish a safe enough environment in collaboration with the members. We did not consider in the beginning stages of this group that certain prompts and exercises (for example: sitting in a circle and being seen by everyone in the room) that seemed benign to us might be experienced as threatening, exposing, and perhaps even dangerous by group members.

In our next session we entered as a foster mother and child deeply engaged in an argument. My character, the foster mother, was imploring her child (played by my partner) to stop breaking curfew and smoking weed with his friends. Many group members gravitated to my character and instructed me that "Your son is hurting. He smokes to self-medicate." They sat my character down and explained to her, "When you yell at him it makes him want to run away. He needs his friends because they understand what he is going through." My character listened to the group members' words and started to implement their direction into the scene. "You need to listen and try to understand him," they said. Then, one group member who rarely spoke said to my character: "If he ends up at a school like this they are going to give him drugs anyway, and those drugs don't help. Smoking weed makes him feel better . . . it's how he copes."

This scene was one that invited deep sharing of group members' experiences through projection onto the characters. Through this scene, there were powerful moments in which participants were able to console my partner's character (the foster child), telling him, "we understand" and "you will be okay." They also had an opportunity through my character (the foster mother) to speak to an adult who was listening and taking in their feedback and suggestions in earnest.

We continued these break-in scenes for several weeks. As time went on, group members too would take on roles in the play to add to the stories and character development. For example, we explored tensions in a friendship that emerged due to cyberbullying. Group members cast themselves as friends to both my character (who had been bullied) and my partner's character (who participated in the bullying). As group members would take on these roles, we would pause the scene to learn their character's name and hear their thoughts (through their role) regarding the situation. We then resumed with the play as these additional characters helped to guide the scene by advising their respective friends and trying to mediate a constructive conversation between the two. The therapeutic encounter became one of a call and response—my partner and I would call to the group with an issue and they would respond with creative explorations through it. Each week we took on new roles that the members could project onto and work with. The stories that emerged were closely related to participants' own lives but distant enough that it was safe for exploration. The dramatic play became the container to explore challenging themes while group members served as playwrights and directors helping to guide and shift the narratives.

When we as facilitators shifted our idea of what the group *should* be, it made space for the members to imagine what the group *could* be. In reflecting on the group, it became clear that the participants' behaviors were self-protective. Like many adolescents, the participants were reluctant to engage in a group that looked and felt like therapy—a space meant to get them to express and share of themselves (Haen & Weil, 2010). It was through my partner and I accessing our spontaneity and allowing a creative image of what a "successful" group looks like that we were able to engage them in a new way. This working with, or blending, allowed facilitators and group members alike the opportunity to look in the same direction and find our way through.

Conclusion

This chapter outlined ways in which creative modalities can be used to work with resistance in the group treatment process with adolescents. Many creative arts-based interventions were offered as tools for encountering resistance in groups. It is our hope that readers will take away tangible techniques to implement in their practices. The examples and exercises offered herein can be adapted and amended as necessary to fit the needs and uniqueness of each group. It is also important to note that an imperative part of encountering resistant groups is the therapist's stance and viewpoint. The clinician's spontaneity and willingness to welcome and play with resistance is perhaps the greatest tool one can access to help guide the way.

References

Altman, N., Briggs, R., Frankel, J., Gensler, D., & Pantone, P. (2010). *Relational child psychotherapy.* New York, NY: Other Press.

Barker, G., & Crenshaw, D. A. (2011). Honoring masculine strivings in individual psychotherapy with boys. In C. Haen (Ed.), *Engaging boys in treatment: Creative approaches to the therapy process* (pp. 41–62). New York, NY: Routledge.

Bischoff, M. M., & Tracey, T. J. (1995). Client resistance as predicted by therapist behavior: A study of sequential dependence. *Journal of Counseling Psychology, 42*(4), 487–495.

Crenshaw, D. A. (2008). *Therapeutic engagement of children and adolescents: Play, symbol, drawing, and storytelling strategies.* Lanham, MD: Rowman & Littlefield.

Dean, M., & Landis, H. (2017). Creative arts-based approaches with adolescent groups. In C. Haen & S. Aronson (Eds.), *Handbook of child and adolescent group therapy: A practitioner's reference* (pp. 124–136). New York, NY: Routledge.

Doyle, C. (2005). Aikido and drama therapy with families and children. In A. M. Weber & C. Haen (Eds.), *Clinical applications of drama therapy in child and adolescent treatment* (pp. 207–226). New York, NY: Brunner-Routledge.

Drass, J. M. (2016). Creating a culture of connection: A postmodern punk rock approach to art therapy. *Art Therapy, 33*(3), 138–143.

Emunah, R. (1994). *Acting for real: Drama therapy process, technique, and performance*. New York, NY: Bruner-Routledge.

Emunah, R. (2005). Drama therapy and adolescent resistance. In A. M. Weber & C. Haen (Eds.), *Clinical applications of drama therapy in child and adolescent treatment* (pp. 107–120). New York, NY: Routledge.

Fox, J. (Ed.) (2008). *The essential Moreno: Writings on psychodrama, group method, and spontaneity*. New Platz, NY: Tusitala.

Freud, S. (2010). The interpretation of dreams. In J. Strachey (Ed. & Trans.), *The standard edition of the complete psychological works of Sigmund Freud* (Vols. 4–5, pp. 1–627). London: Hogart Press. (Original work published in 1900)

Freud, S. (2010). The dynamics of transference. *The standard edition of the complete psychological works of Sigmund Freud* (Vol. 12, pp. 97–108). London: Hogarth Press. (Original work published in 1912a)

Freud, S. (2010). The ego and the id. *The standard edition of the complete psychological works of Sigmund Freud* (Vol. 19, pp. 3–66). London: Hogarth Press. (Original work published in 1923)

Gans, J. S., & Alonso, A. (1998). Difficult patients: Their construction in group therapy. *International Journal of Group Psychotherapy, 48*(3), 311–326.

Haen, C. (2011). The therapeutic use of superheroes in the treatment of boys. In C. Haen (Ed.), *Engaging boys in treatment: Creative approaches to the therapy process* (pp. 153–175). New York, NY: Routledge.

Haen, C. (2015). Fostering change when safety is fleeting; Expressive therapy groups for adolescents with complex trauma. In N. B. Webb (Ed.), *Play therapy with children and adolescents in crisis* (4th ed., pp. 239–256). New York, NY: Guilford.

Haen, C., & Weil, M. (2010). Group therapy on the edge: Adolescence, creativity, and group work. *Group, 34*(1), 37–52.

Kemper, B. J. (1994). Dealing with resistance in group therapy. *Perspectives in Psychiatric Care, 30*(3), 31–33.

Lang, N. C. (2016). Nondeliberative forms of practice in social work: Artful, actional, analogic. *Social Work with Groups, 39*(2/3), 97–117.

Malekoff, A. (2016). On getting over oneself and creating space for all voices in group work with adolescents. *Social Work with Groups, 40*(4), 364–375.

Moon, B. L. (2016). *Art-based group therapy: Theory and practice*. Springfield, IL: Charles Thomas.

Moreno, J. L. (1987). Spontaneity and catharsis. In J. Fox (Ed.) *The essential Moreno: Writings on psychodrama, group method and spontaneity* (pp. 39–59). New York, NY: Springer. (Original work published 1940)

Nash, E., & Haen, C. (2005). Group drama therapy in a children's inpatient psychiatric setting. In C. Haen & A. M. Weber (Eds.), *Clinical applications of drama therapy in child and adolescent treatment* (pp. 189–206). New York: Routledge.

National Child Traumatic Stress Network. (n.d.). *Trauma types*. Retrieved January 21, 2007, from www.nctsn.org/what-is-child-trauma/trauma-types.

Newman, C. F. (1994). Understanding client resistance: Methods for enhancing motivation to change. *Cognitive and Behavioral Practice, 1*(1), 47–69.

Ormont, L. R. (1990). The craft of bridging. *International Journal of Group Psychotherapy, 40*(1), 3–17.

Rogers, C. R. (1951). *Client-centered therapy: Its current practice, implementation and theory*. Boston, MA: Houghton Mifflin.

Sassen, G., Spencer, R., & Curtin, P. C. (2005). Art from the heart: A relational-cultural approach to using art therapy in a group for urban middle school girls. *Journal of Creativity in Mental Health, 1*(2), 67–79.

Schwarz, B., Mayer, B., Trommsdorff, G., Ben-Arieh, A., Friedlmeier, M., Lubiewska, K., . . . Peltzer, K. (2012). Does the importance of parent and peer relationships for adolescents' life satisfaction vary across cultures? *The Journal of Early Adolescence, 32*(1), 55–80.

Siegel, D. J. (2015). *Brainstorm: The power and purpose of the teenage brain.* New York, NY: Tarcher/Penguin.

Stauss, K. A. (2009). Reflective narrations of female inmates: Dealing with resistance during adolescent mental health treatment. *Journal of Human Behavior in the Social Environment, 19*(7), 843–858.

Twemlow, S. W., Sacco, F. C., & Fonagy, P. (2008). Embodying the mind: Movement as a container for destructive aggression. *American Journal of Psychotherapy, 62*(1), 1–33.

Vickers, E. (2013). "Yes, and": Acceptance, resistance, and change in improv, Aikido, and psychotherapy. Retrieved from www.sfxmachine.com/docs/yes%2C_and.pdf

Williams, B. M. (2017). Role power: Using role theory in support of ethical practice. *Drama Therapy Review, 3*(1), 131–148.

11
Arts-Based Approaches to Fostering Adolescent Affect Regulation

REINA LOMBARDI AND ANGEL DUNCAN

Introduction

Adolescence is marked by rapid changes in social, emotional, intellectual, and physical development. The neurobiological work of this developmental stage is focused on the integration of maturing biological structures of the body and mind, and consequent enhancement of executive and social functioning skills (Ahmed, Bittencourt-Hewitt, & Sebastian, 2015; Blakemore & Choudhury, 2006; Siegel, 2013; Steinberg, 2005). Teens are grappling with understanding their position in this complex puzzle of life: making sense of their maturing bodies; understanding themselves in the context of peers, family-of-origin, and the larger world; navigating complex social relationships; tolerating and managing uncomfortable emotions; asserting independence; making responsible decisions when confronted with exciting risk-taking opportunities; identifying their sexual orientation; and much more.

Stress and emotional vulnerability are heightened, and for some adolescents this may contribute to an impaired ability to effectively regulate their emotional, affective, and behavioral experiences. Likewise, the developmental stage of adolescence is marked by a significant increase in major mental health diagnoses and crises, evidenced by dysregulated states of emotion, affect, and behavior. The prevalence of these problems prompts the need for effective treatment modalities for youth (Centers for Disease Control & Prevention, 2016; Choudhury, Charman, & Blakemore, 2008).

The ability to identify an emotion, reflect on it, and consequently employ a socially appropriate strategy or set of strategies to modulate this internal experience is the process of *emotional regulation*. The outward expression of this process pertains to affect; thus, *affect regulation* refers to modulating the observable state of one's mood. *Behavioral regulation* describes the ability to control or shift one's outward behavioral response to the internal stimuli (emotion) in a socially appropriate manner (Johnston & Olson, 2015). These regulatory processes theoretically can be discussed in isolation, but for the purposes of therapeutic application are best addressed as a single unit. Therefore, the authors will use the term affect regulation within this chapter to describe the entirety of these processes.

This chapter will discuss the benefits of using arts-based group treatment approaches with this population, identify potential challenges and ways to address them, suggest why creative group therapy interventions can produce impactful results, and highlight specific arts-based techniques to which this population appears to be highly responsive. It will provide case examples drawn from a museum-based art therapy group that has been in operation in Naples, Florida, since the fall of 2014. The group has been made possible through collaboration between a local Community Mental Health Agency (the David Lawrence Center [DLC]) and the Artis–Naples Baker Museum, and is facilitated by the authors. The art therapy group meets at the museum one Saturday per month for 90 minutes. The focus of the group is on developing understanding and better management of the participants' affective experiences. This is achieved through members' structured engagement with the art in the museum, rehearsal of skills needed to regulate themselves within the museum space, and the creation and shared processing of personal artwork in response to the professional art on display.

Affect Regulation in Adolescence

The ability to regulate affective experience originates in the context of parent–infant and caregiver–child relationships (Reinstein & Burau, 2014; Schore, 1994; Siegel & Bryson, 2012). Schore (1994) asserted that a child's ability to self-regulate is consistent with experiencing secure attachment and having a caregiver who has this same capacity. Affect regulation is reliant on both socially learned experiences and effective executive functioning. *Executive functioning* is a term used to describe a variety of complex processes the brain undertakes in goal-oriented behavior (Reinstein & Burau, 2014). Affect regulation falls under the umbrella of executive functioning, as do goal setting, directing and maintaining attention, inhibitory control, problem solving, and employing working memory and cognitive flexibility (Reinstein & Burau, 2014). During infancy, babies rely on their caregivers' more mature systems for regulating their own internal states, but in early childhood parents often scaffold a process that might be more accurately referred to as *co-regulation*. These processes foster the child's ability to identify the causes of various affective experiences and what they can do to manage them. As we learn, human brains become more integrated and proficient in organizing experiences with maturation, allowing this process to shift from an external (dependent) to an internal (independent) one (Reinstein & Burau, 2014).

Neuropsychologists have identified two integrative processes occurring in the brain during adolescence that are of particular importance: *pruning* and *myelination* (Blakemore & Choudhury, 2006; Choudhury et al., 2008). Pruning refers to the reduction of neuronal synapses that the brain deems unnecessary, or those connections that have not been used as frequently; myelination attends to reinforcing and optimizing neuronal connections considered to be important, or those that have been used with greater frequency. Both processes are associated with synthesizing and strengthening executive functions needed for decision making, social cognition, big-picture or gist thinking, working memory needed for planning, and effective emotional regulation (Ahmed et al., 2015; Blakemore & Choudhury, 2006;

Romer, Reyna, & Statterthwaite, 2017; Siegel, 2013). They facilitate more accurate and efficient processing of cognitive and sensory information. Some theorists proffer that another consequence of synaptic reorganization during adolescence is that the brain becomes more responsive to experiential learning pertaining to both executive function and social cognition (Blakemore & Choudhury, 2006).

Given the breadth of developmental shifts that teenagers experience, it is not surprising that some struggle with successful emotional regulation and behavior in response. Some adolescents report feeling misunderstood or, worse, invalidated by the adults in their lives. The latter experience can, at times, lead teens to believe that adults can't be trusted. Those who perceive adults as untrustworthy or incapable of understanding their experience will seek guidance and support from the people whom they most relate to: their peers. While this may be developmentally expected, it can result in dissemination of misinformation and myths, as well as use of unhealthy behaviors to manage affective experiences. Many adult caregivers describe a sense of helplessness because their teen resists parental bids for connection and disclosure. Confusion regarding how best to help young people is often a motivator for caregivers to seek clinical treatment for their children and for educators to make referrals to school counselors and social workers.

The Role of Dopamine

Another result of adolescent neuromaturation is an increased activity of the neural pathways using *dopamine* (Siegel, 2013). Its chemical release is so powerful that people will ignore understood risks in order to experience the reward, a phenomenon evident in all addictive behavior. Dopamine is one of the reasons even the most grounded, responsible, or securely attached teens might act 'out of character' and place themselves in high-risk situations. When released, dopamine creates a profound sense of awe, excitement, and deeper understanding of the self within the world. This highly intoxicating reward is responsible for thrill and relief seeking behavior (Siegel, 2013; Steinberg, 2005).

The impact of dopamine will come as no surprise to mental health providers who work with adults experiencing substance abuse or other process addiction problems; many report onset of maladaptive coping strategies during adolescence. While there are additional predictive factors for addiction in adulthood, early onset of this maladaptive behavior during adolescence ranks high on the list (Center for Behavioral Health Statistics and Quality, 2013; Chen, Storr, & Anthony, 2009; Gil, Wagner, & Tubman, 2004).

Siegel (2013) asserted that dopamine affects adolescent behavior and cognition in two other important ways: *impulsive behavior* and *hyperrational thinking*. He argues that teens must learn methods to interrupt dopamine-fueled impulses, and that adults can aid in teaching these skills. Impulsiveness, or acting without considering the consequences of one's actions, leads to risky behavior. Affective regulation and impulse control go hand in hand. An ability to regulate affective experiences is a demonstration of effective impulse control.

Romer and colleagues (2017) suggested that surges in dopamine, in addition to aiding executive functions, are also responsible for increased sensation seeking opportunities. These behaviors may appear impulsive, yet might be better understood as a necessary part of social learning that fosters experiential mastery over risk and reward (Romer et al., 2017). Siegel (2013) posited this process to be a function of hyperrational thinking, which involves the weight the brain assigns to the pros and cons of a given experience. He suggests that during this time period, the brain emphasizes the reward over the risk; therefore, even when adolescents know what they are about to do is dangerous, their brains will disregard or minimize the risk in favor of the reward or the experience. This reward-seeking can result in frustration for loving adults in teens' lives and contributes to the prototypical adolescent assertion that "adults just don't understand."

When teens are regulating in healthy, adaptive ways, their affective and behavioral expression are congruent with cognitive or environmental stimuli. Maladaptive methods of regulating may be expressed by either a hypo- (under) or hyper- (over) reaction to a given stimulus. Symptoms of maladaptive regulation seen in adolescent and teenage development may be, but are not limited to: self-harming behaviors, suicidal ideation, minimization of serious issues, apathy, drug-seeking and use, and rage (Romer et al., 2017). It should be noted that the majority of teens make it through this stressful stage of life without meeting markers of clinical significance. However, teens with ruptured or insecurely attached parent–child relationships, neurodevelopmental delays, those who have experienced trauma, and those with a history of childhood psychiatric diagnoses may be most vulnerable and in need of clinical intervention during this stage of life.

Affect Regulation Strategies

Affect regulation strategies teens may learn and/or practice within arts-based groups are as follows: situation selection, situation modification, attentional deployment, cognitive change, or response modulation (Gross, 1998; Johnston & Olson, 2015). These strategies can be broken into two categories: *antecedent* and *response oriented*. *Situation selection* involves planning ahead. One must first have the understanding that a particular situation will be emotionally triggering in order to decide to either avoid it or alter the method of engagement with the situation. For example, a teen who has been using drugs or alcohol with their peer group may employ situation selection by avoiding people or locations where use has occurred. *Situation modification* is enacted when a situation cannot be avoided. The teen who is using drugs at an unavoidable location, school for example, might instead modify who they associate with (sober peers) during the school day.

Attentional deployment is the process of shifting one's focus and attention to something else, or deliberately distracting oneself from a discomforting emotional situation. In the example above, this may be achieved by investing more time in coursework, singing an uplifting song in one's mind while walking through the hallways, or engaging a peer in conversation about a topic that has nothing to do with the emotional stressor. *Cognitive change*, grounded in cognitive–behavioral theory, is the process of using thoughts to purposefully shift perceptions about a situation to alter the emotional response. This process is also referred to as *cognitive reframing* or *reappraisal*.

Response modulation refers to actions one takes to modulate an emotional response. Distraction methods taught through distress tolerance skills within a Dialectical Behavior Therapy (DBT; Linehan, 2015) framework encompass various types of response modulation techniques. Through focus on something else, one may develop frustration tolerance and self-control, and alleviate emotional suffering. The process of distraction may be achieved through *opposite-action*, a form of expressive suppression, mindfulness or relaxation strategies, activities that change autonomic nervous systems such as diaphragmatic breathing or rigorous exercise, or soothing oneself through sensory activities (Johnston & Olson, 2015; Linehan, 2015).

Arts-Based Affect Regulation

Expressive arts-based group work with adolescents provides opportunities for fostering affect regulation in a variety of ways. Artistic expression, such as drawing, painting, or sculpting, offers opportunities for individuals to emote their affective experience without solely relying on verbal communication. Creating tangible products aids the adolescent in making sense of their experience and provides normalizing opportunities for group participants. They are able to see the artwork and hear about experiences from others that they may relate to and which therefore provide validation. Group treatment approaches are helpful because participants learn to understand that they are not alone in their suffering and that other people resonate with their experience (Yalom & Leszcz, 2005). Affect regulation requires that the individual be able to name or describe their affective experience. Creating an artwork is a nonverbal means of describing an experience and can function as a container for the creator's affective experience. The artwork can tell a story about their experience, yet also can be processed and understood as something outside of oneself. This permits emotional distance which, for some, may be less threatening than traditional talk therapy.

For example: *When creating a collage of how one perceives themselves, using magazine images to illustrate personal strengths and overcome negative thinking, a 14-year-old girl was able to articulate how she felt through her art. She struggled with being bullied and had negative, self-critical thoughts about herself; the images she selected were pictures of stars and confetti. When asked to name the emotion of the stars, she was able to say it felt "free" and elaborated that it was a celebration of being different, with the confetti feeling "confident" and representing having self-confidence in her own unique beauty. Prior to creating this art, she was reluctant to communicate in purely verbal therapy; the art enabled her to have a voice and process with her peers, who also resonated with her experiences.*

Prescriptive engagement with art media/mediums and the creation process itself can contribute to development of affect regulation skills. For example, watercolor painting on quality paper, using slow rhythmic strokes integrated with diaphragmatic breathing, can be used to teach self-calming and grounding skills. In this activity, the emphasis is placed on the experience of doing without the intention of creating an image. Participants are directed to focus on their sensory experience: the feeling of the brush strokes, observing the paint as it morphs and blends on the page, listening to the soft music in the background. It is helpful to play soft music with nature sounds in the background while engaging in the painting. After painting in this manner for 15 minutes or more, the somatic experience of the process is discussed. What, if any, changes were noticed within the body between onset and completion? How difficult was it to sit quietly and attend to the process? Was any delight experienced in the process?

Teens often report listening to music as a coping skill. Response painting to different genres of music promotes experiential understanding of how one can produce various affect changes through external stimuli. Teens are encouraged to paint using only line, shape, and color to reflect the *felt sense* of the music being played. It is helpful to ask the teens what they might typically listen to when attempting to cope with anger or sadness. An example of a playlist for this intervention might be: a violin rendition of a heavy metal song, an Afro-Cuban jazz piece, a Bach concerto, a rap song, a Spanish guitar piece, and an electronic dance music selection. Each piece should convey a different *felt sense*. After the response paintings are complete, discussion is focused on the similarities and differences in the colors, quality of strokes, the *felt sense* of the composition, and any affective shifts they experienced in response to the music. It is important to discuss how they can curate their music more effectively to manage affect regulation, and to discuss times when it may not be helpful to listen to music that mirrors the affective state in need of regulation.

Another technique using watercolors can be used when there is a need to provide containment for emotionally laden content. This can be achieved by first writing on the paper in white or light-colored crayon prior to using the watercolor. The written words become obfuscated with the layering of paint over them. Art therapist Wix (2016) takes this painting process further and creates tiny accordion and meander books out of the individual watercolor paintings, filled with illegible secrets. This artistic process permits the creator to freely express hidden wounds and hurts, as there is safety in knowing that what is revealed will remain concealed. This intervention is well received by adolescents and teens being treated in the children's crisis stabilization unit. These teens have either threatened or attempted to harm or kill themselves or someone else—an extreme manifestation of an unpropitious attempt to regulate their affect. This artistic process allows them to express and contain their feelings within a group lacking cohesion, because their secrets can remain hidden. The secrets, often traumas, are an underlying reason for their struggle with self-regulation.

Museum-Based Art Therapy Groups and Affect Regulation

Published evidenced-based research or even documentation of museum-based art therapy programs for adolescent and teens in need of higher-level mental health services appear sparse; however, clinical papers and some studies in support of museum-based arts and wellness programming for a variety of clinical populations are gaining traction (Camic & Chatterjee, 2013; Canas, 2011; Chatterjee & Noble, 2013; Ioannides, 2016; Kaufman et al., 2014; Linesch, 2004; Morse, Thomson, Brown, & Chatterjee, 2015; Peacock, 2012; Rosenblatt, 2015; Thaler et al., 2017; Treadon, Rosal, & Wylder, 2006; Wilson, Bryant, Reynolds, & Lawson,

2015). Chatterjee and Noble (2013) suggested that hosting mental health groups in museum settings contributes to enhancement of social and emotional health needs in a variety of ways, not limited to: healthy leisure activities, new coping strategies, calming skills, multi-cultural edification, structured peer-to-peer socialization, enhanced communication with treatment providers, opportunities for self-expression, identity development, and increased positive emotions. Other benefits to participating in museum-based protocols have been increased levels of confidence, sociability, sense of personal well-being (Morse et al., 2015), and increased positive self-concept (Kaufman et al., 2014). Camic and Chatterjee (2013) advocated for more partnerships between museums and health care providers and for continued evaluation of the health outcomes of such programming.

Adolescents participating in the outpatient art therapy museum group present with varied types of affect regulation deficits, which change throughout the course of treatment. They must meet the following requirements in order to access this program: 1) a mental health or co-occurring diagnosis, 2) marked impairment in the ability to function in the home, school, and/or community environment, 3) risk for residential placement, 4) family commitment to participate in treatment, and 5) have exhausted lower levels of clinical care. Many of the clients have experienced one or more stays in the children's crisis stabilization unit due to threat of imminent danger to self or others.

Teens may arrive to their first art therapy group angry, depressed and withdrawn, or anxious and may be reluctant to engage.

An older male, resistant to participating, initially presented to the group with flat affect and observed apathy but made positive affective shifts over time. He wore a black hooded sweatshirt and walked or sat with his head down, occluding one's ability to even see his face. Mumbles and other guttural vocalizations were offered in response to attempts to engage him in verbal dialogue. He strategically placed himself as far from the other participants as possible and required much encouragement to engage with the art media. Initially, he declined to speak about the artwork he created, preferring one of the therapists to hold and show his work to the group. Over the course of treatment, he eventually began to slide his hood down, lift his face, make eye contact, and verbalize his emotions and lived experiences with the group. Notable shifts were observed after a peer shared about their own struggle with being bullied and lacking self-confidence. The content of his artwork mirrored his affect. He went from creating imagery of daggers, blood, and other morbid symbols in his first group sessions to creating bright, colorful, happy faces and cute animals. Mid-way through treatment, he began volunteering at a local animal shelter, which appeared to reinforce a healthier assessment of himself as a person of value.

The museum-based art therapy program benefits from the participation of at least one or more behavioral technicians, primary therapists, or therapeutic mentors of the therapy program who attend and support the group in the community. The Artis–Naples Baker Museum, a 30,000 square foot museum emphasizing contemporary and modern art, valued the idea of using their space to host this expressive arts therapy program and welcomed the group into their facility. They host several rotating exhibitions per year and house a robust permanent collection of artwork created by Chihuly, Picasso, Rauschenberg, and Nevelson, among others.

Sessions always begin with an introduction to group expectations and rules followed by an introduction to each participant, facilitator, and support staff in attendance. Group rules are as follows:

- *Be respectful to yourself, each other, the materials provided, and the space we are in.*
- *When moving throughout the museum gallery be mindful of your body in space, use an inside voice, and walk not run.*
- *Don't touch any of the artwork on display unless there are white gloves with a written invitation to touch the art. Oils on our fingers cause the artwork to decay over time.*
- *Phones are to be turned to silent while in the museum and put away.*
- *If you need to use the restroom, let one of us know and we will escort you to the closest facility.*
- *The structure of this group is as follows: we will view and discuss some works of art, then we will go into the studio and you will create. Everyone will be given the opportunity to share a little bit about their work.*
- *Please share to the best of your ability and comfort level.*
- *Whatever is shared in the group will stay in the group and does not go back out into the community.*

This procedure enables participants to experience success in the group, whether it is their first or fifth time attending. Structured, predictable experiences promote the development and reinforcement of internal self-regulation. The museum provides in-vivo exposure opportunities for group participants to practice affect regulation in real-life situations with the support of their therapy team. The group then moves into the selected gallery/galleries where artwork on display is viewed and discussed. Finally, participants make their way into a small studio housed on the second floor of the museum to create and share their artwork.

The museum is a resourceful community-based facility where local to worldly artists are introduced. The facilitators pre-select three pieces from the museum's current exhibit that compliment a DBT skill, affect regulation strategy, or other social–emotional theme. They then design an art therapy directive to match the therapeutic framework or context of the viewed art on display.

Some participants have reported never having visited an art gallery or museum before; therefore, the facilitators consider museum education to be an important aspect of the program. While in the gallery space, participants are introduced to the museum labels that list the artist, the title of the piece, art medium, and origin in the collection (e.g., donated or on loan). When hosted within an art gallery, information regarding sale price and how to identify when a piece is sold are reviewed. When appropriate to the therapeutic theme, participants are prompted to read the larger plaques that provide background information about the artist or additional information regarding the context of the work on display. Questions about their observations of the space and items contained within are invited and answered.

Group participants are taught museum etiquette, which emphasizes the practice of self-regulation within the public space, and are engaged in academic and therapeutic discourse about the selected pieces. They are prompted to describe observations about the formal elements of the art, as well as their interpretation of the possible meanings and emotional expressions that an artist may have been attempting to convey. This imagining about the art, the artist's intentions, the underlying meaning, and the thoughts and feelings viewers experience in response to the image all aid in fostering empathic attunement with the creator and serve to reinforce that viewers are not alone in each of their emotional experiences. It is an exercise in reflexive thinking that permits the viewer to experience and contemplate affectively laden content outside themselves and their experiences. It also serves as a rehearsal for clients to have constructive, non-stigmatizing dialogue about psychological experiences. Prompting questions/statements for encouraging gallery artwork discussion may be:

- *What are your reactions to this piece?*
- *Do you like it or not like it, and why?*
- *Tell us what you do or don't like about it.*
- *What is the felt emotional sense of the painting/photograph/sculpture?*
- *What emotions do you think the artist might be expressing?*
- *What thoughts might the artist have been thinking?*
- *What feelings do you experience in response? Why?*

Often, in the beginning stages of the group's session, participants do not know one another and may feel shy, reserved, or vulnerable in exposing their thoughts, emotions, and problems to the group. With the guidance of the facilitators and DLC staff, participants are provided with a safe environment to openly discuss thoughts and emotions. In lieu of ice-breaker activities, artistic inquiry and dialogue afford opportunities for peers to share and connect. It is through connection that barriers may begin to come down and cohesion starts to form. Exploring meanings of the artwork, postulating intentions of the artist, or explaining solutions to overcoming obstacles within the content or the process build participants' cognitive resources.

Once in the private studio, participants are provided the art directive. Typically, instrumental background music is played while individuals create. Facilitators and DLC staff will assist participants and also engage in art making during this time. The adults are mirroring expected behaviors, providing participants with technical examples of how to use particular media, or utilizing their art making as a bridge of connection with a struggling participant. The creation portion of the group is generally done in silence, unless participants have a question. This is not a rule or expectation set by facilitators, but a by-product of being in the sanctuary setting of the museum, and another example of how the museum space itself promotes affect regulation. It is a time for quiet contemplation and creation, as well as an exercise in using the art process as a self-soothing or self-calming experience. Finally, participants process their artwork with the group.

In the first two years, the program was divided into two separate 90-minute groups. Each was an open-ended, ongoing group; thus, participants in attendance varied each time. One group consisted of children ages 6–12 years of age, and the other of adolescents ranging from 13 to 21 years. In the third year, the two groups

were combined and piloted to see if they could work in achieving the same benefits. To provide greater continuity, a Thursday after-school group was added and is
facilitated at the mental health center. The structure of the groups has remained the
same throughout time and across locations; however, at the mental health center,
digital images of artwork are used instead of viewing in the gallery space. There are
tangible differences in participant affect and engagement between locations; notably, an increased level of affect regulation within the museum space.

Since groups have been combined, it is rare that participants under age 10 or
over age 18 present to the groups. When this does occur, older youth have taken
on a "big sister/big brother" approach with the younger children. Sometimes this
is evidenced through patience or tolerance, and other times by serving as a mentor to their younger peers. Younger youth also appear better able to exude control
over their impulsive behaviors when with teen peers. All are desirable behavioral
outcomes that require implementation of affect regulation. When group members
experience heightened behavioral impulses, the DLC staff in attendance is able to
quietly remove them and provide individual intervention. Once calmed, the member is able to rejoin the larger group, or sometimes may work independently. Mature
topics sometimes arise within the group to include suicidal ideation, sexual assault
or abuse, and exposure to or use of illicit substances. If younger participants are
present, these topics are discussed in a therapeutically appropriate manner. Despite
differences in age, there are many parallels between the underlying challenges the
participants have experienced or been exposed to.

Co-facilitation has been beneficial for various reasons: 1) hosting a therapeutic
group in a community setting requires additional staffing in case of any emergen-
cies, 2) successful planning and debriefing after each group 3) one facilitator may
observe therapeutic outcomes or regressions that the other misses 4) each facilitator brings different perspectives, 5) there is an ability to provide individualized
attention to group participants, especially when a participant is in need of more
attention or guidance, 6) one facilitator can take notes while the other facilitates
processing, and 7) in rare circumstances, one can provide coverage when the other
facilitator is unable to attend, ensuring the group's continuity.

Advantages of Group Rather Than Individual Treatment Approaches

There are many advantages to group therapy, particularly for adolescents as they
can more readily identify with and validate one another, understanding that they
are not alone in the conditions and emotions they are experiencing and learning to
overcome. Riley (1999) pointed out that participation in group treatment promotes
stigma reduction as other kids are experiencing similar challenges. This understanding also provides a sense of relief, an unburdening, for clients. Many times,
teens are overheard saying, "I will come to the next one if you are going to be there."
Such communications are viewed as evidence of supportive alliances and accountability being built within the group.

Yalom and Leszcz (2005) wrote, "Many patients enter therapy with the disquiet-
ing thought that they are unique in their wretchedness, that they alone have certain
frightening or unacceptable problems, thoughts, impulses and fantasies" (p. 6). As

we all are unique in the world, the idea of knowing one is not alone in the struggles faced may bolster a more accepting mindset within a group atmosphere. This mindset may not be as easily achieved using individual treatment approaches with this population because integration of that concept has less to do with the knowledge that one is not alone and more to do with the *experience* of being joined.

Adolescents are motivated by spending time with their peer group. As mentioned earlier, their brains are primed for social learning, and group treatment approaches can be an advantage. Insights, validation, and feedback may be more aptly received by the adolescent client when offered by a friend or peer. It is common for participants to share strategies with another member that has helped them overcome a similar problem. While therapists may have suggested the same strategy in the past and been ignored, those strategies when suggested by a peer who "gets it" may be more easily integrated. The ability to access new ways of thinking about how to respond to a situation is an essential component of self-regulation.

Liebmann (1986) suggested that groups have the ability to incite the development of hidden or unconscious strengths and abilities for participants. Groups provide opportunities for teens to engage in positive ways and view themselves as valuable contributors. Experiencing a mindset shift in group provides them with a positive experience to recall the next time they are struggling to regulate. The experiential knowing that feelings will not last forever, that comes from having their contributions received and valued, provides fodder for reappraisal techniques used to regulate in the face of dark and uncomfortable emotions.

Group treatment also provides participants opportunities to practice and rehearse regulation skills in a safe, supportive environment. Successful implementations of strategies within the group reinforce development of healthy, habitual responses for regulation outside of group. Repeated practice of skills is required for hardwiring healthy responses in the brain. The aforementioned process of creating connections within the brain occurs with both desirable and undesirable responses. The more desirable regulation responses are practiced, the more likely they will become habitual and undesirable behaviors will be extinguished.

Advantages of Creative Arts-Based Approaches

Adolescence is a time for experiential learning. It is also a time in which self-expression supports the growth of personal identity. Using creative approaches in treatment promotes new and novel experiences, driving positive dopamine releases, and connects adolescents with their biological impulse to express and learn from experiential methods (Siegel, 2013). Groups in the museum also take advantage of the neural reward systems and release of dopamine to positive, novel, and exciting experiences. The museum is not a frequented space, enhancing its appeal. The emphasis of the group is on process and immersive experience, not solely on "talking about their problems." Attending a treatment group in a dignified museum may contribute to the teen's sense of being respected and valued, minimize the stigma of attending, and elevate the overall experience to something greater than 'therapy.' The museum itself is an environment that showcases, values, and functions as a container for divergent views and perspectives, making it an exceptional container for therapeutic programming (Chatterjee & Noble, 2013).

One of the greatest benefits of experiential approaches is that individuals are provided opportunities to express themselves using nonverbal methods. Nonverbal expression permits the rise of suppressed information, or things an individual needs to remain hidden, and offers an opportunity for this material to be witnessed and examined from a safe distance. Riley (1999) referred to the capacity of art to provide this as the ability to conceal and reveal simultaneously. Artistic expressions and objects in the museum can serve as tangible objects for projective interventions—bringing unconscious attitudes into the foreground.

Viewing, postulating, and discussing the artwork on display, many of which are created by well-known, respected artists, shifts the felt sense of the group and can facilitate group cohesion and teach regulation skills. The pieces serve as concrete examples of similarities and differences within the human experience. Dialogue provides opportunities to experience different perspectives about the same stimulus and can teach reappraisal skills. Referencing experiences when multiple viewpoints were offered for the same stimulus serve as a reminder that alternative perspectives exist. This technique can be beneficial when one gets stuck in the hyperrational, or rigid, mindset.

Empathy can be said to be the ability to both use imaginative processes to genuinely and accurately understand another's felt experience and also to convey this understanding (Rogers, 1993). Empathy for the self is a requisite for effective affect regulation. Responding empathically to the self may be a struggle for many teens in treatment. As such, they may engage in self-flagellating thoughts and behaviors rooted in an unhealthy belief that they are undeserving of love or forgiveness.

Rogers (1993) suggested that the expressive arts therapies provide great fodder for therapists to be highly empathic to their clients due to bearing witness to their emotionally laden creations. Empathic attunement is used to facilitate the reparative processes in therapy. Creative arts-based treatment groups create multiple opportunities for participants to develop and respond empathically to themselves and others (Franklin, 2010). Viewing, contemplating, and discussing artwork with an emphasis on social–emotional themes cultivates empathic attunement within the viewer by interpreting the emotional experience of another within the context of their artistic expression, including imagining oneself within the emotional experience of the other.

Arts-based group treatment approaches serve as in-vivo containers for developing and practicing attentional deployment and response modulation strategies. The sacred space inside the museum contributes to one's ability to shift focus from the inner self to the outward experience. The museum is designed to command the observer's presence, forcing group members to be in the moment. Viewing and contemplating art can become a healthy recreation and coping tool for participants. Creating in the studio provides opportunities to shift cognitive focus and to learn and practice a wide range of healthy skills for responding to emotions.

Therapeutic Art Intervention Applications

Therapists are well equipped to develop creative strategies for engaging clients, as the process of therapy, regardless of one's modality, is inherently a creative one. The authors use the works on display in the museum as musings for the therapeutic interventions employed in group. Artwork is previewed in advance; based on themes identified within the work, interventions are developed. Therapeutic themes may pertain to imagery content or metaphors therein, artistic style, media, application, or process. Two years ago, there was fashion exhibit that took up an entire floor of the museum. The gallery space was filled with mannequins donning 1970s designs by Yves Saint-Laurent and Halston. The authors used the show as an opportunity to explore the role of fashion, style, and clothing and its impact on personal identity and self-perception. It is a focus we likely would not have explored had it not been for the show, yet the theme touched on a topic of critical relevance in the lives of adolescents. We encourage therapists to find inspiration from themes present in art products/experiences they have access to within their offices, facilities, or communities, and therapeutic applications within the elements of the art media itself.

DBT-informed art therapy interventions afford a wealth of opportunities for adolescents to learn and develop self-regulation skills. The artwork created may serve as meaningful examples to foster understanding of DBT principles or function as an application of a DBT skill (Clark, 2017). DBT skills integrated into art interventions may be, but are not limited to: *dialectics; mindfulness; emotion identification, description, and expression; coping ahead* (pre-planning coping skills); *radical acceptance* (the ability to completely accept the situation for what it is without criticism); *self-soothe with senses; reappraisals or reframing;* and *distress tolerance* (Clark, 2017; Linehan, 2015).

Dialectics, the theoretical foundation of DBT, espouses that reality is composed of opposites, ever changing, and moving through states of balance and tension (Clark, 2017; Linehan, 2015). By developing skills that allow one to accept life's dialectical dilemmas (cognitive change), clients learn to tolerate difficult emotional states and experiences. An intervention using the dialectic theme is described in the case example below.

Case Examples

Therapists selected three works of art employing formal elements of light and shadow from the museum's rotating exhibit. These elements served as a metaphor for dialectical principles. After viewing the selection, participants were prompted to consider: 1) *thoughts, emotions, or experiences that may be represented in the art,* 2) *metaphors or symbolism, if any, that can be gleaned from the images,* 3) *personal meaning or associations to the images,* and 4) *any learning that can be applied to their lives by understanding the paradox of light and dark.* Every participant was given the opportunity to share their thoughts on the aforementioned and their opinions about the art—whether they liked it, didn't like it, or were indifferent. They were also asked to identify their favorite among the works discussed. Facilitators explained that all opinions were welcomed as long as they were expressed respectfully. Those whose opinions differed from the majority were not judged but instead accepted for their differing perspectives and preferences. Encouraging this style of discourse provides opportunities for validation of the client's ideas, as well as practicing interpersonal effectiveness skills, which are core DBT skills (Linehan, 2015). What is often discovered is that a participant's favorite work of art is one that has cognitive and empathic resonance.

Case Example One

Once in the studio, the participants were asked to reflect on the selected works and create an image using charcoal and chalk pastels, identifying dark and light contrasts in their thoughts and emotions. Participants were able to identify how contrasting emotions can be felt, contained, and accepted at once. Each participant created an image that contained a wealth of insight. Themes that emerged during processing of the imagery were: the importance of telling oneself that difficult feelings will not last forever; finding balance is a constant process; light can be found even in the darkest situations. An older adolescent boy drew an image of a Buddha-like figure in a meditative pose and emphasized the figure using charcoal shading techniques. He shared how he is learning to be calm and collected while surrounded by negativity, and was able to acknowledge that things would get better. His statements were a reflection of cognitive change strategies being employed to regulate affect.

Case Example Two

There are many different distress tolerance skills taught within DBT. A variety of artistic media lend themselves to sensory self-soothing skills (response modulation); depending upon the process, one can engage all of the senses, except perhaps taste. Self-soothing skills are activities that engage one or more of the five senses. They typically elicit feelings of safety and comfort, and bring awareness from the mind to the body. Clay may be one of the most underused materials by art therapists, yet it has a multitude of therapeutic properties, including engaging four of the five senses for self-soothing interventions. The case example below describes such an intervention.

In a small exhibit featuring rare ceramic plates, vases and statues created by Picasso were on display. Participants were prompted to consider the roles of culture, nationality, and family in individual identity as expressed within the ceramic oeuvre. A repeated image of a woman, Jacqueline, was observed by one of the participants, which led to inquiries about her significance. It was postulated by a participant that she must be an important figure in the life of the artist. This shifted the group dialogue to focusing on supportive relationships in group members' lives and their role in client self-perception. Just as in the previous example, each member was prompted to share in the dialogue, identify their favorite object, and have their contributions validated.

A preteen male verbalized struggling to not touch the displays and asked if he could sit on the floor instead. He was able to identify that his emotional response (overly excited) required an emotional regulation strategy (attentional deployment) and appropriately requested to engage in a possibly socially inappropriate behavior (sit on the floor in the middle of the gallery). The museum and its precious contents offered a highly motivating stimulus for him to rehearse affect regulation.

Once in the studio, each participant was provided with a very moist lump of clay. It was unintentional that the clay was overly moist, making it particularly challenging to model. Participants were prompted to draw their attention to their senses, with the prompts "What does the clay: look like, sound like, feel like, and smell like?" They were also encouraged to consider how they could use clay or other clay-like substances as self-soothing tools at home. Paper towels were provided to absorb moisture from the clay; they were encouraged to play with it until it became more malleable and to focus their attention on the sensory experience. This was challenging for some and highly engaging for others. The overly wet clay created a frustrating situation and also served as a medium for self-soothing to work through the frustration.

Working through what feels challenging in life via tolerance or employing self-soothing techniques was emphasized during the processing of the experience. One client remarked, "I learned you have to work with the challenge, to bond with it and be patient because it'll work out in some way." Her reflection demonstrates rehearsal of cognitive reappraisal as a method of regulation. Another participant shared, "Even though at first I didn't enjoy how it felt, I couldn't stop playing with it. It ended up being a positive experience." Her reflection suggests being able to use the materials as response modulation. The repeated tactile engagement with the materials provided a soothing response.

Addressing Challenges

One of the inherent and expected challenges when working with adolescents is resistance (see Landis & Williams, this volume). There are many possible reasons for teens feeling resistant: not knowing other participants or facilitators, feeling shy, struggling with social anxiety, feeling angry about coming to therapy on a Saturday morning, not being able to play video games on their cell phones, feeling depressed and apathetic, or simply not believing therapy may be of benefit to them. As cohesion develops within the group, participants usually begin to open up and freely express themselves. If resistance persists, Franklin (2010) advised the art therapist to create artwork demonstrating a nonverbal empathic connection to the teen using visual metaphors. This is achieved through thoughtful selection of imagery that employs symbolism that connects to the teen's affective experiences. This approach can be an effective method of breaching the walls of resistance with this population.

The authors suggest Franklin's approach be considered when selecting artwork within the gallery for discussion, by focusing on content and expressions that might resonate with the adolescent experience. For example, the facilitators selected an image created by a Mexican painter whose piece depicted a shadow figure weighted down and hunched over carrying a large bale of hay on his back. The metaphor depicted having the weight of the world on your back, shoulders, or mind. The teens related this image to the pressures of daily life, growing responsibilities and expectations, and the impact of stressors on affective functioning.

Another challenge that emerged within the group was the occasional parent perceiving this group to be a "fun play time" as opposed to a therapy group. They failed to recognize the benefits of art therapy and its relation to mental health (i.e., if their child was acting up during the week, parents would punish him or her by prohibiting them to attend the group as a result of being able to "not have any fun"). With educational discussions and family meetings provided by the participant's primary therapy team, parents were taught the value of what these types of therapy groups provide, such as learning effective coping strategies for reducing the undesirable behaviors. Another avenue currently being explored to address this challenge is including parents and siblings for a family art therapy group, so that all parties may experience the therapeutic value of the group. The group will also provide opportunities for developing healthier interactions with one another within the family system.

Summary

This chapter discussed affect regulation during adolescent development and how experiential approaches may facilitate healthy affect regulation. The case examples illustrated were pulled from a museum-based art therapy group whose focus is to provide opportunities that foster and enhance participant effective affect regulation skills through artistic exploration and self-expression. The authors postulate that other immersive experiential approaches would be similarly beneficial when working with this population. Each teen is an individual with preferred methods of self-expression; thus, he or she will respond differently to the types of modalities used. Confirmation that teen participants value the group experience is evidenced when they independently drive themselves to attend the groups. The authors speculate that creative treatment approaches that capitalize on adolescents' desire for self-expression and novel experiencing via community partnerships would achieve similar buy-in and results.

In summary, the advantages for arts-based therapy groups with adolescents are multiple as they: 1) provide an opportunity for greater sense of control through artistic expression and discourse about it, allowing for concealing and revealing simultaneously (Riley, 1999), 2) meet teens' developmental need for self-expressive outlets and desire for novel experiencing within a social framework (Siegel, 2013), 3) model and promote the use of healthy, prosocial recreation skills, 4) permit participants to create solutions to their problems via autonomous self-discovery within the safety of a peer group, 5) teach skills that challenge a hyperrational mindset, 6) provide plentiful opportunities to develop empathy for self and others, 7) allow participants to try on new strength-based roles in a supportive environment, and 8) teach various strategies for promoting affect regulation.

References

Ahmed, S. P., Bittencourt-Hewitt, A., & Sebastian, C. L. (2015). Neurocognitive bases of emotion regulation development in adolescence. *Developmental Cognitive Neuroscience, 15*, 11–25.

Blakemore, S. J., & Choudhury, S. (2006). Development of the adolescent brain: Implications for executive function and social cognition. *Journal of Child Psychology and Psychiatry, 47*(3–4), 296–312.

Camic, P. M., & Chatterjee, H. J. (2013). Museums and art galleries as partners for public health interventions. *Perspectives in Public Health, 133*, 66–71.

Canas, E. (2011). Cultural institutions and community outreach: What can art therapy do? *Canadian Art Therapy Association Journal, 24*(2), 30–33.

Center for Behavioral Health Statistics and Quality. (2013, August 13). *The TEDS Report: Marijuana admissions aged 18 to 30: Early vs. adult initiation*. Rockville, MD: Substance Abuse and Mental Health Services Administration.

Centers for Disease Control and Prevention. (2016). *1991–2015 high school youth risk behavior survey data*. Retrieved from http://nccd.cdc.gov/YouthOnline/App/Default.aspx

Chatterjee, H. J., & Noble, G. (2013). *Museums, health and well-being*. Farnham: Ashgate Publications.

Chen, C.-Y., Storr, C. L., & Anthony, J. C. (2009). Early-onset drug use and risk for drug dependence problems. *Addictive Behaviors, 34*(3), 319–322.

Choudhury, S., Charman, T., & Blakemore, S. J. (2008). Development of the teenage brain. *Mind, Brain and Education, 2*(3), 142–147.

Clark, S. M. (2017). *DBT-informed art therapy: Mindfulness, cognitive behavior therapy, and the creative process.* Philadelphia, PA: Jessica Kingsley.

Franklin, M. (2010). Affect regulation, mirror neurons, and the third hand: Formulating mindful empathic art interventions. *Art Therapy: Journal of the American Art Therapy Association, 27*(4), 160–167.

Gil, A. G., Wagner, E. F., & Tubman, J. G. (2004). Associations between early-adolescent substance use and subsequent young-adult substance use disorders and psychiatric disorders among a multiethnic male sample in south Florida. *American Journal of Public Health, 94*(9), 1603–1609.

Gross, J. J. (1998). The emerging field of emotion regulation: An integrative review. *Review of General Psychology, 2*(3), 271–299.

Ioannides, E. (2016). Museums as therapeutic environments and the contribution to art therapy. *Museum International, 68*(3–4), 98–109.

Johnston, E., & Olson, L. (2015). *The feeling brain: The biology and psychology of emotions.* New York, NY: Norton.

Kaufman, R., Rinehardt, E., Hank, H., Wilkinson, B., Tush, P., Mead, B., & Fernandez, F. (2014). The effects of a museum art program on the self-concept of children. *Art Therapy: Journal of the American Art Therapy Association, 31*(3), 118–125.

Liebmann, M. (1986). *Art therapy for groups: A handbook of themes and exercises* (2nd ed.). New York, NY: Brunner-Routledge.

Linehan, M. M. (2015). *DBT skills training manual* (2nd ed.). New York, NY: Guilford.

Linesch, B. (2004). Art therapy at the Museum of Tolerance: Responses to the life and work of Friedl Dicker-Brandeis. *The Arts in Psychotherapy, 31*(2), 57–66.

Morse, N., Thomson, L. J. M., Brown, Z., & Chatterjee, H. (2015). Effects of creative museum outreach sessions on measures of confidence, sociability and well-being for mental health and addiction recovery service-users. *Arts & Health, 7*(3), 231–246.

Peacock, K. (2012). Museum education and art therapy: Exploring an innovative partnership. *Art Therapy: Journal of the American Art Therapy Association, 29*(3), 133–137.

Reinstein, D. K., & Burau, D. E. (2014). *Integrating neuropsychological and psychological evaluations: Assessing and treating the whole child.* New York, NY: Routledge.

Riley, S. (1999). *Contemporary art therapy with adolescents.* Philadelphia, PA: Jessica Kingsley.

Rogers, N. (1993). *The creative connection: Expressive arts as healing.* Palo Alto, CA: Science & Behavior Books.

Romer, D., Reyna, V. F., & Satterthwaite, T. D. (2017). Beyond stereotypes of adolescent risk taking: Placing the adolescent brain in a developmental context. *Developmental Cognitive Neuroscience, 27*, 19–34.

Rosenblatt, B. (2015). Museum education and art therapy: Promoting wellness in older adults. *Journal of Museum Education 39*(3), 293–301.

Schore, A. N. (1994). *Affect regulation and the origin of the self: The neurobiology of emotional development.* Hillsdale, NJ: Erlbaum.

Siegel, D. J. (2013). *Brainstorm: The power and purpose of the teenage brain.* New York, NY: Penguin.

Siegel, D. J., & Bryson, T. P. (2012). *The whole-brain child: 12 revolutionary strategies to nurture your child's developing mind.* New York, NY: Bantam.

Steinberg, L. (2005). Cognitive and affective development in adolescence. *TRENDS in Cognitive Science, 9*(2), 69–74.

Thaler, L., Drapeau, C. E., Leclerc, J., Lejeunesse, M., Cottier, D., Kahan, E., & Ferenczy, N. (2017). An adjunctive, museum-based art therapy experience in the treatment of women with severe eating disorders. [Abstract] *The Arts in Psychotherapy, 56*, 1–6.

Treadon, C. B., Rosal, M., & Wylder, V. D. T. (2006). Opening the doors of art museums for therapeutic processes. *The Arts in Psychotherapy, 33*(4), 288–311.

Wilson, L., Bryant, W., Reynolds, F., & Lawson, J. (2015). Therapeutic outcomes in a museum? "You don't get them by aiming for them." How a focus on arts participation promotes inclusion and well-being. *Arts & Health, 7*(3), 202–215.

Wix, L. (2016, November 11). *Books by hand: Holding secrets.* Master class presented at Expressive Therapies Summit, New York, NY.

Yalom, I. D., & Leszcz, M. (2005). *The theory and practice of group psychotherapy* (5th ed.). New York, NY: Basic Books.

12

Who Am I to You? Using the Creative Arts to Build Interpersonal Relationships
A South African Perspective

PAULA KINGWILL, LESLEY PALMER, AND SIAN PALMER

Adolescence is a time of radical change when increasing importance is placed on social relationships. In this chapter, we seek to answer the questions: How can group leaders enable interdependence as a resource for adolescents? How can they strengthen and encourage supportive interpersonal relationships that enhance health and well-being? And how can the creative arts help group leaders to achieve this? We find our answers by exploring the use of drama processes specifically and their relevance more generally in collaborative group process. We will offer ways that group leaders can capitalize on these art forms and their potential for forging connections within their own groups.

> *I have learnt how to share things with my team mates, how to trust myself, I have also learnt how to prove to myself that I can do it. Its great work, I love it!*
> (15-year-old learner, 2012)[1]

Who Am I to You? Shifting From Parents to Peers

"Look at me!" These are words that parents and other adults in the lives of small children hear many times a day. Every victory and disappointment experienced by the child is shared with primary caregivers as part of the process of making experiences real and understood. As children grow into adolescence, they no longer look to parents as often for emotional support, approval, or guidance. Now peers begin to play that role (Haen & Weil, 2010; Tousignant, Sirois, Achim, Massicotte, & Jackson, 2017). Parents shift from being the center of adolescents' worlds, and peers instead become the reference point for how the teen should behave.

At the same time that adolescents are shifting from parent to peer, they are also undergoing massive physical, emotional, and cognitive changes (Carr, 2016; Crocket & Crouter, 1995). For teens, it may feel like nothing is stable or known. This can be a very treacherous landscape through which to journey toward adulthood. During this new and challenging life stage, one of the most important areas of development is that of social connections. The ability to develop and maintain relationships supports adolescents in their present and future resilience (Schonert-Reichl, 1993).

However, the tricky part is that social cognitive abilities are linked to a part of the brain that is still developing during the teen years (Blakemore, 2008; Haen & Weil, 2010). When we speak of *social cognition* we include the ability to *mentalize* (to see ourselves as others see us and others as they see themselves), the ability to recognize others' emotions, and the ability to read social situations (Tousignant et al., 2017). As these skills develop, adolescents are better able to understand and predict the behavior of others so that they can respond appropriately (Nilsen & Basco, 2017; Tousignant et al., 2017). Appropriate responses to social situations are the ticket to accessing acceptance within peer groups. This seems to be the critical factor that contributes to a happy adolescence and long-term healthy social adjustment.

Life is much easier for the teenager who finds a peer group in which to belong. This peer group becomes the laboratory where the individual can experiment, discover, and understand how to create and maintain healthy relationships (Nilsen & Basco, 2017).

It is possible to predict which adolescents will have an easier time building and maintaining a peer group that will provide opportunities to develop healthy interpersonal relationships. These adolescents tend to have: *more finely developed empathy skills* (so they can have better quality relationships; Schonert-Reichl, 1993); *better self-esteem*, which results in higher status among peers (Carr, 2016); *functional social cognitive abilities* (Tousignant et al., 2017); and *healthy early attachment relationships* (which we will discuss in more detail later in the chapter). These assets have a cumulative effect, as those who have high status in their peer groups evaluate themselves more positively, which can in turn result in the confidence to take initiative, leading to lowered anxiety and lessened risk for developing mental illness in the long term (Carr, 2016; Kenny, Dooley, & Fitzgerald, 2013; Lenz, Holman, & Dominguez, 2010).

For me, it also made me overcome my shyness and build teamwork with the people I'm with . . . now I'm encouraged to want to know [my friends] and to communicate with them.

(15-year-old learner, 2013)

The price of exclusion is high, both during adolescence and into adulthood. The teenager who is rejected from belonging to a group not only feels loneliness and isolation but also misses out on practicing important social relationship skills during adolescence (Kenny et al., 2013, Nilsen & Basco, 2017). With these high stakes, it is easy for teenagers to make choices that may be seen to compromise their values and their sense of identity in service of belonging to a peer group (Carr, 2016; Espelage & Holt, 2001). Those that are excluded are highly vulnerable to being bullied, while others may choose bullying behavior as a means to gain status (Espelage & Holt, 2001). It can be a treacherous journey for teenagers, whose future is predicated upon building strong interpersonal relationships, but whose brains haven't quite finished developing those very skills.

Sometimes I was tired to come upstairs [to the group], and I would listen to my friends that don't want to come and I would also not want to come. But later

I realized, it's not going to help me. When I'm old I might have a job and I don't want to finish it in the middle. It taught me a lot, I learnt to finish what I started.
(13-year-old boy living on the streets)

Engaging with social media is something that teenagers are required to navigate without the help of parents who have traveled that way before them. While we cannot do justice to this topic in this chapter, it deserves a brief mention here, as this generation will be the first to have grown up surrounded by these communication technologies. Adolescents are found to be the most prolific users of social network sites (Ahn, 2011). An American study showed that 94% of teens are online daily (Christofferson, 2016). This has a significant impact on the way that social relationships are formed and maintained, as it appears that social media is used by adolescents to manage their social interactions (Rajeev & Jobilal, 2014). While it is too early to draw conclusions of the positive or negative impacts of social media on adolescent development, it appears that similar dynamics are at play as in the offline world. Studies show that those who are popular and confident online and offline use social media to strengthen their self-concept and can benefit from the additional positive reinforcement. However, those who struggle with confidence and popularity offline can find that same negative self-image reinforced online, increasing the risks of harm to long-term mental health (Ahn, 2011; Khan, Gagné, Yang, & Shapka, 2016).

Who Am I to You? The Struggle for Power

Bullying has been defined as "when an individual uses goal-directed behavior that causes significant harm to another individual within the context of a power imbalance" (Volk et al., 2016, p. 167). Bullying is the bane of the teenager's existence, being both pervasive and extremely damaging. In a South African study of school dropouts, 52% of boys and 37% of girls who had dropped out had been involved in bullying behavior (Townsend, Flisher, & Chikobvu, 2008). A more recent study revealed that 30% of adolescents are affected by bullying annually worldwide (Volk et al., 2016).

This statistic is staggering when one considers the serious implications of being exposed to dominance and harassment. Bullying can negatively affect the psychosocial functioning, academic competence, and mental health of the victims (Volk et al., 2016) and is strongly related to suicide attempts (Jimerson et al., 2009). It has also been shown to have a long-term negative impact on both victim and perpetrator (Bhui, Silva, Harding, & Stansfeld, 2017; Espelage & Holt, 2001). Bullies and victims are more likely to suffer symptoms of depression and anxiety and are also more likely to be at risk of serious psychological adjustment problems than those who have not been involved (Espelage & Holt, 2001). There is no denying that bullying is a serious cause for concern for anyone who wishes to support young people into a healthy and fulfilled adulthood.

At the center of the bullying problem lies power. Bullies use the power they have to obtain and maintain status among peers, and they do so by disempowering others. This situation is even more extreme in contexts where the power imbalance is institutionalized and historical, like in South Africa. The struggle for power and resources is at the heart of the South African story. For the last 400 years, the people of South Africa have been either the victims or the perpetrators of violence and intimidation in a battle for power and ownership of resources. Oppression has taken place in both the public and private domains. Our long relationship with violence has resulted in its internalization as one of our central tools for survival (Das-Munshi et al., 2016). It is no surprise, then, that bullying, victimization, and violence are widespread in South African schools.

School-based violence is multi-directional, with both teachers and students being victims and perpetrators. In many South African schools within communities where gangs are active, teachers and students are justified in fearing for their safety as students carry and use weapons, including guns. (Mncube & Harber, 2014). These schools reflect the consequences of historical and current violent oppression which is seen in: acts of racism, sexual harassment, violence in the home and community, poverty and unemployment, overcrowded classrooms, lack of recreational facilities, and lack of teaching resources (Mncube & Harber, 2014). The challenges to a South African teenager making it through to adulthood unscarred are significant.

Anti-bullying programs using the creative arts therapies can make a valuable contribution toward changing attitudes and building resilience. In a program designed by one of the authors, high school learners identified two strategies to end bullying:

1. Make bullying "uncool."
2. Build self-esteem in students, which both reduces the need for and lessens the impact of bullying.

During one workshop we used a sculpting exercise to deepen insights about the causes and effects of bullying. To warm the group up, I (PK) asked them to get into pairs. One member of the pair pretended to be a lump of clay and the other took on the role of a sculptor. The "clay" was not allowed to talk or move (except to keep themselves safe or say if something was uncomfortable) and was asked to hold the position the "sculptor" put them in. Once they had played with sculpting and got a good idea of how it worked, I asked half the sculptors to create an image of someone who would be at high risk of bullying at the school and the other half sculpted someone who would be considered "popular" and unlikely to be bullied. We then had a look at each of the sculpts and discussed what each image represented.

Then I asked the 'sculptors' and 'clay' to swap places. The new sculptors were then asked to create an image of the same person in ten years' time. In the new images, all of those who were bullied were transformed into successful individuals in the future. Among the 'popular' kids, some were happy and fulfilled and others were still trying to recreate their school success.

This exercise had a very powerful impact on the group and inspired a lively conversation. Members recognized that peers who are considered "unpopular" may well have skills and talents that will be valued in their future. The group also saw that some of these individuals might have been driven to prove themselves because they had been bullied at school, and that this drive may be a cause of unhappiness in the long term. They spoke about the idea that being "good at school" does not mean being good at life.

I asked the group to rate whether bullying was a problem for them at this school by standing on an imaginary measuring tape. Those that thought that it interfered significantly with life at the school stood at one end and those who believed there was no problem at all stood at the other. Group members could arrange themselves along the continuum respective of their own opinion. The majority of group members rated the problem of bullying at the school as fairly high (around 8 out of 10). Several had experienced bullying themselves.

Using the arts in this way helped students to engage actively and gain valuable insights that were personally applicable. However, they did not need to expose their personal stories before they were ready to do so. Group members also discovered that they had many beliefs about bullying in common. This subject had not been openly addressed at the school, as individuals speaking out about bullying made them vulnerable to bullying themselves. In this group context, members discovered they had each other's support to lobby against bullying and thus could be effective in changing attitudes and behavior without putting themselves at risk.

I learned that I am me and I have my own value.

(15-year-old learner, 2011)

Who Am I With You? The Power of the Facilitator's Identity

When addressing power imbalances within the context of the adolescent group, it is critical that the facilitator enters the space with the adolescent with a deep awareness of who she is and what effect that has on the members. In South Africa, with our particular sociopolitical history and ongoing differential around who has access to power and resources, the 'otherness' of the facilitator has a significant impact, which must be dealt with consciously and upfront. When therapists are White, and group members Black (as has most often been the experience of the three authors), the therapists must recognize the projections that their skin color invites and work with this complexity as part of the work of the group.

Since identity formation is a key adolescent developmental endeavor, supporting an empowering construction of how the individual sees herself in relation to another is of fundamental importance. As group therapists, we are challenged to see the effect that our power, race, and privilege have on the therapeutic relationship. We need to engage in ongoing reflective practice that takes us out of our comfort zone and asks us to see others and ourselves differently (Hadley, 2013; Meyer, 2014; Sajnani, 2012).

While facilitators must engage with these issues personally and professionally, the arts provide a useful technology to explore these dynamics in the group. When working with a large group of teenagers, we use *sociometry* exercises to discover the demographics of the group in a way that reveals both their rich diversity and the reality that belonging to some groups confers higher status than others. The facilitator introduces a sense of playfulness and urgency into the exercise, encouraging group members to find others who meet the same criteria as quickly as possible: same birth month, same birth place, same birth order, same mother tongue. To start with, we keep it light, reflecting on how random it is that we have such a large group born in October and only one lonely February child. With time we let things go a little deeper. We consider how 'first-borns' see 'last-borns' (e.g., as "spoilt brats") and vice versa (e.g., as "bossy boots"), but also how the reality is beyond the perception (such as lots of responsibility for first-borns; last-borns always having to wear hand-me-downs), and what it feels like to be a middle child (e.g., stuck in between or overlooked).

We allow those who speak a different mother tongue from the majority to express what it's like to always be communicating in a second language and allow those in the majority to wonder what it would be like to swap places. In doing so, previously marginalized voices are given space while similarities and differences among and between group members are held side-by-side in the group consciousness. This helps to develop both individual and group identities. Critically, the facilitator can then also name her own differences and limitations around language and lived experience due to culture and race, even if already noticeable to the group. Voicing the apparent differences enables a more conscious processing of how these differences impact the therapeutic relationship and models an upfront approach to talking about diversity.

With time, the group is able speak honestly about feelings of exclusion based on race, religion, or sexual orientation. The facilitator holds the process respectfully, ensuring all members feel heard and understood. When group members feel seen, they are no longer holding the tension of trying to appear different on the outside from how they feel on the inside. They regard one another with deepened respect and begin to draw on the resources held within the group, rather than relying on narrow perspectives and ways of relating. The therapist also makes space for dialogue around how she is seen in her difference, in an attempt to bring to light unconscious or unspoken feelings, assumptions, or projections, which impact the therapeutic relationship.

> *[Our facilitators] came this year and we're getting to know each other better and now we can express our feelings very well, they're not like the teachers in the class, they don't say shut up and listen, they listen to you, your point of view and correct you in some places and make you feel safe, not like in class*
>
> (15-year-old learner)

Group members need to feel safe in the group if any authentic dialogue is to emerge around racial and cultural identity and difference. Historic trauma still has a powerful effect on how we see one another and the assumptions we hold and projections we make. The arts can provide a way of addressing these themes indirectly to keep the conversation from becoming personal. It can be useful for the group facilitator to bring a traditional story, myth, or fairytale for the group to explore in which themes of difference and acceptance are explored (Gersie & King, 1990).

Who Am I Without You? The Role of Attachment

There is another factor that plays a critical role in the adolescent's capacity to develop healthy interpersonal relationships: the childhood attachment relationship with the primary caregiver. The quality and style of caregiving is a key predictor of the adolescent's capacity to form healthy interpersonal relationships (Dubois-Comtois, Cyr, Pascuzzo, Lessard, & Poulin, 2013). According to Carr (2016):

> If the child does not experience the parent as a secure base from which to explore the world, the child learns to mistrust others and this underpins a view of the world as threatening. This may lead the child to adopt a detached position during later years, and difficulties with making and maintaining peer relationships may occur.
>
> (p. 26)

Bowlby (1969/1982), the leading figure of attachment theory, found that a child's sense of self-worth and belief in others' helpfulness is formed through the supportive encouragement of his parents, which also models positive future relationships.

Attachment theory's relevance in adolescent work is multi-layered. Not only does early attachment have a significant impact on the adolescent's developing socioemotional capacity, but its relevance to the formation of autonomy (which we know is a key developmental task of the adolescent) must be appreciated. Furthermore, the intensity and volatility of adolescents' emotional states can trigger their attachment system, adding to the vulnerability of this period and feelings of powerlessness (Dubois-Comtois et al., 2013). *Attachment security* is indicated by a child's capacity to be comforted by important others when upset and to experience this comfort as soothing, which in turn enables the child to continue to explore their environment and learn new things. When big changes or stresses impact on the developing individual, attachment relationships offer the needed support and consistency (Dubois-Comtois et al., 2013). The enormous changes experienced by adolescents in both their internal worlds and their physical bodies cry out for the support of their attachment relationships. However, the way that support is given and received must be renegotiated to match the changing individual. The point is for the parental attachment relationship to be internalized in order to give the developing human a template for other relationships they will form in later life (Dubois-Comtois et al., 2013).

> *I learn[t] to be honest, love each other and not to be selfish. I trust my group.*
> (16-year-old learner, 2012)

Rutter's (1981) iteration of attachment theory proposed that *privation* (the complete lack of an attachment bond) would most likely lead initially to indiscriminate friendliness, clinging, and dependency, but would later evolve into an incapacity to form lasting relationships, as well as result in a variety of other behavioral issues with cascading impact on all levels of development (McLeod, 2007; Rutter, 1981). As attachment theory has developed, an increasingly hopeful outlook on the possibility of repairing the capacity to attach has been offered. For example, Hodges and Tizard (1989) found that

> children who in their first years of life are deprived of close and lasting attachments to adults can make such attachments later. But these do not arise

automatically . . . they depend rather on the adults concerned and how much they nurture such attachments.

(p. 96)

Group therapy offers an ideal opportunity to work with adolescents on developing the capacity for secure attachment at an opportune developmental period in which peer relationships become prioritized over parental ones. The newness of peer and loving relationships in adolescence offers the possibility for the attachment system to be revised when previously unmet needs can be fulfilled by a larger range of figures than were previously available. The therapeutic relationship can be built on this expanding capacity for new attachment relationships (Dubois-Comtois et al., 2013).

> We've known [our facilitators] for months by now, we know how they act and how they express themselves, and when they express themselves, it makes us want to give that expression back, and that creates this whole feeling when that's really safe and we just go with the flow, when they're pushing, we push too and we'll come up with something and just get it done, we're so with each other that we will not be shy to say something like if something's not right in the play, they will listen to our point of view and use it.

(15-year-old learner, 2013)

Where a constant attachment figure has not been present, the endeavor of the therapist must be to encourage this security and develop the resultant *internal working models* to connect meaningfully with others. The internal working model provides a framework for understanding the world, one's self, and others. It is guided by memories of the healthy attachment relationship (in this case with the therapist), which provides the standard against which other relationships can be measured. Our case history reviews show that adolescents who have been referred for group therapeutic work by schools and other places of institutional care in South Africa often have experienced some disturbance to their primary attachment. In some cases, these teens have not attached at all, which is common in instances of early orphanhood and neglect.

The effects of early and current attachment systems must be acknowledged in working toward the development of healthy social relationships in group therapeutic work with adolescents. The attachment system of each member will play out within the group, both with the therapist and with other members, and is a significant aspect for the therapist to contain and seek to repair.

Case Vignette: Working in a Children's Shelter (LP)

After an introductory presentation to the adolescent boys, who had been living on the streets, the majority decided they wanted to join the group, which seemed to indicate a core desire to be part of something. The lived experience of the weekly group, however, revealed a multi-layered complexity, which at its heart seemed to be an extremely powerful inner programing to reject relationships, both with the therapist and other group members. The entire process of the group had to focus on finding a creative *approach that would not threaten the survival strategies hardwired to defend against yet another broken attachment. All the boys in the group, between the ages of 14 and 17 years, had suffered one or another broken or missing primary attachment due to death, abuse, or neglect. Therapeutic aims and expectations had to be drastically reimagined to suit the reality of what would be achievable.*

It was clear that group cohesion would best be maintained by a focused and contained activity, where individuals in the group would be in a parallel process and come together to share and reflect. I chose the making of a Photo Journal as a piece of short-term work. Each group member was given a disposable camera and took photographs of his life between sessions. This was offered as an opportunity to explore life story, relationships, living context, and future dreams. Group activities were included in the book such as painting self-portraits, writing captions for photos, and providing pieces of prose ("I see a boy who . . ."; "I dream one day . . ."). The editing of the photo journal was done online with each boy during an individual session, which became an important piece of the work. The process involved choosing the thread that the individual wanted to communicate, choosing to discard or incorporate images, and the ordering of the images. Perhaps most significant of all was having the opportunity to choose 'how I will be seen,' as opposed to the labels and assumptions most often layered onto children who live on the street. The photo journal, once printed and bound, became a precious object for each boy to keep. The sharing of them was also a significant moment of interpersonal relating, where the group could not help but be excited by their own and each other's books.

It was good when I was taking photos, but I didn't realize it would make a book. I thought it was a fake camera. I'm proud of my book. I didn't know it was going to happen in my life, to have my own book.

(14-year-old boy living on the streets)

I think my book is great, I like it and I'm sure my friends will also like it
(15-year-old boy living on the streets)

The therapist engaging in group work in these circumstances can consider how she might encourage members to form attachments with each other instead of with herself. Also, group members can 'attach' to the arts techniques themselves (or art object as described above), thus experiencing the technique rather than the therapist as the agent of healing. Thus, the dependence on the individual is reduced, and the group member might carry the arts practices themselves away as a transitional object when treatment ends. For example, one client in a girls' group at a children's home discovers a love of art making and ease in creating with her hands. She enjoys being able to express herself in this new way and finds pleasure in the results. When the group ends she has formed an important relationship with this new skill and has learned that she can take refuge in it when she needs to.

Who Are We to Each Other? Finding Myself Through You

I learned that there is potential in me for everything and that I should never tell myself that I cannot do something—just try and see.

(14-year-old learner, 2011)

Although adolescence is a time of rapid change, it is also a time when behavior patterns become set. Thus, it is an ideal period in which to support young people to make healthy choices and orient them toward their best potential (Crocket & Crouter, 1995). It is clear that they can do with all the support they can get!

Groups such as those described above provide a space in which individuals can practice being themselves and safely discover who they are. They can play with roles and try out different ways of responding to situations. They can do so in a context where there is no punishment for being awkward or uncomfortable in their new bodies and stretching skins.

> *When I'm acting I'm brave.*

> (14-year-old learner, 2011)

Anxiety causes cognitive processing to slow down: when we are anxious, we don't perform at our best. Adolescents who are struggling in their social landscape will constantly be in a state of anxiety, which will undermine their cognitive processing, as well as their abilities to interpret and understand interactions and respond appropriately. In the creative art group space, teens can experience mastery over a social situation, which will raise their confidence, lower their anxiety, and ultimately improve their ability to interact with their peers in a socially acceptable manner (Haen & Weil, 2010; Lenz et al., 2010; Rousseau et al., 2005).

Case Vignette: Drama Group in a Primary School (PK)

In a group of young adolescents, members were almost paralyzed by the fear of "getting it wrong." When asked to contribute to the group process, the members would look to the others for help and then would be given the "correct" answer by the group. In a game where the teens were invited to introduce themselves with a physical gesture that indicated how they were feeling that day, everyone gave a version of the gesture offered by the facilitator. Group members could not risk expressing their individuality.

The use of the creative arts in this context can feel very threatening, as the perceived risk of being exposed as a failure is so much higher than in the traditional verbal or written group processes. And yet, it is also the ideal way in which to challenge fears and to allow group members the satisfying experience of expressing themselves without being judged. In this context, group members are most afraid of judgment from their peers. Through the process, though, they discover that in fact their most cruel critic is themselves.

In an exercise in which a repeated movement is passed around the circle, with each member altering it and then passing it along, one shy girl adds a sassy rhythm and the group shrieks with delight. In another exercise, one group member starts doing a simple activity in the middle of the circle in silence. Once other group members guess what the first is doing they must join the scene, contributing in some way to the activity. The emphasis of the game is not on performance but on guessing. Thus, to get it "right," group members must "guess" by getting on stage and performing! The actions are known and familiar, and so the chance for success is high. The experience of applause and support at the end of the scene affirms the individual's choice to take a risk to be seen and heard. The group members experience the support of the others as they all risk being "fools together," lowering the potential threat of judgment and failure. As the overwhelming fear of judgment by other group members is reduced, the adolescents discover that they do in fact have some good ideas, they're able to respond spontaneously, and the consequences of not being perfect are not in fact total annihilation, as they had secretly feared.

With time, the culture of the group changed and group members' growing ability to be spontaneous and playful gave others permission to do the same. Group members were able to reveal a little more about who they were, and were therefore prepared to trust one another more easily. A natural consequence of this is that the teens were able to form deeper bonds with one another and find the peer support that they so desperately needed.

Case Vignette: School Therapeutic Theater Project (SP, LP, PK)

When working with a group of adolescents, creating something together is a powerful way to foster group cohesion and strengthen interpersonal relationships. Between 2006 and 2014, the authors of this chapter were involved in a school-based therapeutic theater project for adolescents. The project took place at various schools throughout South Africa in partnership with a number of NGOs and donors. The groups were offered as an extra-curricular activity at underprivileged schools and care centers in communities affected by poverty, conflict, and HIV. The aim of the work was to provide a safe and creative space for the development of healthy relationships, fostering confidence and self-esteem, and developing the potential for mastery, power, and purpose.

SP shares her experience below.

The following describes a 20-week process run by myself (a drama therapist) together with an applied theater practitioner. We worked with 16 adolescents of mixed gender between the ages of 14 and 16 years. Apart from a one-off nativity play, this was the first experience of drama and theater making for many of these young people.

The ongoing process of finding both the individual and collective voice became one of our key therapeutic aims, and we focused on bringing games and stories that supported expression both through the body and voice. This enabled group members to speak up about the injustices and challenges they faced, as well as giving them the space to share their hopes, dreams, and aspirations.

As the group journeyed together over the weeks, my co-facilitator and I reflected on the significance of the innate creativity, health, and capacity for transformation that had been activated in the group through the use of art making and performance. Group members made creative offers with confidence and gleefully played with characters that pushed back against the status quo. As the group became comfortable with the medium of storytelling, they were able to share some of their more deeply rooted struggles with power imbalances and safety.

A shared struggle for many was the absence of their fathers, who were either physically or emotionally unavailable. A third of the way through the process we introduced the Native American story "The Twin Warrior Heroes" in order to enable the group to work more deeply with the theme of absent fathers as well as to continue to find creative expression and voice (Pearson, Smail, & Watts, 2013). The teens used their own experiences to rework the characters and plot of the original story, making it more relevant to them and their context.

The process of selecting the cast and crew proved to be a useful therapeutic opportunity for identity development through trying out new roles. For example, we decided to offer the role of the father in the story to a group member who was often scapegoated by the group and bullied at school. He usually adopted the role of the clown; however, he accepted our suggestion of a new role in the story, which enabled him to try out a different way of being. We witnessed a significant shift in his relationships within the group over time. By the end of the process, he seemed to be treated with more respect by his peers. He reveled in the opportunity to transform that was given by his role as the ill father who receives his heart back and rises as the sun.

The sense of pride and purpose in their work was visible from the way the group took the stage and performed with confidence, focus, and collective support. The invaluable power of witnessing was evident in the group's celebrations and reflections post-performance. The process of workshopping, rehearsing, and performing this piece encouraged each individual to bring their best selves forward and to invest their focus and creativity in the product. Through bearing witness to one another, and making their offering public, we saw that both their interpersonal and intrapersonal relationships were strengthened. This was evident in the group cohesion that had been achieved by the end of the process.

Our overall aim in the theater making was for individuals and the group as a whole to recognize their own and one another's value in the world and the importance of their creative contribution. This process can be deeply satisfying to the adolescents for whom group belonging and individual identity are of utmost importance. It provides enough emotional distance from their own personal material that it allows them to actively engage, transform, and integrate those experiences into a new version of themselves (Emunah, 1994).

With reference to exploring identity, it is useful for the group leader to identify a full spectrum of possible roles that are already both conscious and latent in the group in order to encourage role flexibility and experimentation. There are many playful ways to evoke these roles through role cards, myth or fairytale characters, or group-made story characters. For example, in one exercise we selected two characters and placed a chair for each in the space. We then created a scenario for the characters. Group members were invited to sit on the chairs and offer a line that one of the characters might say, think, or feel. A number of group members made offers and tried out playing the two characters. Playing different characters and roles helped the group members to see the world through another's eyes, which developed their appreciation of diversity and, in turn, supported individual inclusion within a group.

Creative arts groups offer group members an opportunity to work through relationship conflicts within the safety of therapeutic space. Orienting the group toward the specific goal of performance or a collaborative arts project offers an acute focus that enables group dynamics to surface more quickly than in a more traditional therapy group. The pressure of a deadline or performance date provides an opportunity to work through possible difficulties and conflicts that surface interpersonally. Conflicts around different viewpoints, ideas, or opinions need to be grappled with and resolved in order for the process to move forward. This group can be a model of a functioning, communicative, supportive, and co-creative family unit where individual expression and identity is celebrated, and supportive interpersonal relationships are essential.

Along with the goal of performance or completed collaboration comes the creative process and development of specific skills and tools. Focus, self-discipline, a healthy amount of group cohesion and interpersonal support, and a number of artistic skills related to the craft are encouraged as part of this creative process. The theater performance creates space for ensemble work, which enables a more fluid and dynamic landscape for interpersonal relationships to develop. In ensemble work, the act of moving beyond oneself in order to be of service to the performance can be incredibly empowering and healing, especially for the adolescent who spends a lot of time worrying about whether she will be accepted or rejected.

I learned that I can be myself and not to be afraid of what people think of me.
(14-year-old, 2011)

If the group is going to show their completed projected to an invited audience through an exhibition, presentation, or performance, group members learn more important lessons for dealing with life's stressors: when they step on stage they discover that everything they need to perform and to succeed they have within themselves and the ensemble (Emunah & Johnson, 1983). The performance can support a change in perspective as to how the adolescent performers are viewed by their communities.

I realized that I'm really good at performing when I have self-confidence.
(15-year-old, 2011)

Therapists need to take great care when they expose the work of their group members to an audience. This process can have a powerful healing effect if carefully managed and supported. However, this exposure can also be harmful if the groundwork has not been sufficient. As part of the rehearsal and post-performance process, it is helpful to work with performers around expectations (pre-performance) and experiences (post-performance) of the audience–performer relationship. Facilitators can communicate possible feelings that group members may experience pre- and post-performance, bearing in mind the possibility of post-show letdown. It is useful to prepare the ground for the audience–performer relationship by offering a written invitation or a pre-performance introduction to the work. It is important that the facilitator has a good sense of how the audience may respond to the work and that the group is prepared appropriately for an audience of their peers who may laugh at the wrong time or struggle to pay attention. If the work is very intimate and personal, then it is important the audience is carefully selected and has the capacity to hold and honor the work.

Pendzik (1994) emphasized the sacred space of the theater and how performance enables both the performers and the audience to move beyond the bounds of everyday experiences into the realm of imagination and possibility; through the suspension of disbelief in this sacred space they enter into the *imaginary-real*. This dimension is likened to the *transitional space*, the play space that Winnicott (1971) referred to in which healthy relationships can develop through playing.

Pendzik (1994) described how group members transition together onto the stage, which is a ritualized, set-apart environment that is conducive to supporting and encouraging individual and collective creative expression and experimentation. It is this liminal space that allows for healthy alternatives to be explored, fostering an environment that is conducive to growth. Taking to the stage requires the courage to show up and be seen; it asks of performers to be bold enough in their voices and connected to their bodies and feelings. Indeed, any group process that requires group members to work together, support one another, and present their results at the end has this effect on the participants.

> *This journey has been very inspiring, I enjoyed it a lot . . . it empowered me. [This] is something that no one can now ever take away from me. I have learnt to accept myself for who I am, and I have also found myself during this journey. And I've met some new people. Like before this, we weren't even a group, and now I like have some people to talk to, and I know that they have my back. Today I also met a lot of people from other schools and it was just an amazing experience . . . they can actually accept me for who I am, and we don't get that a lot.*
>
> (15-year-old learner, 2011 commenting on the public performance of their show)

Speaking for Ourselves: Case Study (PK and LP)

In 2005, we worked with a group of adolescents who lived in an informal settlement near Cape Town. These learners experienced extreme poverty. Most were raised by single parents, and all were at risk of violent crime, both at school and in their neighborhoods. The focus of this group was to create a piece of theater together. Over the course of a year, we watched as these individuals stepped more fully into their own skin, took more responsibility for themselves in relation to one another, and recognized their capacity to make a new path in the world.

Through the use of improvisation and play, group members laughed with one another, let down their defenses together, and discovered new things about one another. They had to let go of their restrictive notions of how they were supposed to behave and open up to new ways of relating that allowed for a greater range of expression of emotion and possible responses to situations.

Movement exercises, collaborative art making, and trust games allowed for non-sexual, safe physical contact, which in turn allowed group members to soften and deepen their relationships with one another in a way that they had never experienced before. As the pressure of rehearsals and performances mounted, each member of the cast had to recognize their own importance. If one of them missed a rehearsal, all the members were affected. They needed one another and had to learn the responsibility that comes with interdependence.

Many of these young people had grown up with the message that they were not valued or seen, that they were invisible to the rest of the world. (This was clearly illustrated when only one parent came to witness the performance of the show that had been arranged in the township community hall where the families were residents.) The teens also had to learn that while on stage the audience could see them, and each move they made had an impact.

However, the ultimate reward of being seen and applauded for telling their story was transformative in a deep and lasting way. The fact that relationships between the group members outlasted the group and continue into the present is a testimony to repairing broken attachment relationships. A moment that stands out for us is the time we went to perform the show at an exclusive, all-girls school in the wealthy suburbs of Cape Town. The group was very anxious about how they would be received and perceived. Being seen as 'poor' was an identity the group members rejected, and they would go to great lengths, under difficult circumstances, to avoid being labeled as such.

The performance took place in the plush, custom-built auditorium to a rapt and deeply appreciative audience. Afterward the cast and members of the school's drama group all joined together for a drama workshop. The group members' reflection after the whole experience revealed how, through this process, they felt 'seen,' not as poor, or different, or bad, but as equally human.

The growth and transformation in the group members was due to a number of things: the long-term process of working together; the fact of their stories being seen and acknowledged through performance; the trust and connection that built between the group members; but most of all the use of the arts, which opened the door to a whole new world of possibility and served as a container for the complexity of their adolescent experience.

Conclusion

It is clear that adolescence can be a very tough time for those who are making the journey through that life stage. We know that life can be made easier for those who belong to a healthy and supportive peer group. However, teens are presented with the double bind that the skills they need to be accepted into a peer group are often only learned within the peer group they wish to be accepted into! This is made even harder in a world where the temptation to interact with screens rather than people pulls them even further away from one another. We also hope this chapter has convincingly shown how a collaborative group process can create the environment where teens can learn the crucial skills they need to form healthy and supportive peer relationships and heal the wounds made by broken primary attachments. We hope that the reader has been shown that the use of the arts is a powerful ally on this journey as it strengthens the sense the creator has of who she is and her own potential.

The Southern African concept of *Ubuntu* was articulated beautifully by Archbishop Desmond Tutu when he wrote,

> We shrivel when we are not able to interact . . . We depend on the other in order for us to be fully who we are. A person is a person through other persons. Because, after all, none of us came into the world on our own.
>
> (Dalai Lama, Tutu, & Abrams, 2016, p. 60)

We need relationships with other people in order to be fully human. Collaborative group processes are a wonderful route to healthy relationships.

Note

1. Throughout the chapter we use quotes of group participants from a theater making process, taken from feedback given during semi-structured interviews and on individual feedback forms. To preserve the authenticity of their voices, we have not edited for grammar or tense.

References

Ahn, J. (2011). The effect of social network sites on adolescents' social and academic development: Current theories and controversies. *Journal of the Association for Information Science and Technology, 62*(8), 1435–1445.

Bhui, K., Silva, M. J., Harding, S., & Stansfeld, S. (2017). Bullying, social support, and psychological distress: Findings from RELACHS cohorts of East London's white British and Bangladeshi adolescents. *Journal of Adolescent Health, 61*(3), 317–328.

Blakemore, S. (2008). Development of the social brain during adolescence. *The Quarterly Journal of Experimental Psychology, 61*(1), 40–49.

Bowlby, J. (1982). *Attachment and loss. Vol. 1: Attachment* (2nd ed.). New York, NY: Basic Books. (Original work published 1969)

Carr, A. (2016). *The handbook of child and adolescent clinical psychology: A contextual approach.* London: Routledge.

Christofferson, J. P. (2016). How is social networking sites effecting teen's social and emotional development: A systemic review. *Master of Social Work Clinical Research Papers*, 650. Retrieved from https://sophia.stkate.edu/msw_papers/650/

Crocket, L. J., & Crouter, A. C. (Eds.). (1995). *Pathways through adolescence: Individual development in relation to social contexts.* Hillsdale, NJ: Psychology Press.

Dalai Lama, Tutu, D., & Abrams, D. (2016). *The book of joy: Lasting happiness in a changing world.* New York, NY: Penguin.

Das-Munshi, J., Lund, C., Mathews, C., Clark, C., Rothon, C., & Stansfeld, S. (2016). Mental health inequalities in adolescents growing up in post-Apartheid South Africa: Cross-sectional survey, SHaW study. *PLoS ONE, 11*(5), e0154478.

Dubois-Comtois, K., Cyr, C., Pascuzzo, K., Lessard, M., & Poulin, C. (2013). Attachment theory in clinical work with adolescents. *Journal of Child and Adolescent Behavior, 13*(9), 1–8.

Emunah, R. (1994). *Acting for real: Drama therapy process, technique and performance.* New York, NY: Brunner/Mazel.

Emunah, R., & Johnson, D. R. (1983). The impact of theatrical performances on the self-images of psychiatric patients. *The Arts in Psychotherapy, 10*(4), 233–239.

Espelage, D. L, & Holt, M. K. (2001). Bullying and victimization during early adolescence. *Journal of Emotional Abuse, 2*(2–3), 123–142.

Gersie, A., & King, N. (1990). *Storymaking in education and therapy.* London: Jessica Kingsley.

Hadley, S. (2013). Dominant narratives: Complicity and the need for vigilance in the creative arts therapies. *The Arts in Psychotherapy, 40*, 373–381.

Haen, C., & Weil, M. (2010). Group therapy on the edge: Adolescence, creativity, and group work. *Group, 34*(1), 37–52.

Hodges, J., & Tizard, B. (1989). Social and family relationships of ex-institutional adolescents. *Journal of Child Psychology and Psychiatry, 30*, 77–97.

Jimerson, S. R., Swearer, S. M., & Espelage, D. L. (2009) *Handbook of bullying in schools: An international perspective,* London, England: Routledge.

Kenny, R., Dooley, B., & Fitzgerald, A. (2013). Interpersonal relationships and emotional distress in adolescents. *Journal of Adolescence, 36*, 315–360.

Khan, S., Gagné, M., Yang, L., & Shapka, J. (2016). Exploring the relationship between adolescents' self concept and their offline and online social worlds. *Computers in Human Behavior, 55,* 940–945.

Lenz, S., Holman, R. L., & Dominguez, D. L. (2010). Encouraging connections: Integrating expressive art and drama into therapeutic social skills training with adolescents. *Journal of Creativity in Mental Health, 5,* 142–157.

McLeod, S. A. (2007). *Bowlby's attachment theory.* Retrieved from www.simplypsychology.org/bowlby.html

Meyer, K. (2014). Making fires: Rethinking the possibilities of creative arts therapy practice in South Africa. *Journal of Applied Arts & Health, 5*(3), 303–318.

Mncube, V., & Harber, C. (2014). Violence in South African schools: What is external and what is internal to schools? *Mediterranean Journal of Social Sciences,* 5(3), 203–211.

Nilsen, E., & Basco, S. (2017) Cognitive and behavioural predictors of adolescents' communicative perspective-taking and social relationships. *Journal of Adolescence, 56,* 52–63.

Pearson, J., Smail, M., & Watts, P. (2013). *Dramatherapy with myth and fairytale: The golden stories of Sesame.* London: Jessica Kingsley.

Pendzik, S. (1994). The theatre stage and the sacred space: A comparison. *The Arts in Psychotherapy, 21*(1), 25–35.

Rajeev, M. M., & Jobilal (2015). Effects of social media on social relationships: A descriptive study on the impact of mobile phones among youth population. *International Research Journal of Social Sciences, 4*(2), 11–16.

Rousseau, C., Gauthier, M., Lacroix, L., Alain, N., Benoit, M., Moran, . . . Bourassa, D. (2005). Playing with identities and transforming shared realities: Drama therapy workshops for adolescent immigrants and refugees. *The Arts in Psychotherapy, 32*(1), 13–27.

Rutter, M. (1981). Stress, coping and development: Some issues and some questions. *Journal of Child Psychology and Psychiatry, 22*(4), 323–356.

Sajnani, N. (2012). Response/ability: Imagining a critical race feminist paradigm for the creative arts therapies. *The Arts in Psychotherapy, 39*(3), 186–191.

Schonert-Reichl, K. A. (1993). Empathy and social relationships in adolescents with behavioural disorders. *Behavioral Disorders, 18*(3), 189–204.

Tousignant, B., Sirois, K., Achim, A. M., Massicotte, E., & Jackson, P. L. (2017). A comprehensive assessment of social cognition from adolescence to adulthood. *Cognitive Development, 43,* 214–223,

Townsend, L., Flisher, A. J., & Chikobvu, P. (2008). The relationship between bullying behaviours and high school dropout in Cape Town, South Africa. *South African Journal of Psychology, 38*(1), 21–32.

Volk, A. A., Farrell, A. H., Franklin, P., Mularczyk, K. P., & Provenzano, D. A. (2016). Adolescent bullying in schools: An evolutionary perspective. In D. C. Geary & D. B. Berch (Eds.), *Evolutionary perspectives on child development and education* (pp. 167–191). Basel, Switzerland: Springer.

Winnicott, D. W. (1971). *Playing and reality.* London: Routledge.

13

Teen Bodies

The Problem of Adolescent Embodiment, and How the Arts Can Help

WENDY ALLEN AND T. THOMAS

The word *embodiment*, like most language, has layers of meaning that reflect cultural values, beliefs, and biases. This chapter suggests that the problem with teen embodiment is due to the unexamined history and meanings of the term, the privileging of certain bodies, and how these factors interact with the developmental tasks associated with adolescence. Through investigating the impact of sociocultural and institutional norms on intra- and interpersonal dynamics, this chapter hopes to offer new perspectives on embodiment and propose ways a creative arts-based approach to group work can support embodiment in adolescent treatment.

The Problem With Embodiment

Body–Mind Dualism and a Somatophobic Culture

Most definitions of embodiment include: *self-awareness; the centralization of the body; its inherent intelligence;* and *its participation in cognition* (Caldwell, 2014; Cohen, 1993; Johnson, 2018; Kossak, 2015). By establishing arguments for integrated functioning, such definitions of embodiment attempt to challenge the culturally embedded belief that the body and mind are separate entities. Yet the very use of this term indicates the persistence of a dualistic perspective. This dualism is found across centuries of Western thought, from early Greek to modern philosophers such as Descartes.

Descartes' well-known version of body–mind dualism posited that the mind and body were of distinctly different materials and functions, making unity an impossibility (Descartes, 1641/1991). The body was regarded as some "configuration of accidents" (Descartes, 1641/1991, p. 74) and given secondary status. Descartes' introduction of mind–body dualism has had a lasting impact on Western ideology. These ideas run through all aspects of Western culture, and their lingering influence has contributed to the establishment of a *somatophobic culture* (Caldwell, 2014); that is, a culture in which the body is not only devalued and marginalized but also actively avoided and feared because it holds the sensuous, nonlinear, potentially messy, uncomfortable, inconvenient, and uncontrollable aspects of vitality.

This belief system is evident in what is given value or status in Western culture. For example, education and research tend to favor cognitive ways of knowing, perceiving knowledge gained through other, potentially 'bottom-up' means such as the arts as inferior. Caldwell (2014) contended that the marginalization of the body can be seen "in the devaluing of the body itself as a source of identity and authoritative knowledge about our direct, lived experience of the world" (p. 80). This devaluation of the body is the first challenge to embodiment. When working clinically with teens through expressive and somatic means, often the first hurdle is related to deconstructing the patterns of somatophobic culture that contribute to lack of awareness, understanding, and trust of their own embodied experiences.

In addition, adults in the teen's life, such as parents, caregivers, clinicians, and teachers, whose thoughts have likely been shaped by the same dominant norms, often unintentionally perpetuate somatophobia by casting the body in a negative light. Haen and Weil (2010) pointed out that many group facilitators tend to minimize the role of activity and embodied expression in their groups, suggesting the presence of an unspoken "fear that adolescents' actions lie on the precipice of disaster, and that being in the room with them is only possible if they refrain from being their fully embodied selves" (p. 38). This observation is shared by Malekoff (2014), whose reflections on his work with adolescents often include anecdotes about how others perceive the messy vitality that is characteristic of embodied, expressive approaches to group work with teens. He reflected, "The road for group workers who work with kids is clogged with those who insist that the only worthwhile group is one that speaks politely and insightfully" (Malekoff, 2014, p. 22).

In an environment where cognitive, verbal approaches are seen as more valuable, groups that "make noise and move about, vibrate and explode, laugh and have fun" (Malekoff, 2014, p. 22) are regarded as less deep, less transformative, less serious approaches to therapy. The result, Malekoff (2014) suggested, is that group workers using active, expressive approaches with kids do not receive much respect from their professional peers. This disregard or disrespect is a common challenge facing those who work in the field of expressive therapies, as many creative, embodied approaches to treatment are understood by clinicians from other disciplines to be recreational or adjunctive at best. The presence of these perspectives and challenges are further evidence of the pervasiveness of the ongoing division of mind and body, a separation that has particularly negative implications for adolescents, whose bodies often seem to be leading their developing minds.

Oppression and Othering Dynamics

The second problem with embodiment stems directly from the separation of mind and body and has to do with how this separation creates conditions for oppressive dynamics and exclusion. According to researchers in the fields of somatics and social justice, mind–body dualism enables systemic oppression and perpetuates privilege through its objectification of the body and its sanctioning of sensory detachment (Carmichael, 2012; Delgado & Stefancic, 1997; Johnson, 2011; Klein, 2016; Sherrell, 2018). When these two factors (objectification of the body and non-feeling) function in cooperation with one another, they set the stage for *othering*. Historically, differences in physical appearance, presentation, and expression have been the means through which othering and domination could be legitimized and enacted (Caldwell, 2014; Johnson, 2014; Sherrell, 2018).

Caldwell (2018) links othering with her notion of somatophobia by explaining that *somatophobia* is "both internalized as self-criticism of one's [own] body and externalized by critiquing others' bodies for deviating from a restrictive norm" (p. 36). What is understood and referred to as "normal" is the experience, expression, appearance, and world-view of the dominant culture. What does not conform to or fit this mold, whether it is in one's own body or another's, is pathologized or made wrong (Caldwell, 2018; Jensen, 2011; Klein, 2016). Those bodies at the margins of the dominant group are assigned limited and often stereotypic social identities. Adolescents are particularly susceptible to these stereotypic messages because they are at a crucial stage in identity development (Erikson, 1980) and may lack experience with the diverse range of normal human variation in body types, thereby "unconsciously tak[ing] this misinformation as truth" and feeling self-conscious about "flaws" in their own bodies (Dow, 2006, p. 302).

Dosamantes-Beaudry (1997) asserted that children learn "what to exalt or denigrate about their bodies" (p. 132) in accordance with the nonverbal social matrix of the environment around them. This view is affirmed by recent research in the field of body psychotherapy acknowledging that development is bodily based, with information being taken in from one's surroundings through sensory and somatic means (Grand, 2015). These interactions are the ground from which representations of self and other are formulated. These representations are, in turn, the basis for the feelings, postures, and enactments that both express and continue to create one's daily lived experience.

Given that dualistic perspectives on the mind and body make all bodies suspect and particular bodies wrong or pathological, the invitation to experience or inhabit one's body is a complex proposition. This is particularly true for teens, who may be more impacted by pervasive social perspectives on the body due to the significant physical changes and identity development that occur during adolescence. However, these same characteristics and developmental tasks are precisely what make embodied group work so essential in adolescent treatment.

Clinical Considerations

In a historically somatophobic environment, teens have few models and little guidance around how to listen to, celebrate, enjoy, and protect their bodies. In this void, adolescents tend to create their own structures for interacting with the body, using, for example, substances or sexual activity as a means for engaging somatic experience. Clinicians working with teens can use the arts to help teens explore and develop healthy relationships with their bodies.

Whether clients are molding and pounding clay, banging drums, or moving through a dance sequence, they are actively using their bodies during therapeutic explorations (Kossak, 2015). The arts, then, offer a means for experimenting with and practicing embodiment under conditions that do not carry the risk of real-life consequences. This imaginal realm, particularly when held in an inclusive way, can become a place to play with and explore one's relationship to their body.

As clinicians employ the arts to encourage exploration of the body and its experience, they need to keep in mind the ways that socially constructed views of the body can create resistance to active, embodied therapeutic approaches. In addition, group workers using embodied approaches need to be conscious of the ways othering and the idealization of some bodies impacts individual group members, as well as the overall group culture or climate. Finally, clinicians need to be cognizant of the ways their own biases and sociocultural locations may become embodied and unintentionally enacted. The following section explores the clinical implications of embodiment in more detail. Included are suggestions for approaches to supporting and developing embodiment with teens in a group context.

Self-Consciousness and the Impact on Teen Embodiment

Awareness of Self and Other

The messages that adolescents receive and internalize about their bodies inform not only how they sense, experience, and express themselves, but also how they believe others see them. This internal/external awareness is referred to respectively as *private body consciousness* and *public body consciousness* (Miller, Murphy, & Buss, 1981). Private body consciousness refers to an awareness of oneself gained through internal felt sense and *interoception*, or an internal experience of the state of the body (Duschek, Werner, Reyes del Paso, & Schandry, 2015). Public body consciousness refers to an individual's tendency to perceive self from an external point of view. Because evaluation of one's body is based on how it might appear to others, public body consciousness is vulnerable to the dominant social narrative, potentially resulting in self-objectification and negative self-image (Ainley & Tsakiris, 2013), particularly for teens in marginalized locations.

Developmental perspectives suggest that the awareness of self in the eyes of the other is particularly heightened during adolescence because it is a time of such dramatic physical change (Ryan & Kuczkowski, 1994), and the body, with its appearance, movements, and expressions, is always on display. As a result of socialization, teens might consciously or unconsciously recognize that the observing gaze of the other holds judgments and comparisons that reflect mainstream norms and ideals, creating an inhibitive self-consciousness, especially when they are among peers. For adolescents in marginalized locations, this consciousness may be significantly heightened because of their awareness of the dangers of not fitting into dominant social norms. Here, perceiving oneself from an external point of view is not simply developmental; it is, by necessity, perpetual. The impact of ongoing consideration of oneself from this external perspective can create a sense of internal disconnect. DuBois (1903/2009) described this as *double consciousness* or a quality of "twoness" resulting from "a sense of always looking at oneself through the eyes of others, of measuring one's soul by the tape of a world that looks on in amused contempt and pity" (p. 7).

Body Shame

Body shame "involves a state of self-consciousness [in which] individuals perceive their body shape or physical appearance as inferior in relation to the ideal [body] represented by the society" (Silva, 2013, p. 37). In an era of pervasive technology, teens are constantly bombarded with images of "perfect" bodies; images that are arbitrary yet pervasive in their portrayal of the norm. Media images in the current era are not just limited to magazine photos or film/TV images, but include 'selfies' and photos of real people on social media sites such as Facebook (FB) and Instagram. One study found that "the amount of FB time allocated to photo activity . . . is associated with greater thin ideal internalization, self-objectification, weight dissatisfaction, and drive for thinness" (Meier & Gray, 2014, p. 4). Other research noted that negative body image is closely associated with peer comparison on social media (de Vries, Peter, de Graaf, & Nikken, 2016; Fardouly, Diedrichs, Vartanian, & Halliwell, 2015; Ferguson, Muñoz, Garza, & Galindo, 2014).

Body shame can occur when adolescents constantly find fault with their own body in comparison to images of dominant bodies, enhanced bodies, or the bodies of their peers on social media. Clinicians need to be aware that negative body image has been linked to non-suicidal self-injury (Brausch & Muehlenkamp, 2014; Muehlenkamp & Brausch, 2012) and therefore remain sensitive to internalized, negative messages of individuals within a group. Due to the increase in body shame experienced by marginalized groups (Mason & Lewis, 2016; Menon & Harter, 2012), this is particularly important when working with youth-of-color, LGBTQ adolescents, and disabled youth.

Redefining Embodiment

In an environment where particular physical traits, qualities, and culturally bound behaviors or expressions are neither acceptable nor desirable, adolescents are "ultimately rejecting or being asked to reject a fundamental part of themselves" (Gullan, Hoffman, & Leff, 2011, p. 29) in order to fit in with their peers. In some situations, the unacceptable aspects of self may be pushed aside in favor of traits that are perceived to be more desirable. For survival, those in marginalized locations may create brilliant strategies for simulating socially acceptable appearances and behaviors that allow one to *pass*. Social-justice scholar Sherrell (2018) wrote:

> I am systematically and systemically pressured to simulate white bodies in white spaces . . . I am reminded everyday that my livelihood, and indeed my life, may depend on simulating well. Severe negative consequences are levied against those from other communication style backgrounds that are not carried in perceived (phenotypical) whiteness.
>
> (p. 148)

Little of the current literature on embodiment considers how dominant social norms and the resultant coping strategies may challenge current understandings or notions of 'being embodied.' As mentioned earlier, the word 'embodiment' often conjures ideas about sensation, connectivity, and authenticity. Sherrell (2018) contends that the term is problematic because it has been co-opted by Whiteness, suggesting that it assumes a sameness in bodily habitation and expression without consideration of social location and the influence of power, domination, and oppression. Sherrell went on to assert: "The term, [embodiment], as typically employed in dance movement therapy and body psychotherapy is code for white bodily processes and states" (2018, p. 149). The idea that there are normative standards for embodiment is further supported by feminist theorists who note how embodiment has historically been described by binary norms— male/female, well/ill, heterosexual/homosexual, Black/White (Johnson, 2011)—and their stereotypic characterizations.

Clinicians using art-based approaches with adolescents might consider how variation from these norms could influence embodiment. For example, how does having a body that has been deemed (at best) unacceptable influence the way one inhabits that body? What aspects of internal, sensate experience may be inaccessible because they are unacceptable? And which aspects of this internal experience may remain intentionally guarded and unexpressed? How are all of these possibilities also forms of embodiment? In a discourse that frequently equates embodiment with internal sensing and authentic expression, variations from this in the form of inhibition or avoidance are often pathologized as being "disembodied" (Sherrell, 2018). What may be more accurate is that embodiment takes many forms and shapes due to social location and the context a body is in. The next section looks at ways to approach embodiment in clinical work with this expanded understanding of the term.

Addressing Embodiment in Groups

Given that the current dominant discourse on the body can result in body shame, increased self-consciousness, and disconnection with aspects of self, the indicated clinical response is to support a state Grosz referred to as "embodied subjectivity" (1994, p. 22). Through interoception, a client can reestablish a sense of body-as-self that is rooted in self-awareness rather than self-objectification. The opportunity to connect with the body on one's own terms becomes, in the context of dominant social norms and the intensity of external pressure, a form of resistance or reclamation of self (Johnson, 2011; Sherrell, 2018).

Approaching embodiment from this subjective stance involves supporting teens to reconnect to their private body consciousness, to navigate the complex internal terrain of identifying and acknowledging authenticity—not as determined by external measures but through their own felt experience. Because the body is the site at which othering and the enactment of power and trauma occurs, entering into this private space, particularly in a group context, can be daunting and requires special care. Through self-awareness and attending to the dynamics of the group through an inclusive lens, group facilitators can invite embodied experience.

"Therapist, Know Thyself"

A space that is safe enough for adolescent group members to explore embodied clinical work necessitates the clinician's examination of their own identities and areas of privilege and marginalization. This needs to be an ongoing exploration that is both personal and professional. For example, a Native American, cisgender, heterosexual, art therapist has gender, sexuality, and class privilege. What does this mean for clinical work? What are the differences in this therapist's experience of body from that of their White, queer, working-class group member? How might these differences impact the member's ability and willingness to be vulnerable in a group setting? Social identity categories are intersectional in nature; clinicians and clients alike will likely belong to both dominant and marginalized groups. Within one group therapy session, clients and clinicians could both interact in ways that reinforce oppressive norms; therefore, it is an ethical necessity to apply an inclusive lens to clinical work with all populations, not just those who are perceived as marginalized.

In addition to the ongoing examination of personal privilege and implicit biases regarding social identity categories, clinicians need to understand their own body biases and the impact of such tendencies on the health of a group. As discussed earlier, the current mainstream culture of the United States is entrenched in body shame toward anyone whose body falls outside normative standards. For example, the medical model of physical health allows people to believe their biases against overweight people stem from concern for those people's health (Ratcliff & Ellison, 2015), when this is simply one of the most pervasive forms of body shaming (Gilbert & Miles, 2002). Current research tends toward a more inclusive approach to body size, noting that people who were formerly considered overweight and therefore "unhealthy" may be in better shape than people whose body types and Body Mass Index (BMI) are lower (Afzal, Tybjærg-Hansen Jensen, & Nordestgaard, 2016). Due to deeply ingrained attitudes *toward* fat people and subsequent messages internalized *by* fat people, it is vital that clinicians examine and challenge their own beliefs about a diverse range of body types.

Implicit body biases also have the capacity to extend beyond body type, and clinicians need to reflect on their assumptions about embodiment and expression when working with adolescents in a group setting. For example, what biases and implicit assumptions are present in a mixed-gender, mixed-race group? Does the clinician assume that cisgender young men are less likely to engage in dance/movement therapy than cisgender young women? Is there an assumption that Black male adolescents are going to be more physically aggressive than White ones? Or that youth of color will have an affinity for dance? These are uncomfortable beliefs to consider, but if clinicians avoid examination of ingrained prejudices and social messages, they miss an opportunity to deconstruct them, which is a necessary process for the ethical practice of arts-based groups with teens.

Furthermore, without considering how institutional influences become embodied and then enacted through interpersonal dynamics, the therapist might easily miss the social or historical significance of the exchanges occurring between group members. Catching these dynamics and the assumptions that enable them requires finely honed attention to and awareness of how one's own perception has been patterned by dominant social norms. The ability to hold this meta-level of awareness is crucial to the construction of an inclusive group climate.

Creating an Equitable Space Through the Arts

Part of what makes group work effective is its ability to evoke habituated relational patterns that are then addressed and worked through in the context of the session.

This potential is also what can make group work difficult in terms of inclusivity. Because participants enter group therapy carrying not only their family histories but also their sociocultural histories, the group environment can easily become a setting where pervasive social and institutional norms are re-enacted. People who identify as members of marginalized groups may experience more challenges in a group therapy setting due to "nonverbal asymmetry between individuals with differing social [statuses]" (Johnson, 2014, p. 83).

The arts, with their long history of serving to interrogate social and political norms, improve cognitions, cultivate social resilience (Dissanayake, 1988), "foster cooperation and obviate individual competitiveness" (Brown & Dissanayake, 2009, p. 46), can support cohesion and disrupt power structures and the re-enactment of "othering" in group therapy. The use of the arts as an inclusive practice involves understanding how institutional power dynamics occur through interpersonal relationships and in relationship to the arts materials themselves. For example, how might a client who holds more social privileges dominate artistic space? Do they play music louder, dance bigger, or horde art supplies? Does their silence or stillness control the group's development or momentum? Do they comment on the bodies of their peers, highlighting nondominant traits and behaviors?

It is the job of the group therapist to recognize the manifestation of such power structures and disrupt them in order to create an equitable space. Doing so literally means that more space is created for the presence of differences in embodiment and expression so that those in marginalized bodies are included in the emerging group culture. Such space means that one doesn't have to reject or leave part of oneself behind in order to belong (Gullan, Hoffman, & Leff, 2011).

An environment that can support someone's entirety also creates conditions for present-centered awareness and focused attention. As adolescent clients engage with artistic processes, they may enter a state of *flow* (Nachmanovitch, 1990; Nakamura & Csikszentmihalyi, 2014), an experience in which artists find themselves completely absorbed in the present moment while working on a creative task. Flow states are characterized by immersion, intense concentration, deep focus, present-moment awareness, distortion of time, and a merging of response, action, and awareness (Nakamura & Csikszentmihalyi, 2014). The increased value this places on the body and its sensations can act as a measure of resiliency against negative external messages (Milkman, Wanberg, & Robinson, 1995) and sociocultural conditioning. By learning to tune in to the body's intelligence through art making, adolescents begin to gain the resilience of a deep self-knowing that can support them in navigating the challenges of adolescence. In this way, an inclusive group environment supports all participants to make contact with and enter their creative somatic experiences, thus encouraging embodied participation.

The following warm-up is an example of the use of movement as an introduction to embodied, artistic work. It provides participants with an opportunity to tune in to their own bodies and engage in self-reflective processes.

Facilitator: *Begin by walking in the space. Move at any pace that feels comfortable to you. If it feels comfortable to do so, keep your gaze softly focused on the floor and your attention inward. Try not to worry about anyone else in the room.*

Facilitator:

[Participants walk around the room for several moments in silence, attention directed inward.]

Facilitator: *Notice the air moving in and out of your lungs. Do you breathe through your nose or mouth? You do not have to change anything, just notice how you breathe.*

[Some participants may pause in order to breathe fully, others will continue to walk while paying attention to their breath.]

Facilitator: *Feel your feet on the ground. How do you know the bottoms of your feet are there?*

[Participants continue to walk around the room, some may stop and examine their feet before continuing to walk.]

Facilitator: *Now, if it feels comfortable, bring your gaze up and out. Notice the environment. What objects do you see?*

[Participants continue to walk and look up at the walls, ceiling, and objects in the room; some may make eye contact with other participants. Reactions and responses will naturally occur.]

Facilitator: *Can you remain connected to your breath while you look around the room? How about the bottoms of your feet?*

Walking is an example of a pedestrian movement, or a movement that is done by people on a regular basis without a focus on aesthetics or performative aspects. The range of pedestrian movements is vast and, in this case, walking is only one way that movement through space may occur. The exercise can be adapted for people who use a wheelchair or need to sit down (bringing attention to hands or head instead of feet, same focus on breath). The slow, scaffolded approach to somatic awareness allows everyone to begin from the same place, which levels the playing field between people who have extensive experience with movement (for example, dancers) and those who do not. Finally, the simultaneous movement of all participants limits opportunities for witnessing one another, a process designed to decrease self-consciousness and feelings of body shame, while increasing group cohesion. As group cohesion and trust build, participants in the group can be challenged to see and be seen more. Although observation of another can potentially lead to objectification and the re-enactment of oppressive dynamics, seeing another through an inclusive lens has the potential to affirm identity and reestablish connection to self and other. This will be explored further in the next section.

Attunement and Affirmation

Attunement is a central tenet in dance/movement therapy methodologies and is defined as a form of "kinesthetic identification" (Loman & Foley, 1996, p. 345) that results in a deep, body-based recognition of another. The acknowledgement of another's internal state is often demonstrated through reflection. In the expressive arts, this reflection can be expressed through many forms such as sound, image, and movement. Dance/ movement therapy emphasizes the use of physical mirroring as a way to convey such understanding and acceptance (Chace, 1975; Levy, 2005). In form, mirroring involves the therapist moving in the same way as the client. However, rather than being purely imitative, the movement is 'taken in' by the therapist, allowing them to feel and sense the client's movement as they are doing it with them. The therapist's reflection may contain intentional variations in the size, shape, intensity, and pace of the movement as a way to support expression and avoid the appearance of mimicking.

By acknowledging and reflecting marginalized aspects of a client's experience, the therapist can offer what media and other purveyors of dominant social norms cannot: an external reflection of expression and identity that is neither stereotypic nor idealized. Such a reflection communicates acceptance of socially and personally rejected traits (Chace, 1975). Because identity formation is such an important task in adolescent development, validation of aspects of identity that are systematically negated or made invisible can be deeply healing.

Mirroring can be used to support the development of trust and empathy between members of the group as well. Participants in the group can be asked to "try on" one another's movements through various expressive, arts-based activities. One example frequently used in dance/ movement therapy is to have group members mirror back a movement from each person in the group. This action not only communicates to the mover that they have been received, but also provides those who are reflecting an opportunity to explore a different perspective through somatic means.

A note of caution: by making what may be held as private more visible and public, mirroring can be unintentionally intrusive or even oppressive across difference. It is therefore important for the clinician to consider the role that power and sociocultural locations can play in the dynamic. One way to address this is to titrate the experience by offering opportunities for mirroring that are less personal or at a greater distance from private consciousness, gradually moving toward more personal reflections as trust is built. Play and the imaginal realm provide ways to do this, as demonstrated in the following example of a familiar drama therapy warm-up game.

Facilitator: *Line up on the diagonal with everyone facing the same direction. The first person in the line will turn to face the person behind them and do some kind of movement or sound. The second person will repeat this sequence back to the person they received it from. Then they will turn to face the person behind them and they will do a new movement or sound. This will be repeated all the way down the line.*
[Participants line up with some giggling and chatter. The first person in line faces the person behind her and makes a high trilling sound accompanied by a small hand gesture. The person smiles and mirrors back. The second person then turns and faces the next person. There is a long pause as they appear to be thinking of what to do.]

Facilitator: *Try not to think too much! Keep it moving down the line! It's okay if it's silly or weird, it's a game!*
[The pace and energy of the group picks up. There is more laughter and sound as the movements and sounds travel down the line.]

This game can be varied and changed to meet the particular needs of the group. In this case, a diagonal line was used to minimize the amount of visibility and exposure while still providing an opportunity to be seen. More cohesion or trust in the group may make it possible to use other, more intimate spatial configurations such as a circle. The prompt to respond spontaneously without a lot of planning or thinking helps teens to stay with their experience rather than self-consciously considering how they may appear. Finally, the game-like context and permission to be silly allows teens to play with somatic expression without it being directly attributed to their private internal states.

In this and other movement activities with teens, it is important to establish boundaries around personal space and particular movements. For example, participants may be instructed that they are not allowed to touch each other or use movements that mimic violence toward the person mirroring them. Finally, it is important to allow the person mirroring to make adaptations that account for the state and needs of their own body. The activity can be closed with an invitation to participants to check in with their own internal state to notice how they are feeling. Have there been any changes in their energy level? In what it feels like to be in the group that day? In their mood?

Case Study

As we have now discovered, the problem with adolescent embodiment stems primarily from oppressive cultural norms that shame somatic experiences and expressions. Moreover, the developmental period of adolescence is characterized, in part, by feelings of insecurity and a desire to 'fit in' with peers (Eccles & Roeser, 2011; Schall, Wallace, & Chhuon, 2016). For these reasons, many adolescents will be timid about engaging in embodied work because they may feel less vulnerable sitting and talking than they do moving and feeling. However, as much as embodied arts-based approaches might intimidate, they also have enormous potential to counteract and heal the dominant social narratives around the body, its role, and the narrow confines that allow it to be acceptable. The following case study, which took place at a public high school on the west coast of the United States, explored embodiment with a group of adolescent participants. While the program was psychoeducational rather than clinical, parallels can be drawn between this project and clinical work. Forty-two adolescents (split into two groups), ages 16–18 years, participated in two 90-minute sessions that utilized an arts-based approach to explore the topics of depression, anxiety, and self-harm. Dance and drama were the primary modalities used, but visual art was also included.

Establishing the Space—Introductions

As mentioned earlier, establishing a safe enough space for artistic exploration through the body is about establishing a space that does not perpetuate the same unjust social dynamics that exist outside the group. This requires the therapist to be aware of the group's process at both the interpersonal and institutional levels and to offer interventions that disrupt oppressive dynamics without shaming or spotlighting participants. This process can begin immediately through the way introductions happen in the group. In the case study below, the facilitators introduced themselves by stating their names and gender pronouns, inviting participants to do the same if they felt so inclined.

This gender inclusive practice offers space for both gender conforming and gender non-conforming students to state their identities if they so desire. The risk of such an opening is that youth who may not be ready to share their particular gender location could feel pressured to identify or be identified simply by their choice not to respond to the invitation to share. One way of working with this unintended outcome might be to offer a space where youth are invited to share something about who they are that would enable them to bring more of themselves into the room. This introduction can be modeled by the therapist as a way to provide some guidelines and structure for the sharing.

For example, the therapist might say, "*I'm Wendy, I'm White and I identify as female. I'm excited to be here.*" Since the beginning phases of group work often involve assessing belonging (Corey, Corey, & Corey, 2010), such a process could indicate to participants that difference is recognized and welcomed. Carmichael (2012) suggested that such intentional self-disclosure could even serve as an invitation. "If a client feels that [their] therapist has the courage to step into that conversation, [they] too, may be willing to explore the complex topic" (p. 108).

The creation of group agreements followed introductions on day one of this project. Each participant had an opportunity to verbalize an item that would support them to fully engage with the work. Items included: *respect, open-mindedness, confidentiality, support,* and *cooperation.* Each item was discussed and agreed upon before it was added to the agreements poster. Agreements of this kind provide leverage throughout sessions for group dynamics that move into unsafe territory. For example, if an agreement has been made to respect the opinions of all members and someone makes a comment that is disrespectful or shaming, the agreement can be referenced and clients can be redirected appropriately. Agreement to uphold such values can also serve as a tool to combat other messages adolescents receive from the dominant culture: messages that tell them their bodies and identities are flawed or wrong.

Embodied Exploration of Topics

After the initial warm-up, which included walking, breathwork, and grounding, participants created posters using words and experiences that they personally connected to each of the three topics (depression, anxiety, self-harm). Words written by the students included:

- Depression: *alone, no other way, putting on a cracked mask, shame, quiet, sad, isolation, doom.*
- Anxiety: *can't breathe, heavy, on edge, amped, constant fear, racing heart.*
- Self-harm: *quiet, ugly, comforting, "dumb," justify, numb, regret.*

Following the poster-making session, participants were invited to slowly walk in the space, concentrating on their own body. This format was familiar because it was introduced in the warm-up. The process of focusing on one's own body was intended to decrease self-consciousness and impede the projection of cultural norms onto others' bodies through witnessing. The facilitator explained the structure of the following exercise as participants walked. This structure was designed to allow for movement of emotion; sitting still when one is nervous or fearful causes those feelings to become blocked in the body, whereas gentle movement allows them to release, supporting participants to be more easeful with the exercise.

Facilitators should be aware of different learning styles and know that some participants may need to pause their movement momentarily as they digest verbal instructions or information. After allowing participants a few moments to move in the space, the facilitator spoke several of the words participants had written and asked them to pause their walk in order to create embodied shapes or gestures for each of the words.

During this exercise, it was clear that many participants were hesitant to engage in an embodied way. They giggled, glanced at each other, moved haltingly into shapes, and looked expectantly at the facilitator to see if they were "right." This may have been due to self-conscious feelings, lack of experience with embodiment, and/or lack of experience with artistic expression. The facilitator offered gentle encouragement, acknowledging that shapes and gestures can range from tiny and/or subtle to large and grandiose. Each word was repeated three times by the facilitator with a prompt to change or deepen the shape or gesture after each word. Finally, the participants were asked to speak the word while they held their pose. Once the experiential exercise was complete, participants were invited to sit in a circle for a verbal debriefing of the process. Facilitators asked the simple question, "*What was that like for you?*" Participants noted that the exercise was "*challenging,*" "*refreshing,*" and "*relieving.*" One participant stated that she felt a release of the stigma surrounding the topic when she created an embodied representation of it. Another participant noted that embodying the words allowed them to "get out" of their head.

Following the warm-up and creation of individual shapes, participants were asked to create a group sculpture for each of the three topics. This exercise brought their individual experiences into the realm of interpersonal relationships as they created shapes and gestures that connected to each other. By this point in the session, many participants appeared more at ease with embodied work and freely used their bodies to create poses signifying their experience. This is likely attributed to the use of embodied exercises during the warm-up as well as the constant encouragement and validation from facilitators, who often noted "*there is no wrong way to do this.*" Even so, some participants remained hesitant and needed support from group members and facilitators to engage in the process. Such diversity of participation is typical for movement-based, experiential group work and highlights the cultural norm of cerebral, verbal processing over somatic, nonverbal processing.

At the end of the session, participants were given a homework assignment to take two photographs: one that depicted their understanding and/or experience with either depression, anxiety, or self-harm and one that depicted their understanding and/or experience with resilience. The photographs were viewed on a projector at the beginning of session two and discussed verbally. Students noted that anxiety was commonly correlated with school and school work, and that animals and music were prominent themes of resilience. The photography homework was offered so that participants had another language through which they might communicate their feelings. While the in-person sessions consisted of embodied work, the photographs offered space for participants to engage with their bodies (if they chose) in a potentially less intimidating way.

Some images that included bodies were: a participant curled in the fetal position amid scattered piles of exams and papers (anxiety), a participant's arm with the word "shame" painted on it (self-harm), a participant's face with the shadow of a noose in the foreground (depression). Images that did not include bodies were: a black and white photo of empty swings (depression), a guitar (resilience), the front of the school (anxiety). Inclusion of bodies in the photos was not mandatory, which allowed each participant to be as creatively expansive as they chose; however, clinicians could choose to make this a required component of the homework if it felt appropriate and productive for the group.

During the final arts-based exercise in session two, participants were divided into three groups, each tasked with the creation of three frozen pictures telling a story of an experience with one of the three topics (depression, anxiety, or self-harm) and how resilience could support the mental health complexity. The story could be fictional or based on real-life experiences, the choice of which was determined by members of each group. At this point, participants appeared more comfortable with the act of embodied work and stepped into the exercise with greater confidence than in previous activities, suggesting that inclusive practices and scaffolded exposure to arts-based exercises are necessary components to reduce adolescent resistance to embodied work. Moreover, engagement with an exercise that included discussion, planning, and presenting within a peer group seemed more supportive of issues of confidence than "fish bowl" type activities in which one person works while the rest of the group witnesses. The groups then presented their frozen pictures to each other and verbally discussed the process following each presentation. Witnesses to the presentations noted specific aspects of the stories, particularly how social pressures were often the reason why an individual might suffer from depression, anxiety, or self-harm. This process supported participants to gain insight into the experiences of others that likely reflected their own.

The session closed with facilitators and participants sitting in a circle. Moving around the circle, one participant at a time was invited to create a sound or movement for how they felt in that moment. Finally, participants were presented with notebooks that had lists of school and community resources that could be accessed for further information, counseling, or therapy.

Summary

While this project was therapeutic in nature, it did not delve into individual or group psychotherapy, which might seek to understand internal and external factors relating to participants' struggles with depression, anxiety, or self-harm. Rather, the project's main goals were to introduce the topic of resilience to high school students, decrease stigma attached to mental health complexities, and connect students to school and community mental health resources. If undertaken in a more clinical setting, facilitators would support participants to engage with cognitive or somatic impulses, ultimately seeking a change in thoughts, feelings, or behavior. However, the problem of adolescent embodiment remains the same in both psychoeducational and clinical formats, requiring facilitators to ask: how can we create a safe enough space for group members to explore their authentic body without feeling overly oppressed by normative values?

References

Ainley, V., & Tsakiris, M. (2013). Body conscious? Interoceptive awareness, measured by heartbeat perception, is negatively correlated with self-objectification. *PLoS ONE, 8*(2), e55568.

Afzal, S., Tybjærg-Hansen, A., Jensen, G. B., & Nordestgaard, B. G. (2016). Change in Body Mass Index associated with lowest mortality in Denmark, 1976–2013. *JAMA, 315*(18), 1989–1996.

Brausch, A. M., & Muehlenkamp, J. J. (2014). Experience of the body. In L. Claes & J. J. Muehlenkamp (Eds,), *Non-suicidal self injury in eating disorders* (pp. 237–253). Berlin, Germany: Springer

Brown, S., & Dissanayake, E. (2009). The arts are more than aesthetics: Neuroaesthetics as narrow aesthetics. In M. Skov & O. Vartanian (Eds.), *Foundations and frontiers in aesthetics: Neuroaesthetics* (pp. 43–57). Amityville, NY: Baywood.

Caldwell, C. (2014). Mindfulness & bodyfulness: A new paradigm. *The Journal of Contemplative Inquiry, 1*(1), 69–88.

Caldwell, C. (2018). Body identity development. In C. Caldwell & L. B. Leighton (Eds.), *Oppression and the body: Roots, resistance, and resolutions* (pp. 31–50). Berkley, CA: North Atlantic Books.

Carmichael, N. G. (2012). Turning towards multicultural diversity competence in dance/movement therapy. *American Journal of Dance Therapy, 34*(2), 99–113.

Chace, M. (1975). *Marian Chace: Her papers.* (H. Chaiklin, Ed.). Columbia, MD: American Dance Therapy Association.

Cohen, B. (1993). *Sensing, feeling, and action: The experiential anatomy of Body-Mind Centering.* Northampton, MA: Contact Editions.

Corey, M. S., Corey, G., & Corey, C. (2010). *Groups: Process and practice.* (9th ed.). Belmont, CA: Brooks/Cole.

Delgado, R., & Stefancic, J. (1997) *Critical white studies: Looking behind the mirror.* Philadelphia, PA: Temple University Press.

Descartes, R. (1991). *Descartes: Selected philosophical writings.* (J. Cottingham, R. Stoothoff, D. Murdoch, Trans.). New York, NY: Cambridge University Press. (Original work published 1641)

de Vries, D. A., Peter, J., de Graaf, H., & Nikken, P. (2016). Adolescents' social network site use, peer appearance-related feedback, and body dissatisfaction: Testing a mediation model. *Journal of Youth and Adolescence, 45*(1), 211–224.

Dissanayake, E. (1988). *What is art for?* Seattle, WA: University of Washington Press.

Dosamantes-Beaudry, I. (1997). Embodying a cultural identity. *The Arts in Psychotherapy, 24*(2), 129–135.

Dow, B. J. (2006). Gender and communication in mediated contexts. In B. J. Dow & J. T. Wood (Eds.), *The Sage handbook of gender and communication* (pp. 263–270). London: Sage.

Du Bois, W. E. B. (2009). *The souls of black folk.* New York, NY: Simon & Schuster. (Original work published in 1903)

Duschek, S., Werner, N. S., Reyes del Paso, G. A., & Schandry, R. (2015). The contributions of interoceptive awareness to cognitive and affective facets of body experience. *Journal of Individual Differences, 36*(2), 110–118.

Eccles, J. S., & Roeser, R. W. (2011). Schools as developmental contexts during adolescence. *Journal of Research on Adolescence, 21*(1), 225–241.

Erikson, E. (1980). *Identity and the life cycle.* New York, NY: Norton.

Fardouly, J., Diedrichs, P. C., Vartanian, L. R., & Halliwell, E. (2015). Social comparisons on social media: The impact of Facebook on young women's body image concerns and mood. *Body Image, 13*, 38–45.

Ferguson, C. J., Muñoz, M. E., Garza, A., & Galindo, M. (2014). Concurrent and prospective analyses of peer, television and social media influences on body dissatisfaction, eating disorder symptoms and life satisfaction in adolescent girls. *Journal of Youth and Adolescence 43*(1), 1–14.

Gilbert, P., & Miles, J. (Eds.). (2002). *Body shame: Conceptualisation, research and treatment.* London: Routledge.

Grand, I. J. (2015). Body, culture, and body-oriented psychotherapies. In G. Marlock & H. Weiss (Eds.), *The handbook of body psychotherapy and somatic psychology* (pp. 264–272). Berkeley, CA: North Atlantic Books.

Grosz, E. (1994). *Volatile bodies. Towards a corporeal feminism.* Bloomington, IN: Indiana University Press.

Gullan, R. L., Hoffman, B. N., & Leff, S. S. (2011). "I do but I don't": The search for identity in urban African American adolescents. *Perspectives on Urban Education, 8*(2), 29–38.

Haen, C., & Weil, M. (2010). Group therapy on the edge: Adolescence, creativity, and group work. *Group, 34*(1), 37–52.

Jensen, S. Q. (2011). Othering, identity formation and agency. *Qualitative Studies, 2*(2), 63–78.

Johnson, R. (2011). The silent wound: Discourse and the non-verbal re-production of oppression. (Unpublished master's thesis). Meridian University, Petaluma, CA.

Johnson, R. (2014). Grasping and transforming the embodied experience of oppression. *International Body Psychotherapy Journal, 14*(1), 80–95.

Johnson, R. (2018). *Embodied social justice.* New York, NY: Routledge.

Klein, S. (2016). *Social justice-oriented dance movement therapy: A new clinical paradigm.* (Unpublished master's thesis). Naropa University, Boulder, CO.

Kossak, M. (2015). *Attunement in expressive arts therapy: Toward an understanding of embodied empathy.* Springfield, IL: Charles Thomas.

Levy, F. (2005). *Dance movement therapy: A healing art.* Reston, VA: The American Alliance for Health, Physical Education, Recreation, and Dance.

Loman, S., & Foley, L. (1996). Models for understanding the nonverbal process in relationships. *The Arts in Psychotherapy, 23*(4), 341–350.

Malekoff, A. (2014). *Group work with adolescents* (3rd ed.). New York, NY: Guilford.

Mason, T. B., & Lewis, R. J. (2016). Minority stress, body shame, and binge eating among lesbian women: Social anxiety as a linking mechanism. *Psychology of Women Quarterly, 40*(3), 428–440.

Meier, E. P., & Gray, J. (2014). Facebook photo activity associated with body image disturbance in adolescent girls. *Cyberpsychology, Behavior, and Social Networking, 17*(4), 199–206.

Menon, C. V., & Harter, S. L. (2012). Examining the impact of acculturative stress on body image disturbance among Hispanic college students. *Cultural Diversity and Ethnic Minority Psychology, 18*(3), 239.

Milkman, H., Wanberg, K., & Robinson, C. (1995). *Project self discovery: Artistic alternatives for high risk youth.* Retrieved from www.cominguptaller.org/report/chapter2-1.

Miller, L. C., Murphy, R., & Buss, A. H. (1981). Consciousness of body: Private and public. *Journal of Personality and Social Psychology, 41*(2), 397–406.

Muehlenkamp, J. J., & Brausch, A. M. (2012). Body image as a mediator of non-suicidal self-injury in adolescents. *Journal of Adolescence, 35*(1), 1–9.

Nachmanovitch, S. (1990). *Free play: Improvisation in life and art.* New York, NY: Penguin.

Nakamura, J., & Csikszentmihalyi, M. (2014). The concept of flow. In M. Csikszentmihalyi (Ed.), *Flow and the foundations of positive psychology: The collected works of Mihaly Csikszentmihalyi* (pp. 239–263). Dordrecht, Netherlands: Springer.

Ratcliff, D., & Ellison, N. (2015). Obesity and internalized weight stigma: A formulation model for an emerging psychological problem. *Behavioural and Cognitive Psychotherapy, 43*(2), 239–252.

Ryan, R. M., & Kuczkowski, R. (1994). The imaginary audience, self-consciousness, and public individuation in adolescence. *Journal of Personality, 62*(2), 219–238.

Schall, J., Wallace, T. L., & Chhuon, V. (2016). 'Fitting in' in high school: How adolescent belonging is influenced by locus of control beliefs. *International Journal of Adolescence and Youth, 21*(4), 462–475.

Sherrell, C. (2018). The oppression of black bodies. In C. Caldwell & L. B. Leighton (Eds.), *Oppression and the body: Roots, resistance, and resolutions* (pp. 141–155). Berkley, CA: North Atlantic Books.

Silva, A. R. D. C. (2013). Evaluating the effect of body dissatisfaction and body shame on eating psychopathology in young adolescence: The role of cognitive fusion, experiential avoidance and fear of self-compassion (Unpublished doctoral dissertation). University of Coimbra, Coimbra, Portugal.

14

Embodied Practices and Queer Anthems

Working Against Risk Discourses With Young People 'At the Margins'

ELLY SCRINE AND CAMILLA STANGER

Introduction

Since its cultural "invention" as a distinct developmental stage in the early twentieth century, adolescence has been a key site for public and private discussion about sex, gender, and sexual identity. While (often inequitable) gender and sexuality norms may intensify during adolescence and can set trajectories for health, wellbeing and social empowerment (Chandra-Louli et al., 2017), contemporary international research reveals how young people are actively negotiating, challenging, and re-writing these scripts (Bragg; Renold, Ringrose & Jackson, 2018). It is therefore crucial for those who conduct therapeutic, educational, or community-based work with adolescents to remain sensitive to the voices and complex identities of young people, and to develop a critical understanding of debates surrounding young people's sexualities when developing practice(s). In this chapter, we discuss some theoretical and practical strategies for doing just this, specifically as arts-based practitioner–researchers who work with young people who are positioned 'on the margins' in regard to their (sometimes imagined) sexualities.

We adopt the position that those who aim to conduct affirmative and inclusive therapeutic or educational work with young people must develop approaches that are mindful of how young people's sexualities are regulated and policed by adults and institutions, with a critical awareness of one's own position as often privileged adult professionals. We discuss this in specific relation to developing arts-based projects in mainstream urban school settings with young people deemed "at risk" (and doing so as White, middle class, neuro-typical, adult practitioner–researchers, both socialized as women).

Working to confront and challenge exclusionary processes with a diverse cohort of young working-class Black British[1] women in an inner-city London college,[2] dance teacher Camilla develops and evaluates a feminist and anti-racist dance–voice pedagogy (Brown, 2009; hooks, 1994; Sears, 2010). In the outer suburbs of Melbourne, Australia, music therapist Elly approaches group work as an anti-oppressive practice (Baines, 2013), where young people engage creatively in exploring gender, sexualities, and experiences related to power and violence. Through discussions of our respective work and its points of overlap, we invite group clinicians/practitioners/facilitators to develop a critical understanding of the relevant issues that contextualize adolescent sexualities, while offering some ideas for critical and creative practice with young people 'at the margins.'

Thinking Critically About Adolescent Sexualities

The question of what constitutes a "healthy" sexuality for young people has been critiqued across the fields of gender studies, psychotherapy, and the sociology of education as an act of control, and one that manifests in rigid gender and sexuality norms. Early sociological research in this respect demonstrates a fraught history of medicalization and pathologizing of the transgression of gender and sexuality norms (Foucault, 1990), while contemporary literature problematizes, for example, our tendency to see Lesbian, Gay, Bisexual, Transgender, Queer, Intersex and Asexual (LGBTQIA+) youth as inherently vulnerable (Bryan, 2017), or their gender identities as symptoms of mental ill health (McNeil et al., 2012). Researchers also discuss how questions around the "health" of a young person's sexuality can center upon particular raced, classed, and gendered identities. For example, Weekes (2002; 2004) explored the ways in which young working-class Black British women can be positioned through ideas of hypersexuality and deviance, and therefore adopt their own compensatory strategies of sexual conservatism and respectability to avoid such labeling. This critical literature suggests that when sex is understood as a site of moral, physical, and economic 'risk' for a young person, their pleasure and personal choices come to matter less, and their bodies and what they choose to do with them become a matter for intervention and (sometimes self-directed) control (Keller, Mendes, & Ringrose, 2016; Renold & Ringrose, 2011).

Alongside these discussions are equally important considerations of the ways in which sex and sexuality can indeed be a site of harm for young people, especially when it comes to particular relations of power. For example, schools have been widely acknowledged as spaces where girls and young women commonly experience sexual harassment, which is typically normalized as a part of adolescent social–sexual development (Conroy, 2013). There is substantially less research into how violence intersects with queer and gender diverse identities, and even less so investigating intersections of 'race' with gender and sexuality, despite evidence indicating that LGBTQIA+ young people and communities of color endure disproportionately rates of violence in this respect (Grant et al., 2011; Smith et al., 2014). Overall, however, the literature widely suggests that adolescent sexualities develop and operate within sometimes oppressive relations of power, both interpersonal and institutional.

From Harm and Control, to Agency and Creative Practice

Leading authors in LGBTQIA+ adolescent literature elucidate how, in positioning certain groups of young people as being 'at risk' of harm, we may institutionally (re)position these groups as vulnerable, powerless victims (Bryan, 2017; Rasmussen et al., 2017). Concurrently, Ruth Nicole Brown (2009) has explored how well-meaning, White, liberal interventions into the lives of young Black women, even with a goal of empowerment, can serve to sideline young women's agency. These concerns require expanding from an approach that seeks to single out and *help* marginalized groups, to focus on the structures and effects of normativity to which *every* young person is subjected, sometimes referred to in queer youth literature as an *after-queer* approach (Talburt & Rasmussen, 2010). Such an approach comes to focus on diversity of experience, possibilities, and capacity for joy, pleasure, agency, and creativity. Indeed, the importance of young people's (often very creative) agency in directing and re-writing their sexual identities in the face of public discourses of 'risk' (Hickey-Moody, 2013; Sears, 2010), and in creating alternative spaces of relative 'safety' from sexual violence (Kearney, 2007), should not be underestimated.

Anti-oppressive practice (AOP) provides therapists and other practitioners with a helpful framework for viewing the roots of people's problems not as their personal failings, but as related to power structures and relations (Baines, 2007). The premise of AOP is that intersecting structures of oppression such as patriarchy, racism, ableism, heterosexism, and colonization are *relevant to* and *part of* our practice and the lives of the people with whom we work. In this sense, the therapeutic space should not be seen as separate from these power relations, but rather a space for transforming them. AOP is utilized as a key methodological and theoretical paradigm in social work and, more recently, has been developed as an approach for music therapists (Baines, 2013). In general, the creative arts have been posited as fitting therapeutic spaces for working against deficit models of 'risk' and 'vulnerability' because they are inherently strengths-based and participatory, and emphasize therapy as something clients 'do,' as opposed to something that is done 'to' or 'for' them (Bain, Grzanka & Crowe, 2016; Baines, 2013; Sajnani, Marxen, & Zarate, 2017).

Why Arts-Based Group Work?

Guattari (1995) proposed the vitality and unique capacity of artistic creation to "engender unprecedented, unforeseen and unthinkable qualities of being" (1995, p. 106). Renold (2017) drew on the work of Guattari (among others) to explicate the emancipatory potential of arts-based methodologies to foster new forms of thinking, feeling, and voicing with young people across contexts and identities. Renold and her colleagues' research (e.g., Renold, 2017; Renold & Ivinson, 2015; Renold & Ringrose, 2016) views art-based group practices such as visual arts, music, dance, sculpting, photography, filmmaking, and more as offering dynamic and powerful opportunities to support young people "to safely and creatively communicate and potentially transform oppressive sexual cultures and practices" (Renold, 2017, p. 1). The literature also illustrates ways in which the creative arts therapies—including art therapy (Visser & du Plessis, 2015), drama therapy (Haen, 2007), dance/movement therapy (Pierce, 2014), and music therapy (Fairchild, Thompson, & McFerran, 2016)—may be used to support young people who have experienced violence and/or abuse.

Fittingly for our research contexts, the creative arts therapies literature also reveals a corollary interest in critical, feminist, queer-affirming, anti-racist, and anti-oppressive approaches. In developing a 'radically inclusive' queer music therapy framework for adolescent contexts, Bain et al. (2016) argued that, rather than positioning such work as 'therapy for queer clients,' we instead consider 'queer therapy,' where young people are not assumed to be vulnerable, in need of fixing, or encouraged to adjust to an oppressive culture. Evaluating the queer music therapy model, Boggan et al. (2017) noted how such an approach may be considered an 'intervention' itself, but into the systems that position particular communities on the margins.

Sajnani (2012) has also argued for extending the central tenets of feminist therapy into a critical race feminist paradigm to consider how the body is a gendered, racialized, and classed site of political and social struggle, and where creative arts therapists have not only the capacity but also a *responsibility* to utilize the arts as a site for social justice. Since then, authors such as Wright and Wright (2017) and Sajnani et al. (2017) have explored the significance of critical approaches to the creative arts therapies in de-pathologizing marginalized identities, reshaping therapeutic relationships, and situating social justice as central to healing.

Introducing Our Contexts and Practical Approaches

Camilla's research explores the ways in which her research participants, as young Black British women who study for vocational courses in a 16–19 college, face processes of implicitly racist, sexist, and classist moral panic (Cohen, 1999) around their bodies and their sexualities. These young women were West African and/or African Caribbean in heritage, and despite mobilising their 'Blackness' 'Britishness' and 'woman-ness' in diverse ways, they encountered an essentialising and pathologising positioning common to the experiences of young women identified as 'Black' in UK schools (Weekes, 2002; 2004; Youdell, 2006). For example, on three separate occasions during her research, senior staff members approached Camilla in her role as dance teacher to request that Black female students either "cover up" or "wear more clothes" during dance rehearsal, with one of these requests occurring during the college's open evening for prospective students and parents. In these instances, and within this institutional sphere, it seems that a young Black woman could not simply enjoy and direct her own body, for example in the production of an art form or an aesthetic ideal: her body was a sexualized item of public property, with the power to harm—the girl it belonged to, the institution it belonged in, or even, implicitly, the staff member who was looking at it. A practice of 'risk management' around young Black women's bodies (and sexualities) was also enacted in how Black working-class young women were discussed in staff meetings as being "at risk of pregnancy" (more so than other students in the college). These findings resonate with research around young Black women's bodies becoming objects for "punishment and consumption" (Brown, 2009, p. 93) and for intervention and 'healing' (Mirza, 2010; Youdell, 2006) within schools, raising a question: where are young Black women's *own* experiences of their bodies and their sexualities?

For the purposes of this chapter, we suggest seeking communal, creative spaces and embodied practices in which young women can articulate, explore, and draw pleasure from their sexualities "outside of oppressive discourse" (Mirza, 2010, p. 5). However, we also propose that there is no singular way to set up or evaluate arts-based group work, and to suggest so might in itself be harmful. In this respect, Camilla takes a pedagogical rather than therapeutic approach, in which mutual processes of deeply embodied and emotionally engaged learning, and therefore (ex)change, take place between members of a learning community, in service of liberation within a world marked by racial, gender, and class inequalities (hooks, 1994). We argue that for Camilla to have developed an explicitly therapeutic approach within this particular context, especially as a White, middle-class woman, would have been to potentially reinforce discourses around the excessive and deviant sexualities of young Black women in need of treating/healing. The aim would therefore be to strive to co-develop a space in which young women can articulate and explore their sexualities on their own terms, in resistance to the pathologizing White, patriarchal gaze of the institution. It is in this respect that we turn to dance as an empowering practice.

Research suggests that dance, a practice that uniquely occupies an overlapping space between the athletic cultural production of sport and the aesthetic cultural production of art, can deconstruct the physically debilitating norms of patriarchy for the young woman, freeing an embodied space for her to do and to create (Paechter, 2013; Stinson, 1998). Dance has also been discussed as a powerful practice through which Black women direct their subjectivities in the face of controlling discourses (Gottschild, 2003; Stanger, 2016; Stanley Niaah, 2010), with Sears (2010) suggesting that through dancing *together*, young Black women can experience a deeply corporeal sense of "Black female bodies as sites of beauty, pleasure, agency and power" (p. 134). In this respect, Sears (2010) foregrounded dancing that centers around and emanates from the pelvis and buttocks, as a bodily site of cultural signification and remembering that comes to be experienced through dance as intensely sensual *and* transcendent, in ways that simultaneously embrace but also go beyond sexuality.

Brown (2009) has also explored this, but in relation to the power of the Black girl dance cipher, or freestyle circle. This is a lively communal space, in which dancer–participants move together in a close-knit circle and take turns to enter its center. Once at the center of this energized space, the dancer–participant, using whatever movements they choose/feel in that moment, dances—for their fellow Black girls, and for themselves. Brown (2009) argued that the dance cipher "provides the possibility of creating a narrative of the self in communal company that insists on complex identities. . . [regarding] who we are and what we want to be" (2009, p. 101). Drawing on this research and the artistic offerings of her students, Camilla worked with groups of young women to explore practices that moved away from dance as an individualized (and institutionalized) performing art form and toward dance as a social, meaning-sharing, and meaning-making practice that might challenge institutional discourses of 'risk' and deviance.

Music Therapy Research

Two overarching aims of Elly's research and practice run in parallel: 1) to locate music therapy within broader health, education, and community contexts as an engaging, liberatory space for young people to explore, examine, and communicate their experiences related to gender and sexuality, and 2) to develop and deepen creative arts therapists' understanding of critical issues related to adolescents, gender, and sexuality. Elly seeks to contribute to empirical understandings of critical and anti-oppressive practice in music therapy, emphasizing the ways in which young people's participation in the creative arts can allow for interrelated experiences of therapy and activism. Underpinning this kind of group work are contemporary approaches to collaboration with young people, particularly the work of scholars who focus on intergenerational feminist activism (Brown, 2016), attend to intersecting notions of race, class, dis/ability, and sexuality (Ahmed, 2017; Renold & Ringrose, 2011; Showumni, 2017; Stanger, 2016), and disrupt discourses of postfeminism and neoliberalism with girls in schools (Retallack et al., 2016).

When commencing an action research project in a public high school, Elly conducted preliminary interviews with staff, asking their impressions about whether the school was a safe place for LGBTQIA+ young people, to which she received a range of conflicting responses. Two teaching staff and one of the school social workers described the school as *"extremely open and tolerant,"* with a sense of inclusion between students: *"boys, girls, nothing's off limits,"* said one staff member. Contrastingly, another said, *"I don't think we're quite there yet . . . it's not like you're just going to be seeing people be super open about their sexuality, or their gender."*

During these interviews, Elly noted how teaching and well-being staff regularly referred to the "cultural" aspect of these issues, and how exploring them would be most helpful for particular groups of students. Ward (2017) described a common view among Australian teachers that 'Western' ideas and values fundamentally clash with those from Islamic cultures. In this instance, the teachers were referring to students from particular cultural backgrounds, as well as those who were Muslim, upholding the prevailing narrative around supposedly progressive 'Western values' that meant exploring oppressive gender and sexuality constructs was *most* important for those students who were not White. This sits within a context of deeply embedded colonial and assimilatory narratives in the Australian education system (Patrick & Moodie, 2016) and a complex culture of racism and xenophobia in Australian schools (Mansouri & Jenkins, 2010). Reflecting on this culture further contextualizes processes of 'risk management' and panic that operate in regard to young people's gender identities and sexualities. Within an institutional context that both denies and perpetuates racist and heterosexist discourses, Elly's research and practice examines music therapy as an inclusive, engaging, and critical space for young people in school to explore gender and how it relates to power, sexuality, and their lived experiences.

Complications and Risks

In setting up a liberating pedagogical/therapeutic space, where members of a community feel ready to share and "create a [dancing/talking/writing/singing] narrative of the self in communal company" (Brown, 2009, p. 101), the matter of trust and "safety" always emerges as a complication. Indeed, we are setting up spaces for young people to share and explore their gender and sexual identities: spaces that are never entirely free from the discourses of judgment, shame, and 'risk' that operate within the world 'outside' the pedagogy/therapy space. However, we also adopt the position that tensions within this space can be drawn upon as important sites of healing, learning and (ex)change (hooks, 1994). In this respect, some shared reflections have emerged from these two separate research projects, especially regarding the points of difference that emerge between us as raced, gendered, and classed professionals, and the young people we conduct our research with. These differences in many ways cannot and should not be minimized, despite how critically we draw upon anti-racist and intersectional theories.

These complications invite a particular kind of reflexivity in navigating points of difference and remaining attendant to relationships, how these relationships play out through bodies and feelings, and how these relationships imply and enact processes of power. We aim to demonstrate this form of reflexivity throughout our practice and in disseminating our reflections through the rest of this chapter.

Case Material

Case Example 1: "Let's Play One Black Girl in the Middle!" (Camilla)

Within my (CS) Ph.D. project, I worked with a class group of 17 young British women aged 16–19 years who were studying for a vocational qualification in Health and Social Care. The different ethnic and national heritages within the group, as articulated by the young women, included Black West African, Black African Somali, Black Caribbean, Turkish, and Iranian. I had initially spent a few weeks getting to know the group in the context of their classroom lessons, in which we discussed our personal, cultural, and national identities as a group of (very different) women—discussions in which I named and attempted to de-center my privileged position as a White, middle-class adult. After this initial period, we moved our weekly sessions to the college dance studio. In our first session together in this new space, we sat on the floor with blankets and cushions, curtains drawn over the windows, watching YouTube clips of dance chosen by the group and discussing what dance means to women from different cultures. This session erupted into a spontaneous final free-style dance session after the lesson time was officially over, in which some of the students showed off their moves in dancehall and bellydance.[3] In all this, I was hoping we had started to (co)create something of a radical yet caring 'home' space (Brown, 2009; Sears, 2010). However, despite this initially promising start, it took some time for the sessions to develop toward a liberating group pedagogy.

A key intention was to co-develop a space that belonged as much as possible to the young women, shaped by their styles of embodiment, as part of a goal of de-centering hegemonic, institutional norms (hooks, 2003), allowing "us to create a space that is all our own" (Brown, 2009, p. 4). For the first few weeks, however, there were tangible and palpable challenges to this. First, the young women would wait for me to direct the sessions, perhaps in alignment with the routines of school, but also in response to, as one participant put it, the "*awkwardness . . . you know, with everyone there in the room.*" Indeed, these young women experienced uneasy and fractured relationships at times, marked by friendship rifts and peaceful, yet still visible and palpable divisions between the different ethnic groupings in class. I also experienced my own initial and ongoing uncertainty of how to bring the group together in ways that were non-exposing for them. However, over time certain embodied practices, or even rituals, started to form that moved this space into one that was (still imperfectly) "all our own."

One subtle yet key development emerged around four weeks into the dance studio project, after small groups of young women started arriving 20 minutes or so early for the session. Rather than waiting until the whole group was present, I allowed these early arrivers into the studio without me. The outcome was that by the time the rest of the class arrived, the studio was often already filled with loud music and rather loose and organic arrangements of dancing bodies—arrangements certainly not overtly directed by me. Even though making the transition from this partially populated space to one that embraced the whole group wasn't always easy, I noted an increasing sense of ease, liveliness, and indeed creativity to the sessions that started this way.

This developing practice came to be more formally consolidated during what I initially feared would be a moment of tension. As context, some of the young Black women within this class had shared with me that they often felt judged more harshly by teachers (including me) than, as they put it, *"the White girls"* in the group, meaning the Turkish students. This was specifically for *"our loud personalities"* but also in respect to dancing (*"even though their dancing is more explicit than ours, you know, Miss"*). On one particular day, a group of Turkish girls had arrived early and were filling the room with the sounds, movements, and energies of bellydance. Five minutes or so later, a small friendship group of Black girls arrived, also early, and all while I was in the corner of the studio organizing some paperwork. As this new group of girls entered this space, one set up by dancing young women rather than by a staff member who might *favoritize* some students over others, cries of seeming appreciation burst out at what their fellow, yet different, group members were doing. After a while I decided to also enter the dynamic communal space that was emerging and encouraged us to all join together in the center of the room. We joined hands, moving to the beat, and sent a wave or ripple around the circle with our arms, with me at this point still unsure as to what might (or should) happen next. Indeed, this 'game' seemed to run its course fairly quickly, but one young woman, Winter (a pseudonym of her choice), kept the momentum going in asking rather tentatively, *"Miss, can we play One Black Girl in the Middle?"*

The game Winter suggested was a British version of the Black girl dance cipher or freestyle circle discussed earlier (Brown, 2009). After Winter explained to me and *"the White girls"* the rules of this game, we all took it in turns to come into the middle and dance to the Afrobeats and Bashment music that Winter and her friends were choosing on the stereo. Winter held back from entering the circle until everyone had taken a turn, and then at last walked boldly into the center, turned at a 90-degree angle to her initial entrance and proceeded to *brukkout*[4] to rapturous cheers and applause from the rest of the group.

It seemed that in this space, and in this moment, this Black girl's body was no longer an object for judgment, nor was it 'at risk,' an object for institutional protection or disciplining. Instead, I suggest, this young woman deployed her moving body as a form of "cultural and political expression" (Sears, 2010, p. 123) that, rather than being "inappropriate" or in need of "covering up," was both skilled and powerfully erotic (hooks, 1994; Lorde, 1984) in a way that moved "outside of oppressive discourse" (Mirza, 2010, p. 5). Indeed, in a space marked by moving feminine bodies engaged in communal acts of cultural and artistic production, the young Black woman's embodied sexuality might be experienced by the girl herself, rather than caught in an institutional, White patriarchal gaze.

In order to enrich the quite electric feeling of this moment, one in which a particular gaze had been momentarily punctuated, I left the circle to turn the studio lights all the way down, to even louder cheers from the room as Winter continued to dance. Just as Sears' participants experienced a deeply embodied sense of "Black female bodies as sites of beauty, pleasure, agency and power" in their dancing (Sears, 2010, p. 134), in *this* enclosed, dark, intimate, all-girl/woman dancing space, Winter's final dance quite clearly marked the pinnacle of the game. For that moment, the Black girl "shaking her butt" (Sears, 2010, p. 134) was instructive to the rest of the group and was a (new) form of embodied success in the college—one that also served to address and smooth over institutionally situated rifts between groups of young women.

As emphasized by Brown (2009) however, the dance cipher is a site for learning not only for young women but also for the adults who dance with them. As Brown (2009) put it, "the adult-girl dance cipher transforms typical binary power relationships" (p. 89), in no small part because "to understand what dance does, you have to dance" (p. 102). Indeed, the sensations of my own body moving to the repetitive and inviting beat of the music, accompanied by the visceral feeling of pleasure and celebration in the room (the cheering, the clapping, the laughing, the bodies moving in close proximity to each other), along with what felt like caring acts of instruction and support from these young experts, was an important learning experience for me. I now experience myself as having less concern around and more respect for the embodied practices of the young women I am working with. Brown (2009) has asserted that "while we dance, we also theorize" (p. 69), and in all this, I suggest that the Black girl dance cipher is a powerful space for unlearning institutional racism and sexism and embracing young women's own articulations of their bodies, sexualities, and art forms.

Case Example 2: Creating Queer-Affirming Spaces (Elly)

Before data collection began at the primary site for my music therapy action research project, I (ES) ran a series of pilot workshops with different groups of young people across a range of school settings. A colleague put me in touch with a school in the outer suburbs with a group of students in a drama class, who were described as having "an interest in the arts and LGBT issues."

I entered the room and met the group of eight young people, who were all 17 years old. The first thing we did after seating ourselves in a circle was a call-and-response drumming game, each introducing ourselves by name and pronouns (such as he, she, or they) and playing a beat, for the rest of the group to echo back. I explained that names and pronouns are a good way to start off, because it gives us all the opportunity to tell everyone how we'd like to be referred to on that day, but that they were welcome to skip the pronouns if they didn't feel comfortable sharing. We moved around the circle, and around half of the group openly identified themselves as queer (including myself), trans, and/or non-binary, using a range of pronouns that I would not have known had we not addressed them. Directed by the young people, we next constructed a group agreement for the workshop, writing out ground rules to support everyone to feel respected and safe to contribute, and I hung it on the wall. It included a wide range of principles: *No "isms"* (sexism, racism, ableism and much more); *respect people's pronouns*; *respect and acknowledge the land we're on* (a reminder that our group was taking place on colonized and unceded lands of the Wurundjeri people); *"stay in your lane"* (a reminder to speak only for your own lived experience, not for other people's).

We moved into the main activity for the workshop: writing a song, based around the theme of the future. I knew based on information from their teacher and my colleague that this was a group of young people who could easily be positioned through a lens of risk, vulnerability, and deficit: the school community was located by low socioeconomic identifiers, many of the young people were in foster care, many identified as queer and/or trans, and there was a high youth suicide rate in the community. However, anti-oppressive and after-queer approaches require us to resist the temptation to reduce our discussion down to injury or vulnerability as key discursive frames (Bain et al., 2016; Bryan, 2017). I asked the young people to close their eyes, and I walked around the room, beginning a narrative for them to complete. *"I want you to imagine your perfect world. What does it look like? What does gender look like in this world?"* I observed that the young people appeared to be engaged, so I continued. *"How has gender shaped this world? How are people in this world shaped by it? How does gender play into the way people connect with each other . . . as strangers, as friends, in romantic relationships?"* I wanted to pose as many questions as I could think of, to maximize the opportunity for interest and responses, to provide space for the diversity of thought that existed among them, and to have them articulate their own futures and possibilities.

By the end of the session, we had written a song that the young people described as "anthemic." The group told me, *"We want it to be like a catchy pop anthem, so people can't get it out of their heads, and then they have no choice but to take on the message of the song!"* Their expertise and passion for the issues we raised struck me deeply. I asked them what they were working on in their drama class, and they told me about a play they were writing, to perform at an adolescent conference. I left them with a recording of the song, a copy of the lyrics and the chords, and I explained that they could use their 'anthem' in whatever way they liked after that session. *"Perhaps you might even incorporate it into your play?"* I suggested.

A month later, I received an email from their drama teacher, who told me the group had written another two verses of the song, performed it at the school assembly, and were preparing to present it at the upcoming conference. Songwriting is a versatile technique for music therapists, used to foster a therapeutic process or journey; as a medium for a client's emotional expression, or locus of control; for generating artifacts that extend beyond the therapy room, and much more (Baker, 2015). Songwriting is also socially, culturally, and politically informed and connected (Baker, 2015, p. 16). with a queer-affirmative lens, it enables young people such as these to perform and celebrate a range of identities, subvert dominant norms, reimagine, and reconstruct (Bain et al., 2016). Although we were actively rejecting heteropatriarchal systems of power, we did so by deflecting *away* from these cultures of normativity, and simultaneously challenging the singular, universalizing narrative of 'vulnerable queer youth' (Bryan, 2017). These were the lyrics to their *"queer anthem"* (published with the group's permission):

Verse:

In a perfect world
There is so much more to be
Than just a guy or a girl
I can just be me
And if you don't agree
Keep it to yourself
Lock it in a box
And throw away the key

Chorus:

It's a matter of education
We don't need your discrimination
We'll let everyone know who'll hear
You are who you are
Straight, binary, or queer
You are who you are
Straight, binary, or queer

Case Example 3: "Cultivating Dissent" With Girls Across Modalities (Elly)

The Wellbeing Coordinator and Year Level Coordinators at 'South East College' iden-tified a group of girls for me (ES) to run a group with because of recent conflict that was regularly arising. Relational aggression between the girls was often described by staff as "bitchiness," and carried the weight of entrenched narratives about teen girls as pathologically repressive and mean (Ringrose, 2013, p. 37). Then there were the girls who "acted out," whose issues were not of an internalizing nature. Lloyd (2005) refers to these as 'problem girls,' who disrupt norms of feminine aggression.

These girls lived in some of the poorest suburbs of Melbourne and were from a mix of cultural backgrounds, and the ways they were upholding or transgressing conventions of feminine behavior were also coded by unspoken raced and classed dynamics (Lloyd, 2005; Ringrose, 2013). I considered how to navigate building solidarity between girls without promoting an essential nature of femininity tied to the 'good girl,' in which White and middle class are hidden transcripts (Fordham, 1993; Ringrose, 2013). My mind was drawn to Lyn Mikel Brown's (2016) work on intergenerational feminist activism with teenage girls, based on the notion that 'cultivating dissent' is important for not only girls' healthy development but also the development of *all* schools and *all* communities. Within this, Brown (2003; 2016) has emphasized the need to unveil the hidden limiting and damaging constructions of gender, race, class, and sexuality at play in the largely invisible dynamics of girls' relationships, and to replace them with new stories, words, tools, and realities: "The answer is less about the will of adults or the control over kids than about appreci-ating girls' need to have control in their lives to feel important, to be visible, to be taken seriously, to have an effect" (2003, p. 201).

The girls (their preferred gender expression) and I sat in a circle on the floor of the school music room for our first group session. I started off by asking them to choose some background music to play through the speakers I'd brought. "*So, we're doing a group to get us to stop bitching about each other?*" one of the girls directed at me immediately. "*Suits me, we get to skip class,*" another replied, sighing as she lay down on her back, putting headphones in her ears. Another turned the focus to me: "*So, do you have a boyfriend or not, miss?*" I responded, "*Boyfriend? Is that the only option I get?*" and they gasped, two of the girls turning to each other to discuss animatedly. I plugged my laptop into some speakers and interrupted their conversation: "*Hey, can I show you a video I found last night?*"

We began with a music video of my choice and quickly moved into their suggestions. We watched the songs and their accompanying stories, which raised notions of bodily autonomy, sexualization, agency, desire, and more. Discussion began to flow, so I pulled out a big piece of poster paper and colored pens, switching off the computer. I wanted to redirect the conversation from the commodified images of feminine sexuality that teen girls are so expansively surrounded by, and into their own lived and embodied experiences, so often ignored or silenced at an institutional level (Tolman, 2012). "*So, what about in your life?*", I asked." *Are there any times you've felt like being a girl has shaped how people see your identity, your sexuality, your body? How did it make you feel?*"

After only a minute or so of easing into discussion, the girls were excited, talking over the top of each other and recounting each of their individual experiences. I looked around for a way to focus their energy; to represent the affective and "discursive terrain" of their stories (Braidotti, 2002). I asked each of them to grab a large piece of poster paper, lie on top of it, and have someone else trace around their bodies. Drawing on embodied, intra-activist methods of turning data into *da(r)ta*, as described by Renold (2017), I turned to the girls to explain: "*Now you've each got this representation of your own body, so you can write your stories. Inside, outside, wherever they need to be written. However much you want to say, however you want to say it. You don't have to explain anything.*"

Fifteen minutes later, each of the girls had filled the outlines of their bodies on the paper with quotes, stories, symbols, colors, and drawings. At the end of the session, we held them up for each other. I reflected on how many stories they each had, how much they had to say. "*So, what should we do with all this?*" They didn't respond. I'd noticed that at the beginning, when a particular '90s R&B pop song played in the background, each of them had sung along. "*I take it you're all into R&B then?*" I asked, to which they collectively agreed. "*How about before our session next week, I come up with a beat, and we can spend group next week turning these stories into song lyrics?*"

In a way reminiscent of Brown's (2016) avocations around cultivating dissent in developing youth activism, my aim for the girls group at South East College was not to educate the girls about "behaving respectfully," which so often pertains to particularly gendered, raced, and classed expectations. Nor did I approach group as a space to attempt to resolve their past conflict. Even if I were to fully understand the dynamics of their conflict and relationships, I doubt I could come close to solving the untenable position they are placed in, where they gain social power by meeting expectations that still render them precarious and out of control (Brown, 2003). However, by creating opportunities like these for girls to share, to document, to sing, listen, and negotiate, we provide space for them to navigate complex, culturally mediated forms of oppression, offering them our support for their resistance.

During interviews with participants at the end of the project, 14-year-old 'Amelia' described her first impressions of the group: "*At first I thought, 'Oh this is gonna be some boring thing.'*" She went on to explain that her impressions changed, "*It was when we were talking about real world stuff and listening to videos. I really liked that bit, listening to videos. And actually talking about what happens in the real world.*"

Young people's participation in creative practices can work against processes that essentialize and pathologize them, or position them on the margins. In a context where teen girls are constantly met with the expectation that they will deceive and mistreat each other, cultivating dissent against the structures that enable these processes also allows them to forge new relationships, and ultimately challenge the status quo (Brown, 2016; Showumni, 2017). Amelia's reflections speak not only to young people's enthusiasm for this political work, but also to the unique affordances of the arts, the sense of vitality and interactivity inherent in the creative process: "*But we were actually DOING it. Just right there. We were writing stuff down, making music and stuff, we were really doing it.*"

Practice Principles

Our critical arts-based practices challenge the notion that the issues faced by the young people we work with are their "personal problems," instead understanding these "problems" in the context of processes of heterosexism, racism, classism, and more: processes that can be shaken by critical, arts-based approaches. Specifically, we contend that group work creates conditions in which young people are able to imagine and create new possibilities that de-center their "personal problems." By working creatively in groups, as opposed to individually, young people can materially and collaboratively address the power relations that create conditions of harm and restriction in their daily lives, and in doing so refuse notions of the vulnerable, 'at risk' youth (Bryan, 2017) or the 'problem girl' (Lloyd, 2005). This also opens up a space in which the practitioner too confronts the power relations that shape their position and can work with young people to undergo their own transformation: arguably necessary for truly critical and anti-oppressive practice with young people to develop. Through examining our related yet different practices, we have developed some practice principles to support other group leaders in formulating or enhancing their own groups:

Co-Create a Safer Space, a "Home Place":
(Brown, 2009, p. 143; Sears, 2010, p. 63)

- Address pronouns at the beginning of group work, model by introducing your own, acknowledge they are important and that they can change.
- Use gender-neutral language. Instead of gendered terms like "guys," "girls," "ladies," or "boys," opt for terms like "folks," "all," "everyone," "friends," "people," or use names in individual or small group contexts.

- Allow for spontaneity and openness to look across creative modalities.
- Invite personal narratives of experience and young people's raced, gendered (etc.) cultural practices, finding ways for these narratives and practices to construct/define the space.
- Be prepared for power dynamics and personal tensions to shape the space. Embrace the possibilities in this, while establishing agreements for mutual respect.
- Model what it looks like to notice and acknowledge your assumptions and unconscious bias, to cultivate an environment of accountability and normalize taking responsibility.
- Familiarize yourself with best practice guidelines for disclosures of violence/trauma/abuse, and the policies and obligations of your local organization.

From Singling Out Particular Groups, to Exploring Structures That Create and Perpetuate Marginalization:

- Challenge singular, universalizing narratives to focus on the diversity of experience.
- Open up notions of agency, pleasure, joy, celebration, and the future in body and voice.
- Use the terms and ideas that young people use to define and understand themselves and their practices: strive to leave institutional and often pathologizing labels at the door.
- Participate in the processes of un/learning yourself. Find ways to learn with and from the young people and their perspectives, and strive to acknowledge this in the space.

Offer Young People the Opportunity to Build Their Own Critical Consciousness:

- Instead of working to protect or disallow young people from exploring material that you find problematic, open up dialogue and space for their own critical analysis.
- Embrace how the body can be a site for building critical consciousness; for example, experiencing embodied cultural practices as a starting point for confronting bias.

The principles from which practitioners can shift from intervention *into* young people's identities, to arts-based group work *as an intervention* into the processes that pathologize them, are multiple and complex. This list is by no means exhaustive. In order to practice critically and reflectively, we must continually build a consciousness of our own identities and how these play into the power we hold as "helpers" with young people, particularly within institutions. We recognize that for every local context for such work, there are nuanced exclusionary processes that young people face. However, we believe developing and applying a critical understanding of these issues should be part of any group practice that seeks to enrich and support the well-being and agency of young people and their communities.

Notes

1. See case study sections for more specific discussion of this term in respect to the young women the second author developed her work with.
2. This term refers to the final years of high school.
3. Where I describe the dance and music forms and styles engaged in during this project, I use the terminology the young women themselves employ, while recognizing diverse conversations around and manifestations of these styles, in both academic and artistic contexts.
4. The Black British Caribbean girls in the group used this term to refer to the seemingly spontaneous dancing that would "break out" at the high or breaking point of the music and would deploy movements emanating around the pelvis to mobilize and embody this music.

References

Ahmed, S. (2017). *Living a feminist life*. London: Duke University Press.

Bain, C. L., Grzanka, P. R., & Crowe, B. (2016). Queer music therapy: The implications of queer theory for a radically inclusive music therapy, *The Arts in Psychotherapy, 50*, 22–33.

Baines, D. (2007). *Doing anti-oppressive practice: Building transformative politicized social work*. Winnipeg, Canada: Fernwood Publishing.

Baines, S. (2013). Music therapy as an anti-oppressive practice. *The Arts in Psychotherapy, 40*(1), 1–5.

Baker, F. (2015). *Therapeutic songwriting: Developments in theory, methods and practice*. New York, NY: Palgrave Macmillan.

Boggan, C. E., Grzanka, P. R., & Bain, C. L. (2017). Perspectives on queer music therapy: A qualitative analysis of music therapists' reactions to radically inclusive practice. *Journal of Music Therapy, 54*(4), 375–404.

Bragg, S., Renold, E., Ringrose, J., & Jackson, C. (2018). "More than boy, girl, male, female": exploring young people's views on gender diversity within and beyond school contexts. *Sex Education, Sexuality Society and Learning, 18*(4), 420–434.

Braidotti, R. (2002). Metamorphoses: Towards a materialist theory of becoming. Cambridge: Polity Press.

Brown, L. M. (2003). *Girlfighting: Betrayal and rejection among girls*. New York, NY: New York University Press.

Brown, L. M. (2016). *Powered by girl: A field guide for supporting youth activists*. Boston, MA: Boston Beacon Press.

Brown, R. N. (2009). *Black girlhood celebration: Toward a hip hop feminist pedagogy*. New York, NY: Peter Lang.

Bryan, A. (2017). Queer youth and mental health: What do educators need to know? *Irish Educational Studies 36*(1), 73–89.

Chandra-Mouli, V., Plesons, M., Adebayo, E., Amin, A., Avni, M., Kraft, J. M., . . . Garcia-Moreno, C. (2017). Implications of the Global Early Adolescent Study's formative research findings for action and for research. *Journal of Adolescent Health, 61*(4), S5–S9.

Cohen, S. (1999). Moral panics and folk concepts. *Paedagogica Historica, 35*(3), 585–591.

Conroy, N. E. (2013). Rethinking adolescent peer sexual harassment: Contributions of feminist theory. *Journal of School Violence, 12*(4), 340–356.

Fairchild, R., Thompson, G., & McFerran, K. S. (2016). Exploring the meaning of a performance in music therapy for children and their families experiencing homelessness and family violence. *Music Therapy Perspectives, 35*(1), 36–49.

Fordham, S. (1993). "Those loud black girls": (Black) women, silence, and gender "passing" in the academy. *Anthropology and Education Quarterly, 24*(1), 3–32.

Foucault, M. (1990). *The history of sexuality: An introduction* (Vol. I, Robert Hurley, Trans.). New York: Vintage.

Gottschild, B. (2003). *The black dancing body: A geography from coon to cool.* New York, NY: Palgrave Macmillan.

Grant, J. M., Mottet, L. A., Tanis, J., Harrison, J., Herman, J. L., & Keisling, M. (2011). *Injustice at every turn: A report of the national transgender discrimination survey.* Retrieved from www. thetaskforce.org/downloads/reports/reports/ntds_full.pdf

Guattari, F. (1995). *Chaosmosis: An ethico-aesthetic paradigm.* Indianapolis, IN: Indiana University Press.

Haen, C. (2007). Fear to tread: Play and drama therapy in the treatment of boys who have been sexually abused. In S. L. Brooke (Ed.), *The use of creative arts therapies with sexual abuse survivors* (pp. 235–249). Springfield, IL: Charles C. Thomas.

Hickey-Moody, A. (2013). *Youth, arts, and education: Reassembling subjectivity through affect.* New York, NY: Routledge.

hooks, b. (1994). *Teaching to transgress.* London: Routledge.

hooks, b. (2003). *Teaching community: A pedagogy of hope.* New York, NY: Routledge.

Kearney, M. C. (2007). Productive spaces. *Journal of Children and Media, 1*(2), 126–141.

Keller, J., Mendes, K., & Ringrose, J. (2016). Speaking 'unspeakable things': Documenting digital feminist responses to rape culture. *Journal of Gender Studies,* 1–15.

Lloyd, G. (2005). Introduction: Why we need a book about "problem girls." In G. Lloyd (Ed.), *Problem girls: Understanding and supporting troubled and troublesome girls and young women* (pp. 1–8). Abingdon: Routledge Falmer.

Lorde, A. (1984). *Sister outsider: Essays and speeches.* New York, NY: Ten Speed Press.

Mansouri, F., & Jenkins, L. (2010). Schools as sites of race relations and intercultural tension. *Australian Journal of Teacher Education, 35*(7), 93–108.

McNeil, J., Bailey, L., Ellis, S., Morton, J., & Regan, M. (2012). *Trans mental health study 2012.* Edinburgh, Scotland: Scottish Transgender Alliance. Retrieved from www.gires.org.uk/wp-content/uploads/2014/08/trans_mh_study.pdf

Mirza, H. S. (2010). Plotting a history: Black and postcolonial feminisms in new times. In H. S. Mirza & C. Joseph (Eds.), *Black and postcolonial feminisms* (pp. 1–10). New York, NY: Routledge.

Paechter, C. (2013). Girls and their bodies: Approaching a more emancipatory physical education. *Pedagogy Culture and Society, 21*(2), 261–277.

Patrick, R., & Moodie, N. (2016). Indigenous education policy discourses in Australia. In *Global learning in the 21st century* (pp. 165–184). Rotterdam, The Netherlands: Sense Publishers.

Pierce, L. (2014). The integrative power of dance/movement therapy: Implications for the treatment of dissociation and developmental trauma. *The Arts in Psychotherapy, 41*(1), 7–15.

Rasmussen, M. L., Sanjakdar, F., Allen, L., Quinlivan, K., & Bromdal, A. (2017). Homophobia, transphobia, young people and the question of responsibility. *Discourse: Studies in the Cultural Politics of Education, 38*(1), 30–42.

Renold, E. (2017). "Feel what I feel": Making da(r)ta with teen girls for creative activisms on how sexual violence matters. *Journal of Gender Studies,* 1–19.

Renold, E., & Ivinson, G. (2015). Mud, mermaids and burnt wedding dresses: Mapping queer assemblages in teen girls' talk on gender and sexual violence. In E. Renold, D. Egan & J. Ringrose (Eds.), *Children, sexuality and sexualization* (pp. 239–255). Buckingham: Palgrave Macmillan.

Renold, E., & Ringrose, J. (2011). Schizoid subjectivities?: Re-theorizing teen girls' sexual cultures in an era of "sexualization." *Journal of Sociology, 47*(4), 389–409.

Renold, E., & Ringrose, J. (2016). Pin-balling and boners: The posthuman phallus and intra-activist sexuality assemblages in secondary school. In L. Allen & M. L. Rasmussen (Eds.), *Handbook of sexuality education* (pp. 631–653). London: Palgrave Macmillan.

Retallack, H., Ringrose, J., & Lawrence, E. (2016). "Fuck your body image": Teen girls' Twitter and Instagram feminism in and around school. In J. Coffey, S. Budgeon & H. Cahill (Eds.), *Learning bodies* (pp. 85–103). London: Springer.

Ringrose, J. (2013). *Postfeminist education? Girls and the sexual politics of schooling*, London: Routledge.

Sajnani, N. (2012). Response/ability: Imagining a critical race feminist paradigm for the creative arts therapies. *The Arts in Psychotherapy, 39*(3), 186–191.

Sajnani, N., Marxen, E., & Zarate, R. (2017). Critical perspectives in the arts therapies: Response/ability across a continuum of practice. *The Arts in Psychotherapy, 54*, 28–37.

Sears, S. (2010). *Imagining black womanhood: The negotiation of power and identity in the Girls Empowerment Project*. Albany, NY: State University of New York Press.

Showumni, V. (2017). The role of the Black Girls Club: Challenging the status quo. In J. L. Martin, A. E. Nickels & M. Sharp-Grier (Eds.), *Feminist pedagogy, practice, and activism: Improving lives for girls and women* (pp. 230–246). New York, NY: Routledge.

Smith, E., Jones, T., Ward, R., Dixon, J., Mitchell, A., & Hillier, L. (2014). *From blues to rainbows: Mental health and wellbeing of gender diverse and transgender young people in Australia*. Melbourne, Australia: The Australian Research Centre in Sex, Health, and Society. Retrieved from www.glhv.org.au/files/From-Blues-to-Rainbows-Report-2014.pdf

Stanger, C. (2016). "Let me change it into my own style": Cultural domination and material acts of resistance within an inner city dance class. In A. Hickey-Moody & T. Page (Eds.), *Arts, pedagogy and cultural resistance* (pp. 113–132). London: Rowman & Littlefield.

Stanley Niaah, S. (2010). *Dancehall: From slave ship to ghetto*. Ottawa, Canada: University of Ottawa Press.

Stinson, S. (1998). Seeking a feminist pedagogy for children's dance. In S. Shapiro (Ed.), *Dance, power and difference: Critical and feminist perspectives in dance education* (pp. 23–47). Champaign, IL: Human Kinetics.

Talburt, S., & Rasmussen, M. L. (2010). "After-queer" tendencies in queer research. *International Journal of Qualitative Studies in Education, 23*(1), 1–14.

Tolman, D. (2012). Female adolescents, sexual empowerment and desire: A missing discourse of gender inequity. *Sex Roles, 66*(11–12), 746–757.

Visser, M., & du Plessis, J. (2015). An expressive art group intervention for sexually abused adolescent females. *Journal of Child and Adolescent Mental Health, 27*(3), 199–213.

Ward, R. (2017). 'I just want to be myself': How we can challenge homophobia, transphobia, and racism in Australian Schools. *Journal of Intercultural Studies, 38*(4), 469–479.

Weekes, D. (2002). Get your freak on: How black girls sexualise identity. *Sex Education, 2*(3), 251–262.

Weekes, D. (2004). Where my girls at? Black girls and the construction of the sexual. In A. Harris (Ed.), *All about the girl: Culture, power and identity* (pp. 141–154). New York, NY: Routledge.

Wright, T., & Wright, K. (2017). Exploring the benefits of intersectional feminist social justice approaches in art psychotherapy. *The Arts in Psychotherapy, 54*, 7–14.

Youdell, D. (2006). *Impossible bodies, impossible selves: Exclusions and student subjectivities*. Dordecht, The Netherlands: Springer.

15

The Benefits and Challenges of Using the Creative Arts in Adolescent Groups

NANCY BOYD WEBB

The preceding chapters have testified to both the effectiveness of creative arts-based approaches in stimulating and exploring the expression of feelings and the positive results of engaging adolescents in therapy groups that use various forms of these arts. This process is often complicated and challenging but, despite the difficulties of engaging adolescents in therapy, numerous reports in the group work and mental health literature attest to the effectiveness of the arts in engaging and helping adolescents who are unhappy and involved in problematic behaviors and interactions (e.g., Dean & Landis, 2017; Drapeau & Kronish, 2007; Haen & Weil, 2010; Mapp & Koch, 2004). This chapter will review both the challenges and the benefits of using the arts in group therapy with adolescents, summarizing and highlighting many of the points raised in previous chapters while also hoping to convince students and clinical practitioners that involving adolescents in creative arts-based groups results in many benefits for the teens that would not occur in other forms of therapy.

The Daunting Struggles of Adolescence

The process of navigating the perilous journey of the adolescent years involves perhaps the greatest challenge in normal human development. During the period from ages 13–20, an individual must accommodate to a changing physical body with increasing sexual awareness, an as-yet-immature brain, hormonal imbalances, increasing educational expectations, and growing independence with accompanying freedom to make choices. It's a paradox that at a time when the waters are tumultuous and shifting under them, the sailors are expected to not only keep the boat afloat but also steer it successfully to shore!

Erikson (1959) emphasized the task of identity development as the primary focus of adolescence. Many young people, with increased freedom and time on their hands in their teen years, choose to experiment with smoking and using alcohol and other substances, while spending hours listening to music and engaging with electronics to play games and communicate with peers. They may neglect their school work and family obligations, such as routine chores. Other teens focus on their school work and sports activities and obsessively monitor their grades and rankings among their peers. Gender identity and development can take different paths in adolescence, and some teens decide to experiment with sexual partners of different genders, while others are aligned with the gender of their birth and committed to heterosexuality. Some may disparage youth who identify as LGBTQ.

Malekoff (2014) summarized the major developmental tasks of adolescence as follows:

- Separating from family.
- Forging a healthy sexual identity.
- Preparing for the future.
- Developing a moral value system.

These tasks must be accomplished in the context of an environment that often presents considerable risks and dangers. More is expected at a time when physical, emotional, and cognitive development is changing at a rapid pace, and therefore energy may be depleted. Various psychological conditions are common in adolescence, such as anxiety and depression, and these may lead to the tendency to withdraw and mistrust any efforts of adults to help. About 10% of adolescents will be diagnosed with major depression during their teen years and some will receive medication and therapy, while others may decline or not be offered treatment (Grover, 2017; Swartz, 2018). Suicide may be a sad result of the reluctance to reach out for help or for adults to identify there is a problem. Suicide rates for adolescents are reported to be steadily rising, according to the United States Centers for Disease Control and Prevention (Holmes, 2017), with the rate for girls doubling from 2007 to 2015, and that of boys increasing 30% over the same period.

These realities make it quite understandable that some practitioners are uncomfortable and avoid working with adolescents. Their unpredictability and reluctance to cooperate makes it hard for clinicians to formulate a realistic treatment plan that will meet the youth's needs. Practitioners who persist and manage to engage adolescents have found ways to look beyond the surface presentation of a teen's bravado, with the realization that often this behavior is the product of their individual backgrounds. When their development involves inadequate parenting, the unfortunate result is that the teen does not know productive ways to interact with others when they are upset.

Malekoff (2014) acknowledged that "group work with teenagers is a tricky business and an important calling" (p. 34). He encouraged practitioners to "hang in there for the long haul and not bail out as too many an adult already has. There are too many kids who need people like us" (p. 34). Hopefully, this book will inspire and inform therapists about the many ways the creative arts can provide a strong enticement for engaging adolescents in group therapy and encourage therapists to make a commitment to help young people who are struggling to find acceptance.

How Creative Arts Can Produce Positive Interactions for Teens

As demonstrated in the various chapters of this book, the fields of art, music, drama, dance/movement, play, and poetry therapy, as well as journal writing, all fall within the category of 'creative arts.' The range of creative arts activities is quite extensive, and many group leaders tend to focus on the area with which they are most familiar. Regardless of the activity, however, the fact that it involves input from the group participants makes it drastically different from a classroom situation, and participants quickly perceive that the leader's role is different from that of a teacher. The leader may make certain items available, such as markers and paper, or drums and cymbals, but the decisions about how these will be used depends on the preferences of each group member. Offering choices to the group members appeals to teens who are resistant to being told what to do.

When a young person becomes involved in a group project in which he or she has an active role, the experience can build self-confidence and the realization that everyone in the group contributes to a successful outcome. For example, a 14-year-old who has a reputation as a misfit in his class can convert that perception through being funny in a drama production invented by a group of peers who are all struggling for acceptance among their classmates.

The Benefits of Using Creative Arts in Adolescent Groups

Participation in an arts activity in a group for adolescents can bring with it many benefits, among which are the following:

- The opportunity to try (express) some new ideas/ identities/ experiences in a 'safe' environment.
- The experience of interacting with peers who do not 'fit in' with the larger group.
- The experience of producing something of which the creator is 'proud.'
- The experience of interacting and bonding with an adult (or two) who are fair and accepting.

This volume clearly demonstrates the many ways in which the arts permit the expression of feelings through the various media of music, drawing, dance, and drama, which can occur without the extensive use of words. As a play therapist with over 30 years of experience with young children, I have witnessed countless examples of young people expressing great relief from anxiety after drawing pictures that symbolize their feared or actual traumatic experiences. Although adolescents have a far greater capacity to describe feelings verbally than do younger children, they often feel blocked and reluctant to do so when the experience is emotionally charged. For example, a teenager who has been bullied and ostracized by peers will feel shame and reluctance to verbally admit his feelings of anger and hurt, but in a group of peers who are using drums and other percussion instruments to express anger, this boy can experience great relief through active drumming, followed by listening to other group members discuss examples of how they have been bullied and humiliated (Currie, 2011). The boy learns that his experience is not unique, his anger is justified, and that the perpetrators, not the victim, are at fault.

Adolescents are eager to experiment and try new things. This inclination can have positive or negative results. In the process of moving toward an adult identity, teens may be eager to experiment with activities that were not a part of their families of origin. Thus, many will become involved in peer groups that engage in behaviors that are 'new' to them, such as using alcohol, trying marijuana and other substances, and watching pornography on their devices or with others. The influence of peers can be strong, and teens will do things in a group that they would not have the courage to try alone. This reality speaks to the value of using groups for therapy with adolescents. Whereas a young person typically feels uncomfortable and resistant to engage one-on-one with an adult therapist, most will be far less negative about meeting in a group. Every group has its own dynamics, and each teen must find his or her own way to fit in and find acceptance. Malekoff (2014) described how groups can help adolescents learn to form healthy relationships and feel a sense of worth as a person. These potential benefits serve to inspire the leader to plan interesting activities that will engage adolescents and help them to achieve positive results from participating.

The Challenges of Using Creative Arts Therapy Groups With Adolescents

Despite the good planning and enthusiasm of the group leader, adolescents typically do not engage voluntarily in any kind of therapy. They often do not want to admit that they have any problems and, instead, project and blame any difficulties on the circumstances or on someone else. This means that many teens enter treatment with a chip on their shoulders, and the group leader needs to find a way to overlook this defensive stance and reach out in a manner to entice them. Use of the creative arts can accomplish this when it is introduced with choices of activities for the teen, and without any expectations. A leader who responds with humor to an adolescent's negative behaviors can often break through the resistance with a joke and effectively involve the teen. This was demonstrated in several chapters in this book.

Because adolescents are in the process of exploring their own identities, they may resist efforts of any adult to help them, viewing their need for support as a sign of weakness. Even though leaders try to be accepting and open to new ideas, teens may not trust this attitude on the part of any adult. After all, they have often grown up in a family environment in which parents have control and set the rules, and in which the teen is expected to comply, with few choices. Or, conversely, they may come from families in which the adults have set few limits and there is a lack of containment. Therefore, in group therapy when the leader invites group members to make decisions, the teens may feel initially mistrustful, and they may repeatedly 'test' the leader to determine if they really will allow the members to set their own rules. This 'testing' process can make the leader feel discouraged and uncertain about how to gain the teens' respect. The leader must be patient and able to look beneath the surface to see these behaviors as the youth's effort to challenge their leadership ability and commitment to the helping role.

The following list documents some of the challenges for the leader in using creative arts in adolescent groups:

- Engaging the reluctant adolescent; understanding that *resistance is a defense.*

- Accepting the reality that *confusion and chaos can be an inevitable phase* of group work.
- *Trusting the process*; avoiding power struggles; being flexible.
- *Tolerating personal distress* when group members respond with sarcasm and put-downs.
- Being able to *improvise and be playful.*
- *Balancing warmth and limit setting.*

One might question whether the challenges for the group worker outweigh the benefits for the group participant. Several examples in Chapter 2 (Haen & Webb) and Chapter 10 (Landis & Williams) illustrate the negativity of adolescent members in beginning groups, thereby necessitating that leaders respond in a manner that defuses, rather than escalates, the power struggle. Group workers who are trained and who have good supervision can respond with humor and inventiveness to outright negative or disparaging comments. A wonderful example of a leader's creative approach to the group members' opening negative statements is illustrated in Chapter 10, in which the leader joined the members' negativity about being a 'terrible leader' by asking the group to give awards to those who were doing the worst job!!! This example illustrates both the leader's inventiveness and her playfulness, in addition to her ability to tolerate the distress of being named a terrible leader.

The creative arts provide group leaders with an appealing range of activities that may stimulate an adolescent's curiosity. Instead of talking about their problems (which is the last thing many teens want to do), involvement in a creative art project can provide an outlet for feelings without making the explicit connection to the participants' own lives. The following are some examples:

Song-sharing. In Chapter 8 (McFerran), the leader invites group members to share and play their favorite songs in an early session, and then asks each to state why they like the song. This song-sharing activity can lead the members to discuss the emotions generated by the song, with the result that some members may talk about their feelings, and others who are more quiet benefit by listening to the ensuing discussion.

Group mural making involves the participation of all the members in an agreed-upon project on which they will work together. The leader may stimulate the group by asking, "*What message do you want to convey?*" (Wolf, Chapter 4), and then helping the group select the type of art materials for creating the mural. Individuals may work alone on part of the mural at the beginning, with selective sharing and combining their creations as the project proceeds.

An example of a group mural project that helped a group of preteens and teens express their grief after the bombing and loss of life following the terrorist attacks in New York City on 9/11 is described in Mapp and Koch (2004). The mural making project involved 17 children (ages 8–15 years) and 17 mentors, based at the Big Brothers Big Sisters (BBBS) organization in New York, close to where the Twin Towers were attacked on September 11, 2001. The group met on Saturday afternoons over the course of four months, working on individual segments of the mural depicting various versions of sadness, anxiety, love, and hope connected with the participants' personal experiences of losses involved in this tragedy. After the mural was completed, a tour was arranged to display it in different corporate lobbies around New York City, following which it was hung permanently at the BBBS headquarters. Those who were involved with the project believe that the experience of working on the mural provided important psychological and emotional benefits to help the participants cope with their fears and stress caused by the attacks. They were able to express their feelings of mourning and compassion through the creation of art that clearly conveyed this.

Examples of the mural include one panel (see Figure 15.1) created by a 12-year-old that shows the Twin Towers with the words 'never forgotten' written on them, together with the words '27 and gone!; too young and loved; brother, son, friend. Good-bye Doug.' There are tear-drops scattered in this scene, which is a very moving and intense depiction of the loss of a 27-year-old man in the attacks.

Another panel in the mural (see Figure 15.2) conveys a sense of hope by showing two open hands with the words written on the fingers: 'the sun will still come out tomorrow.'

Obviously, this project had considerable therapeutic benefits for the participants, who were able to process their own grief and mourning, as they shared their experiences first with the other group members, and later with the community at large, and subsequently with the authors of a chapter for publication about their project (Mapp & Koch, 2004).

The various chapters in this book demonstrate the following creative arts approaches for use with adolescent groups:

- Art Therapy: Chapters 4 and 11.
- Bibliotherapy: Chapter 5.

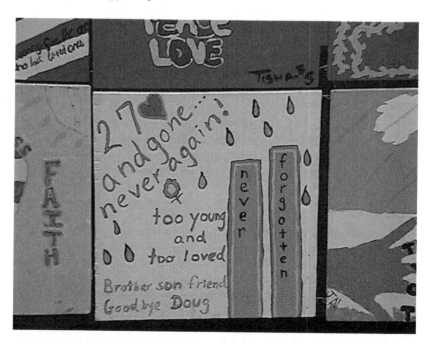

Figure 15.1

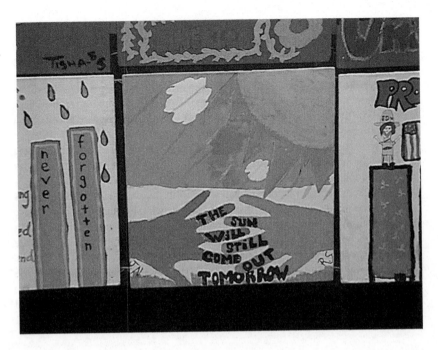

Figure 15.2

- Dance/Movement Therapy: Chapters 6 and 13.
- Drama Therapy: Chapters 7, 10, and 12.
- Music Therapy: Chapters 8 and 14.
- Poetry and Writing Therapy: Chapter 9.

Although Play Therapy employs creative arts in therapeutic interactions with children, the use of the term 'play' therapy is not appropriate with adolescents, who consider play an activity for younger children. However, the importance of symbolic communication through art, music, and movement clearly applies to all ages, including teens.

The chapters in the above list repeatedly illustrate the need for flexibility in the group leader, and the necessity for the leader to tolerate distress in the face of negative behaviors of the members, with the goal to move the group from negativity to problem solving. One chapter demonstrates the positive effects when the therapist shares some of his/her own experiences, including admitting her own mistakes (Chapter 4); this provides a role model for the teens, who observe the leader admitting the problem, taking ownership of her role, and then making a plan to rectify the situation. All the chapters demonstrate the very helpful use of playfulness to lighten an otherwise heavy mood.

Summary

This discussion makes it clear that the role of the group leader in an adolescent creative arts-based group is not easy, and that struggle and disappointment may be an integral component of leadership. The responsibility of dealing with eight to ten angry and/or sullen teens at once may not appeal to therapists who want to have a sense of control and goal-direction in the therapy process. This will not be easy! As Malekoff (2014) wrote, group work is not for the faint of heart. However, the personal reward of witnessing hostility convert into motivated cooperation convinces many therapists that the benefit is well worth the struggle. Group leaders who have seen successful outcomes in groups that began with great resistance have faith in the process and patience to let the events and reactions evolve.

There is no single plan for success, but many of the ideas and experiences described in this book can be adapted for use in other groups, provided the leader is prepared for diverse outcomes. Our hope and expectations are that both beginning and experienced practitioners will learn from the many rich chapters in this book. It is essential that adolescents who are experiencing hurdles in their lives have the opportunity to explore their feelings and their options and to feel accepted even when they may convey hostility or distrust of the process. The creative arts provide many outlets for experimenting, learning, and experiencing successful outcomes, and group leaders who can roll with the punches may watch an exciting sequence of behaviors evolve from negativity to active and enthusiastic participation. The group thus becomes a wonderful learning experience for both the adolescents and the group leader!

References

Currie, M. (2011). Doing anger differently: Working creatively with angry and aggressive boys. In C. Haen (Ed.), *Engaging boys in treatment: Creative approaches to the therapy process* (pp. 197–217). New York, NY: Routledge.

Dean, M., & Landis, H. (2017). Creative arts-based approaches with adolescent groups. In C. Haen & S. Aronson (Eds.), *Handbook of child and adolescent group therapy: A practitioner's reference* (pp. 124–136). New York, NY: Routledge.

Drapeau, M. C., & Kronish, N. (2007). Creative arts therapy groups: A treatment modality for psychiatric outpatients. *Art Therapy: Journal of the American Art Therapy Association, 24*(2), 76–81.

Erikson, E. H. (1968). *Identity, youth and crisis.* New York, NY: Norton.

Grover, S. (2017). Depressed adolescents. In C. Haen & S. Aronson (Eds.), *Handbook of child and adolescent group therapy. A practitioner's reference* (pp. 313–321). New York, NY: Routledge.

Haen, C., & Weil, M. (2010). Group therapy on the edge: Adolescence, creativity, and group work. *Group, 34*(1), 37–52.

Holmes, L. (2017, August 4). Suicide rates for teen boys and girls are climbing. *Huffington Post.* Retrieved from www.huffingtonpost.com/entry/suicide-rates-teen-girls_us_59848b64e4b0 cb15b1be13f4

Malekoff, A. (2014). *Group work with adolescents: Principles and practice* (3rd ed.). New York, NY: Guilford.

Mapp, I., & Koch, D. (2004). Creation of a group mural to promote healing following a mass trauma. In N. B. Webb (Ed.), *Mass trauma and violence: Helping children and families cope* (pp. 100–119). New York, NY: Guilford.

Swartz, K. (2018, February 24). *Adolescent depression: Diagnosis, treatment, and community education.* Keynote presented at the 2018 Duvall Family Studies conference, Sarasota, FL.

Index

Made in the USA
Middletown, DE
07 August 2022

70746033R00166